Psychiatry

THIRD EDITION

Neel Burton
MBBS (Lond.), MRCPsych, MA (Phil.)
Green Templeton College
University of Oxford, Oxford, UK

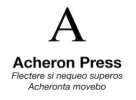

Acheron Press
Flectere si nequeo superos
Acheronta movebo

© Acheron Press 2016

Published by Acheron Press

The right of the author to be identified as the author of this work has been asserted in accordance with the Copyright, Designs and Patents Act 1988.

A CIP catalogue record for this book is available from the British Library.

ISBN 978 0 9929127 4 1

Typeset by Phoenix Photosetting, Chatham, Kent, United Kingdom

Printed and bound by SRP Limited, Exeter, Devon, United Kingdom

Preface

'Psychiatry' derives from the Ancient Greek, *psyche* and *iatreia*, and literally means 'healing of the soul'. *Psyche*—the soul, mind, spirit, ghost, breath, life, understanding—is personified in Greek myth by Psykhe, the beloved of Eros, and often represented symbolically as a butterfly or moth. The butterfly on the cover of this book is also a Rorschach or inkblot test, used to examine a person's psychological functioning, and, at least to me, looks a bit like a brain.

Just as philosophy differs from other academic disciplines, so psychiatry differs from other medical specialties. Psychiatrists train medically because an understanding of the body is integral to the practice of psychiatry, but psychiatry is about more than just an understanding of the body. It is, indeed, about the very essence of what it means to be human.

Like philosophy then, psychiatry faces empirical and conceptual challenges that hinder its progress and leave it exposed to criticism. Yet, it is precisely these challenges that make psychiatry such a satisfying and meaningful pursuit. For in psychiatry each patient is unique, and each patient has something unique to return to the psychiatrist.

I have tried to make this book as readable and relevant as possible: clear and concise yet comprehensive and detailed. I have emphasized important areas such as suicide risk assessment, but have also included a fair bit of material from the arts and humanities that is not on the core curriculum. In so doing, my aim has been to make psychiatry come alive by highlighting some of its more interesting or thought-provoking aspects, and to challenge the stigmatization of mental disorders that continues to prevail even among healthcare professionals.

I want you to excel at your exams, and you will I am sure, but I also want you to reach beyond the core curriculum to the angels and demons of psychiatry.

Let me show you that, of all the medical specialisms, psychiatry is by far the most fascinating, the most exciting, and the most obviously relevant to us as thinking, feeling, and sensing human beings.

Art is long, and Time is fleeting.

Neel Burton
Oxford, February 2016
www.neelburton.com

About Neel Burton

Dr Neel Burton is a psychiatrist, philosopher, and writer who lives and teaches in Oxford, England.

He is the recipient of the Society of Authors' Richard Asher Prize, the British Medical Association's Young Authors' Award, the Medical Journalists' Association Open Book Award, and a 'Best in the World' Gourmand Award.

www.neelburton.com

Contents

Preface to the third edition   v

Part 1

1.   A brief history of psychiatry   3
2.   The psychiatric assessment   11
3.   Mental healthcare   37

Part 2

4.   Schizophrenia and other psychoses   53
5.   Mood disturbances   73
6.   Suicide and deliberate self-harm   95
7.   Anxiety, stress-related, and somatoform disorders   105
8.   Personality disorders   119
9.   Organic disorders (delirium and dementias)   129
10.   Intellectual disability   141
11.   Substance misuse (alcohol and drugs)   147
12.   Eating, sleep, and sexual disorders   161
13.   Child and adolescent psychiatry   173

Self-assessment   184

Index   191

Part 1

'In that direction,' the Cat said, waving its right paw round, 'lives a Hatter: and in that direction,' waving the other paw, 'lives a March Hare. Visit either you like: they're both mad.'
'But I don't want to go among mad people,' Alice remarked.
'Oh you can't help that,' said the Cat: 'we're all mad here. I'm mad. You're mad.'
'How do you know I'm mad?' said Alice.
'You must be,' said the Cat, 'or you wouldn't have come here.'

—Lewis Carroll, *Alice's Adventures in Wonderland*

'Lewis Carroll' was the pen name of Charles Dodgson (1832-1898), a lecturer in mathematics at Christ Church, Oxford, who suffered from classic migraine. Classic migraine is sometimes associated with Lilliputian hallucinations, in which objects, animals, and people appear smaller than they truly are. It has been speculated that Dodgson's inspiration for the Alice stories came from Lilliputian hallucinations, which have since acquired the quixotic sobriquet of 'Alice in Wonderland Syndrome', or 'AIWS'.

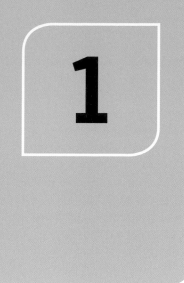

A brief history of psychiatry

Ancient Greece

In antiquity, people did not think of 'madness' (a term they used indiscriminately for all forms of psychosis) in terms of mental disorder, but of divine punishment or demonic possession. Evidence for this comes from the Old Testament, and more particularly the First Book of Samuel, which relates how King Saul became 'mad' after neglecting his religious duties and angering God. Nothing is more revealing of Saul's madness than the story of his senseless slaughter of the eighty-five priests at Nob. That David played on his harp to make Saul feel better suggests that, even in antiquity, people believed that psychotic disorders, or psychosis, could be successfully treated.

> But the Spirit of the Lord departed from Saul, and an evil spirit from the Lord troubled him… And it came to pass, when the evil spirit from God was upon Saul, that David took an harp, and played with his hand: so Saul was refreshed, and was well, and the evil spirit departed from him.
>
> —1 Samuel 16:14, 23 (KJV)

In Greek mythology and the Homerian epics, madness is similarly thought of as a punishment from God—or the gods. Thus, Hera punished Herakles by 'sending madness upon him', and Agamemnon confided to Achilles that 'Zeus robbed me of my wits'. It is in fact not until the time of Hippocrates (460-377 BC) that madness first became an object of scientific speculation. Hippocrates thought that madness resulted from an imbalance of four bodily fluids or humours. Melancholy, for instance, resulted from an excess of black bile (*melaina chole*), and could be cured by restoring the balance of the bodily humours by such treatments as special diets, purgatives, and blood-lettings. To modern readers, Hippocrates' ideas may seem far-fetched, perhaps even on the dangerous side of eccentric, but in the 4th century BC they represented a significant advance on the idea of madness as divine punishment or demonic possession. Aristotle (384-322 BC) and, later, the Roman physician Galen (129-200) elaborated upon Hippocrates' humoural theories, and both men played an important role in establishing them as Europe's dominant medical model.

> Only from the brain springs our pleasures, our feelings of happiness, laughter and jokes, our pain, our sorrows and tears … This same organ makes us mad or confused, inspires us with fear and anxiety…
>
> —Hippocrates, *The Holy Disease*

It is interesting to note that not all minds in Ancient Greece invariably thought of 'madness' as a curse or disease. In the *Phaedrus*, Plato quotes Socrates as saying that madness, 'provided it comes as the gift of heaven, is the channel by which we receive the greatest blessings… madness comes from God, whereas sober sense is merely human.'

The Roman Empire

In Ancient Rome, physician Asclepiades (124-40 BC) and philosopher Cicero (106-43 BC) rejected Hippocrates' humoural theories, asserting, for example, that melancholy results not from an excess of black bile but from emotions such as grief, fear, and rage. Cicero's questionnaire for the assessment of mental disorders bore remarkable similarities to today's psychiatric history and mental state examination (Chapter 2). Used throughout the empire, it included, among others, sections on *habitus* ('appearance'), *orationes* ('speech'), and *casus* ('life events'). Unfortunately, the influence of these luminaries began to decline in the 1st century AD, and physician Celsus (25 BC-50) reinstated the idea of madness as divine punishment or demonic possession, an idea reinforced by the rise of Christianity and the decline of the Roman Empire.

The Middle Ages

In the Middle Ages, religion became central to cure, and, alongside the mediaeval asylums such as the Bethlehem (an infamous asylum in London that is at the origin of the expression, 'like a bad day at Bedlam'), some monasteries transformed themselves into centres for the treatment of mental disorder. This is not to say that the humoural theories of Hippocrates had been supplanted, but merely that they had been incorporated into the prevailing Christian dogma, with older treatments such as purgatives and blood-lettings continuing alongside the prayers and confession.

During the Middle Ages, classical ideas had been kept alive in Islamic centres such as Baghdad and Damascus, and their re-introduction by St Thomas Aquinas (1225-1274) and others in the 13th century once again led to an increased separation of mind and soul, and to a shift from the Platonic metaphysics of Christianity to the Aristotelian empiricism of science. This movement laid the foundations for the Renaissance, and, later, for the Enlightenment.

The Renaissance

The burning of the so-called heretics, often people with psychosis, began in the early Renaissance and reached its peak in the 14th and 15th centuries. First published in 1563, *De praestigiis daemonum* (*The Deception of Demons*) argued that the madness of heretics resulted not from supernatural but natural causes. The Church promptly proscribed the book and accused its author, Johann Weyer, of being a sorcerer.

From the 15th century, scientific breakthroughs such as the heliocentric system of astronomer Galileo (1564-1642) began challenging the authority of the Church. Man, not God, became the focus of attention and study, and it is also around this time that anatomist Vesalius (1514-1564) published his landmark *De humani corporis fabrica libri septem* (*The Seven Books on the Structure of the Human Body*). The *Fabrica* represented the first serious challenge to Galenic anatomy and brought its author considerable fame and fortune. By the age of 28, Vesalius had become physician to the Holy Roman Emperor (neither Holy nor Roman, but in fact the Emperor of Germany), Charles the Quint.

The Enlightenment

Despite the scientific developments of the Renaissance, Hippocrates' humoural theories perdured into the 17th and 18th centuries, to be mocked by playwright Molière (1622-1673) in such works as *Le Malade imaginaire* (*The Imaginary Invalid*) and *Le Médecin malgré lui* (*The Doctor in Spite of Himself*). Empirical thinkers such as John Locke (1632-1704) in England and Denis Diderot (1713-1784) in France challenged this status quo by arguing, in the same vein as Cicero, that the psyche arises from sensations to produce reason and emotions.

Also in France, physician Philippe Pinel (1745-1826) began regarding mental disorder as the result of exposure to psychological and social stressors, and, to a lesser extent, of heredity and physiological damage. A landmark in the history of psychiatry, Pinel's *Traité Médico-philosophique sur l'aliénation mentale ou la manie* (*A Treatise on Insanity*) called for a more humane approach to the treatment of mental disorder. This 'moral treatment', as it had already been dubbed, included respect for the patient, a trusting and confiding doctor-patient relationship, decreased stimuli, routine activity and occupation, and the abandonment of old-fashioned Hippocratic treatments. At about the same time as Pinel in France, the Tukes (father and son) in England founded the York Retreat, the first institution 'for the humane care of the insane' in the British Isles.

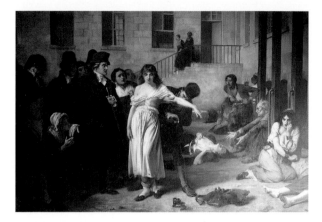

Figure 1.1. Philippe Pinel freeing lunatics from their chains at the Salpêtrière asylum, Paris. By Tony Robert-Fleury.

The Modern Era

In the 19th century, hopes of successful cures led to the burgeoning of mental hospitals in North America, Britain, and many of the countries of continental Europe. Unlike the mediaeval asylums, these hospitals treated the 'insane poor' according to the principles of moral treatment. Like Pinel before him, Jean-Etienne-Dominique Esquirol, Pinel's student and successor at the Salpêtrière Hospital, attempted a classification of mental disorders, and his resulting *Des Maladies mentales...* (*Concerning Mental Illnesses*) is regarded as the first modern treatise on clinical psychiatry. Half a century later, psychiatrist Emil Kraepelin (1856-1926) carried out his landmark classification of mental disorders, the *Compendium der Psychiatrie*, in which he distinguished schizophrenia (or *dementia praecox*, as he called it) from other forms of psychosis. Kraepelin further distinguished three clinical presentations of schizophrenia: (1) paranoia, dominated by delusions and hallucinations; (2) hebephrenia, dominated by inappropriate reactions and behaviours; and (3) catatonia, dominated by extreme agitation or immobility and odd mannerisms and posturing. Kraepelin's *Compendium* is the forerunner of modern classifications of mental disorders such as the *Diagnostic and Statistical Manual of Mental Disorders 5th Revision* (DSM-5) and the *International Classification of Diseases 10th Revision* (ICD-10, Chapter 2).

In the early 20th century, psychiatrist and philosopher Karl Jaspers (1883-1969) brought the methods of phenomenology—the direct investigation and description of phenomena as consciously experienced—into the field of clinical psychiatry. This so-called descriptive psychopathology created a scientific basis for the practice of psychiatry, and emphasized that symptoms of mental disorder should be diagnosed according to their form rather than their content. This means, for example, that a belief is a delusion not because it is deemed implausible by a person in a position of authority, but because it conforms to the definition of a delusion, that is, 'a strongly held belief that is not amenable to logic or persuasion and that is out of keeping with its holder's background or culture.'

Sigmund Freud (1856-1939) and his followers influenced much of 20th century psychiatry, and by the second half of the century a majority of psychiatrists in the US (although not in the UK) believed that mental disorders such as schizophrenia resulted from unconscious conflicts originating in early childhood. As a director of the US National Institute of Mental Health put it, 'From 1945 to 1955, it was nearly impossible for a non-psychoanalyst to become a chairman of a department or professor of psychiatry.'

In the latter part of the 20th century, neuroimaging techniques, genetic studies, and pharmacological breakthroughs such as the first antipsychotic drug chlorpromazine completely reversed this psychoanalytical model of mental disorder, and prompted a return to a more biological, 'neo-Kraepelinian' model.

At present, mental disorders are primarily seen as a biological disorder of the brain, although it is also recognized that psychological and social stressors can play important roles in triggering episodes of illness, and that different approaches to treatment should be seen not as competing but as complementary.

However, critics tend to deride this 'bio-psycho-social' model as little more than a 'bio-bio-bio' model, with psychiatrists reduced to mere diagnosticians and pill pushers. They question the scientific evidence underpinning such a robust biological approach, and call for a radical rethink of mental disorders, not as detached disease processes that can be cut up into diagnostic labels, but as subjective and meaningful experiences grounded in both personal and larger sociocultural narratives.

1

There are more ideas on earth than intellectuals imagine. And these ideas are more active, stronger, more resistant, more passionate than 'politicians' think. We have to be there at the birth of ideas, the bursting outward of their force: not in books expressing them, but in events manifesting this force, in struggles carried on around ideas, for or against them. Ideas do not rule the world. But it is because the world has ideas… that it is not passively ruled by those who are its leaders or those who would like to teach it, once and for all, what it must think.

—Michel Foucault

The philosopher, historian, and sociologist Michel Foucault (1926-1984) argued that 'madness' is a social construct dating back to the Enlightenment, and its 'treatment' little more than a disguised form of punishment for deviating from social norms and expectations.

Foucault is one of the forerunners of the antipsychiatry movement, which took hold in the 1960s and early 1970s. Spearheaded by psychiatrist Thomas Szasz (1920-2012) and others, it claimed that the label of severe mental disorder, especially schizophrenia, was little more than an attempt to medicalize and thereby control socially undesirable behaviour. According to Szasz, 'schizophrenia' does not exist other than as a social construct, a convenient label for the sort of thinking and behaviour that society finds uncomfortable or undermining.

Attractive though it may originally have seemed, the anti-psychiatry claim has been progressively undermined, ultimately, by its reluctance to recognize the distress and suffering of many people with severe mental disorder, as well as the very real risk that they can pose to their safety and prospects.

Of particular note is that Szasz rejected the anti-psychiatry label on the grounds that he did not oppose psychiatric treatment *per se*, but merely held that psychiatric treatment should not be imposed without the consent of the patient.

Today, there can be little doubt that severe mental disorder does, of course, exist, but its nature remains unclear, and an understanding of its place in human affairs—of its meaning—is still sorely lacking.

Sigmund Freud

People with a high level of anxiety have historically been referred to as 'neurotic'. The term 'neurosis' derives from the Ancient Greek *neuron* ('nerve'), and loosely means 'disease of the nerves'. The core feature of neurosis is a high level of 'background' anxiety, but neurosis can also manifest in the form of other symptoms such as phobias, panic attacks, irritability, perfectionism, and obsessive-compulsive tendencies. Although very common in some form or other, neurosis can prevent us from living in the moment, adapting usefully to our environment, and developing a richer, more complex, and more fulfilling outlook on life.

The most original, influential, and polemical theory of the origins of neurosis is that of Sigmund Freud. Freud studied medicine at the University of Vienna from 1873 to 1881, and, after some time, decided to specialize in neurology. In 1885-86, he spent the best part of a year in Paris, and returned to Vienna inspired by neurologist Jean-Martin Charcot's use of hypnosis in the treatment of 'hysteria', an outdated construct involving the conversion of anxiety into physical and psychological symptoms. Freud opened a private practice for the treatment of neuropsychiatric disorders, but eventually abandoned hypnosis for 'free association', which involves asking the patient to relax on a couch and say whatever comes into her mind (Freud's patients were mostly women). In 1895, inspired by the case of a patient called Bertha Pappenheim ('Anna O.'), Freud published the seminal *Studies on Hysteria* with his friend and colleague Josef Breuer. Following the public successes of *The Interpretation of Dreams* (1899) and *The Psychopathology of Everyday Life* (1901), he obtained a professorship at the University of Vienna and began to gather a devoted following. He remained a prolific writer throughout his life. Some of his most important works include *Three Essays on the Theory of Sexuality* (1905), *Totem and Taboo* (1913), and *Beyond the Pleasure Principle* (1920). Following the Nazi annexation of Austria in 1938, he fled to London, where, in the following year, he died of cancer of the jaw.

In *Studies on Hysteria*, Freud and Breuer formulated the psychoanalytic theory according to which neuroses have their origins in deeply traumatic and consequently repressed experiences. Treatment requires the patient to recall these repressed experiences into consciousness and to confront them once and for all, leading to a sudden and dramatic outpouring of emotion ('catharsis') and the gaining of insight. Such outcomes can be achieved through the methods of free association and dream interpretation, and by a sort of passivity on the part of the psychoanalyst. This passivity transforms the analyst into a blank canvas onto which the patient can unconsciously project her thoughts and feelings ('transference'). At the same time, the analyst should guard against projecting his own thoughts and feelings, such as his disappointment in his own wife or daughter, onto the patient ('counter-transference'). In the course of analysis, the patient is likely to display 'resistance' in the form of changing the topic, blanking out, falling asleep, arriving late, or missing appointments. Such behaviour is only to be expected, and indicates that the patient is close to recalling repressed material but afraid of doing so.

Aside from free association and dream interpretation, Freud recognized two further routes into the unconscious: parapraxes and jokes. Parapraxes, or slips of the tongue ('Freudian slips'), are essentially 'faulty actions' that occur when unconscious thoughts and desires suddenly parallel and then override conscious thoughts and intentions, for instance, calling a partner by the name of an ex-partner, substituting one word for another that rhymes or sounds similar ('I would like to thank/spank you'), or combining two words into a single one ('He is a very lustrous (illustrious/lustful) man'). Parapraxes often manifest in our speech, but can also manifest, among others, in our writing, misreadings, mishearings, and mislaying of objects and belongings. Freud reportedly 'joked' that 'there is no such thing as an accident'.

In *The Interpretation of Dreams*, Freud developed his 'topographical model' of the mind, describing the conscious, the unconscious, and an intermediary layer called the preconscious, which, although not conscious, could readily be accessed by the conscious. He later became dissatisfied with the topographical model and replaced it with the 'structural model', according to which the mind is split into the id, ego, and superego (Figure 1.2). The wholly unconscious id contains our drives and repressed emotions. The id is driven by the 'pleasure principle' and seeks out immediate gratification. But in this it is opposed by the mostly unconscious superego, a sort of moral judge that arises from the internalization of parental figures, and, by extension, of society itself. Caught in the middle is the ego, which, in contrast to the id and superego, is mostly conscious. The function of the ego is to reconcile the id and superego, and thereby to enable the person to engage successfully with reality.

For Freud, neurotic anxiety and other ego defences arise when the ego is overwhelmed by the demands of the id, the superego, and reality. To cope with these demands, the ego deploys defence mechanisms to block or distort impulses from the id, thereby making them seem more acceptable and less threatening or subversive. A broad

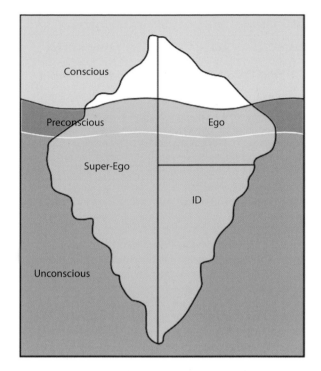

Figure 1.2. Freud's topographical (the ocean) and structural (the iceberg) models superimposed. Only the tip of the iceberg is conscious. In *The World as Will*, philosopher Arthur Schopenhauer, who anticipated Freud, compared the human intellect to a lame man who can see, riding on the shoulders of a blind giant.

range of ego defence mechanisms have since been identified and described (Chapter 8), not least by Freud's daughter, psychoanalyst Anna Freud (1895-1982).

Freud held that the instincts that motivate human behaviour are primarily derived from the sex drive or *libido* (Latin, 'I desire'). This 'life instinct' is counterbalanced by the 'death instinct', the unconscious desire to be dead and at peace (the 'Nirvana principle'). The libido is the primary motivating force in all of us, even in children, who must progress through various stages of psychosexual development before they can reach psychosexual maturity. Each one of these stages (with the exception of the latent stage) is focused on the erogenous zone—mouth, anus, phallus, or genitals—that provides the greatest pleasure at that stage. Ultimately, neurosis arises from frustrations encountered in the course of psychosexual development, and so is sexual in origin. Freud's stages of psychosexual development are outlined in Table 1.1.

1

Table 1.1: Freud's stages of psychosexual development

Name	Age	Principal task
Oral stage	Birth to 18 months	Weaning
Anal stage	18 months to 3-4 years	Toilet-training
Phallic stage	3-4 years to 5-7 years	Sexual identity
Latent stage	5-7 years to puberty	Learning
Genital stage	From puberty onwards	Genital intercourse

The Oedipus complex is arguably the most controversial of Freud's theories. For Freud, the phallic stage gives rise to the Oedipus complex, Oedipus being a mythological king of Thebes who unknowingly killed his father and married his mother. In the Oedipus complex, a boy sees his mother as a love-object and feels the need to compete with his father for her attention. As his father is stronger than he is, he begins to fear for his genitals ('castration anxiety'). In time, he displaces his feelings for his mother onto other girls, and begins to identify with his father/aggressor—thereby becoming a man like him. For girls, the equivalent of the Oedipus complex is the Electra complex, Electra being a mythological princess of Mycenae who goaded her brother Orestes to avenge their father's death by killing their mother. In the Electra complex, a girl sees her father as a love-object because she feels a need to have a baby to substitute for the penis that she is lacking. As her father is unavailable as a love object, she displaces her feelings for him onto other boys and begins to identify with her mother—thereby becoming a woman like her. In either case, the main task in the phallic stage is the establishment of sexual identity.

Although much derided in his time and still derided today, Freud is unquestionably one of the deepest and most original thinkers of the 20th century. Despite the disdain in which doctors often hold him, he is, ironically, the most famous of all doctors and the only one to have become a household name. He is credited with discovering the unconscious and inventing psychoanalysis, and had a colossal impact not only on his field of psychiatry but also on art, literature, and the humanities. He may have been thinking of himself (he often did) when he noted that, 'the voice of intelligence is soft, but it does not die until it has made itself heard.'

Carl Jung

> To be normal is the ideal aim of the unsuccessful.
> —CG Jung

Carl Gustav Jung was born in 1875 in the canton of Thurgau to Paul Jung, a poor rural pastor in the Swiss reformed Church, and Emilie Preiswerk, a melancholic woman who claimed to be visited by spirits at night. His paternal grandfather Carl Gustav Jung, after whom he was named, was a physician who was rumoured to be the illegitimate son of Goethe, and who rose to become Rector of Basel University and Grand Master of the Swiss Lodge of Freemasons. His maternal grandfather Samuel Preiswerk was an eccentric theologian who had visions, conversed with the dead, and devoted his life to learning Hebrew in the belief that it was the language spoken in heaven. He used to make his daughter Emilie (Jung's mother) sit behind him while he composed his sermons so as to prevent the devil from peering over his shoulder. When Jung was three years old, his mother had a nervous breakdown and spent several months in hospital. In his autobiography of 1961, *Memory, Dreams, Reflections*, he wrote, 'From then on I always felt mistrustful when the word 'love' was spoken. The feeling I associated with 'woman' was for a long time that of innate unreliability.' As for his father, he was kind but weak-willed, and all too accepting of the religious dogma in which he had long lost all faith.

Jung was a solitary and introverted child who imagined that he had two personalities, that of a typical school-boy of his time (Personality No. 1), and that of a dignified, authoritative, and influential man from the past (Personality No. 2). He once carved a tiny mannequin into the end of a wooden ruler, which he kept together with a painted stone in a pencil case in his attic. He periodically returned to the mannequin, bringing to it scrolls inscribed in a secret language of his invention. Perhaps unsurprisingly, he was not popular at school. At the age of 12, he received a blow to the head and for a moment was unconscious. He lay on the ground for much longer than necessary and thought, 'Now you won't have to go to school anymore.' For the next six months, he avoided school by fainting each time his parents tried to make him go—an episode which gave him an early insight into hysteria.

Inspired by a dream, Jung entered the University of Basel in 1895 to study natural science and medicine. His father's premature death one year later prompted his mother to comment, rather eerily, that 'he died in time for you'. During his early years at the University of Basel, Jung had a dream in which he was battling against dense fog, with a tiny light in the cup of his hands and a gigantic black figure chasing after him. When he awoke he realized that the black figure was his own shadow, brought into being by the light that he was carrying: '...this light was my consciousness, the only light that I have. My own understanding is the sole treasure I possess, and the greatest.' After presenting a paper on *The Limits of the Exact Sciences*, he spent two years attending and recording the séances of a young medium, his cousin, Hélène Preiswerk. He submitted his observations in the form of a doctoral thesis entitled, *On the Psychology and Pathology of So-Called Occult Phenomena*.

Towards the end of his studies, a reading of Krafft-Ebing's textbook of psychiatry led Jung to choose psychiatry as a career. The preface alone had such a profound effect on him that he had to stand up to catch his breath: 'Here alone the two currents of my interest could flow together and in a united stream dig their own bed. Here was the empirical field common to biological and spiritual facts, which I had everywhere sought and nowhere found.' Jung was taken on at the renowned Burghölzli Psychiatric Hospital in Zürich as an assistant to Eugen Bleuler, who went down in history as the man who coined the term 'schizophrenia'. Bleuler set his new assistant to work on Galton's word-association test, and in 1906 Jung published *Studies in Word Association*, which, he claimed, provided hard evidence for the existence of unconscious complexes. He sent a copy to Freud, and on their first meeting in Vienna the two men conversed without interruption for thirteen hours.

Jung needed a father as much as Freud needed a son, and Freud formally anointed Jung his 'son and heir'. However, as time passed, it became increasingly clear that Jung was unable to accept Freud's assumptions that human motivation is exclusively sexual, and that the unconscious mind is entirely personal. For Jung, sexuality was but one aspect or mode of a broader 'life force', and beneath the personal unconscious there lay a deeper and more important layer that contained the entire psychic heritage of mankind. The existence of this 'collective unconscious' had been hinted at by Jung's childhood dreams and experi-

ences, and confirmed by the delusions and hallucinations of psychotic people which contained symbols and images that occurred in myths and fairy-tales from all around the world. In his book of 1912, *Transformations and Symbols of the Libido*, Jung replaced Freud's concept of libido with a much broader concept of undifferentiated psychic energy, arguing that this energy could 'crystallize' into the universal symbols contained in dreams and myths, for example, into the hero's slaying of the dragon, which represents the struggle of the adolescent ego for deliverance from parental dominance. For Jung, the purpose of life was 'individuation', which involves pursuing one's own vision of the truth, and, in so doing, realizing one's fullest potential as a human being. If this meant disagreeing with Freud, then so be it. In 1913, on the eve of the First World War, Jung and Freud broke off their relationship.

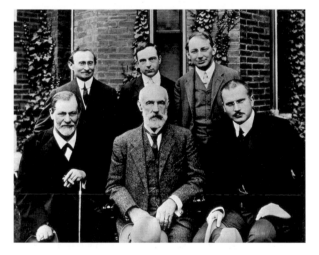

Figure 1.3. Jung (front right) with Freud (front left) at Clark University in 1909.

Once again Jung was alone, and he spent the next few years in a troubled but highly creative state of mind that bordered on psychosis and led him to a 'confrontation with the unconscious'. By then Jung had had five children with his wife Emma Rauschenbach, the daughter of a rich industrialist. Despite being happily married, he felt that he needed a muse as well as a home-maker, observing that, 'the pre-requisite of a good marriage... is the license to be unfaithful.' The marital strife that resulted from his affairs, particularly his affair with a former patient called Toni Wolff, contributed to his troubled state of mind, and Emma accepted Toni as much from a concern for Jung's sanity as from a desire to salvage her marriage.

During his confrontation with the unconscious, Jung gained first-hand experience of psychotic material in which he found a 'matrix of mythopoeic imagination which has vanished from our rational age'. Like Gilgamesh, Odysseus, Heracles, Orpheus, and Aeneas before him, he travelled deep down into an abyssal underworld where he conversed with Salome, a beautiful young woman who was the archetype of the feminine, and with Philemon, an old man with a white beard and the wings of a kingfisher who was the archetype of the wise old man. Although Salome and Philemon were products of his unconscious, they had lives of their own and said things that he had not previously thought. In Philemon, Jung had at long last found the father-figure that both Freud and his own father had failed to be. More than that, Philemon was a guru, and prefigured what Jung himself was later to become: the 'wise old man of Zürich'. At the end of the First World War, Jung re-emerged into sanity, and considered that he had found in his madness 'the prima materia for a life-time's work'. Jung died in 1961, at the age of 85.

The psychiatric assessment

Descriptive psychopathology

Much of the difficulty we face in mental health, whether as users or providers of services, whether as psychiatrists, psychologists, nurses, or advocates, arises from the stigmatization of our discipline as being, somehow, an inadequate also-ran to general medicine. Well, it is easier to run up a small hill than a mountain! The scientific mountain of psychiatry is, partly, the empirical challenge of developing methods of investigating the brain. Psychiatry shares this empirical challenge with neurology. But psychiatric science, in being concerned with the higher functions (of emotion, belief, volition, and so forth) has conceptual challenges as well. These challenges start with the structure of experience and of the disturbed experiences that are the subject of descriptive psychopathology.

—The Oxford Textbook of Philosophy and Psychiatry

Descriptive psychopathology provides a common language to define and recognize the signs and symptoms of mental disorder, and, notably by emphasizing form over content (Chapter 1), can be seen as a scientific basis for the practice of psychiatry.

The psychiatrist and philosopher Karl Jaspers (1883-1969) pioneered the field of descriptive psychopathology, and his *Allgemeine Psychopathologie* (*General Psychopathology*) of 1913 still provides one of the most complete accounts of the subject. The philosopher Edmund Husserl (1859-1938) inspired the thought of Jaspers. Husserl believed that the direct investigation and description of phenomena as consciously experienced, without any theories or preconceptions about their nature or causes, could lead to greater insight into their true essence. Accordingly, one of the central tenets of descriptive psychopathology is to avoid making assumptions about the signs and symptoms of mental disorder, but simply to define, distinguish, and inter-relate them. This section upholds this principle, leaving the causes and consequences of mental disorder to subsequent chapters.

Etymology for descriptive psychopathology

Etymon is Greek for 'literal meaning'. Etymology helps us to understand and remember the terms used in descriptive psychopathology: most are derived from Greek, some from Latin, and a handful from French or German. The short list in Table 2.1 is by no means exhaustive.

Table 2.1: Etymology for descriptive psychopathology

Root term	Meaning	Derivation (definitions to follow)
Agora	Assembly, market place	Agoraphobia
Alucinor (**Latin**)	To journey in the mind or dream	Hallucination
Ambi-	Both, around, about	Ambitendence
Athetos	Unfixed	Athetosis
Athron	Joint	Dysarthria
Campus (**Latin**)	Field	Extracampine hallucination
Choreia	Dance	Choreiform movements
Cryptos	Hidden	Cryptolalia
Eidos	Form, shape	Eidetic image
Eu	Good, easy	Euthymia, euphoria
Horama	View (from *horan*, to see)	Panoramic hallucination
Hypnos	Sleep	Hypnagogic hallucination
Kinesis	Motion	Akinesia
Laleo	Talk	Echolalia, cryptolalia, palilalia
Logos	Word	Neologism, logoclonia, logorrhoea
Nihil (**Latin**)	Nothing	Nihilistic delusion
Opsia	Sight	Palinopsia
Palin	Again	Palinopsia, palilalia
Pathos	Emotion	Apathy
Phasis	Speech	Aphasia
Phonia	Sound, voice	Dysphonia
Praxis	Acting, doing	Dyspraxia
Pseudo-	False	Pseudo-hallucination
Rheos	A stream (from *rhein*, to flow)	Logorrhoea
Soma	Body	Somatic delusion
Stereos	Solid	Stereotypy
Stupere (**Latin**)	To be numbed or stunned	Stupor
Thumos	Temper	Euthymia, cyclothymia

Introduction to the psychiatric assessment

The psychiatric assessment is usually carried out in two parts:

1. Gathering information: the psychiatric history and mental state examination.
2. Assessing and acting upon that information: the formulation.

You will find a sample psychiatric assessment towards the end of this chapter.

The psychiatric history

In psychiatry, the history is of special importance, since the physical examination and investigations are seldom of diagnostic value. The psychiatric history is actually not very different from any other medical or surgical history: its structure is the same, except that *past medical history* is split into *past psychiatric history* and *past medical history*, and there is an additional section for *personal history*. *Drug history, family history, social history,* and *personal history* are accorded a lot of importance, owing to their strong bearing on aetiology, management, and prognosis.

In sum, the psychiatric history can be carried out under ten main headings:

1. Introductory information
2. Presenting problem and history of presenting problem
3. Past psychiatric history
4. Past medical history
5. Drug history/current treatments
6. Substance use
7. Family history

8. Social history
9. Personal history
10. Informant history

Do however keep in mind that your aim is not to rattle through a long list of headings, but to facilitate the patient's telling of his or her story. A rigid and robotic approach damages your rapport with the patient, who is likely to perceive you as cold and distant, and lacking in humanity and wisdom.

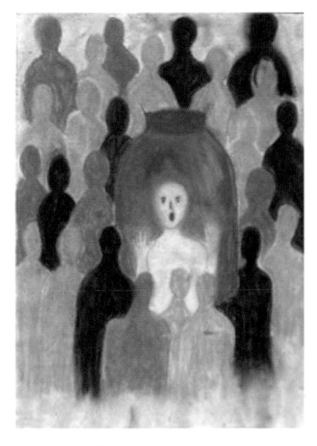

Figure 2.1. A good historian is not one who practices textbook psychiatry, but one who listens for the sake of listening, with respect, interest, and understanding. This in itself is a powerful form of therapy.

The mental state examination

The mental state examination (MSE) is, strictly speaking, a snapshot of the patient's behaviour and mental experiences at or around that point in time. Just as an abdominal examination serves to seek out the signs of

gastrointestinal disorders, so the MSE serves to seek out the signs of mental disorders. In addition, the MSE also serves to seek out the *symptoms* of mental disorders, and in that much also resembles the functional enquiry of a medical history. Being as it is part examination and part functional enquiry, the MSE relies on a firm grasp of descriptive psychopathology.

The MSE is usually carried out after the psychiatric history. Alternatively, it can be carried out during the psychiatric history, immediately after *presenting problem and history of presenting problem* (an approach that often makes more sense, not least to the patient). In practice, the MSE takes place surreptitiously throughout your time with the patient.

The MSE can be carried out under seven main headings:

1. Appearance and behaviour
2. Speech
3. Mood, plus anxiety and risk assessment
4. Thoughts
5. Perceptions
6. Cognition
7. Insight

The role of the MSE is to ensure that important signs and symptoms of mental disorder are screened for and, if present, fully explored.

The MSE can be looked upon as a 'core and module questionnaire', with positive responses to simple screening questions about important psychiatric symptoms prompting further, in-depth questioning around the symptom(s) in question.

The formulation

The formulation is not merely a summary of the psychiatric history and mental state examination, but also an assessment of the case.

Like the MSE, it can be carried out under seven main headings:

1. Case summary or synopsis
2. Further information required
3. Differential diagnosis
4. Risk assessment
5. Aetiology
6. Management
7. Prognosis

Safety (!)

By and large, people suffering from mental disorder are a vulnerable group, and pose no greater threat to safety than the average person. However, a small minority may pose a threat (Table 2.9), and some simple precautions need to be taken.

- Before seeing a patient, ask a qualified member of staff if it is safe for you to do so. In particular, does the patient have a history of violence?
- If it is safe for you to see the patient, tell the staff member where and how long you will be.
- Ask to be accompanied, for example, by another student.
- At least one of you should be carrying a portable alarm.
- Familiarize yourselves with the interview room's alarm system, if any.
- Configure the interview room so that you are sitting closest to the exit.
- At the same time, ensure that you are not blocking the patient's escape route.
- Remove any obvious potential weapons or projectiles.

Think of the bigger picture and trust your instinct. If you feel unsafe in any given situation, calmly and politely extricate yourself. This is, in fact, much more professional than putting yourself at risk. Remember that the vast majority of people suffering from a mental disorder are in the community, and that in-patients are the most ill of the ill. They are not representative of most people with mental disorder.

The psychiatric history

Introductory information

Before introducing yourself, note the patient's:
- Sex, age, occupation, and ethnic or cultural background.
- Mode of referral, and the reason for the referral.
- Mental Health Act status, if detained under a Section of the Mental Health Act (Chapter 3).

Presenting problem and history of presenting problem

- After putting the patient at ease, begin with an open question such as:

  How are you?

  How have you been doing lately?

  Why have you come to see me today?

In general, try to use open rather than closed or leading questions. Then listen. Do not underestimate the power of listening. In normal conversation, people tend to talk at each other, or past each other, but rarely if ever *to* each other. Try really listening to one of your friends and see what happens.

Clinical skills: Open, closed, and leading questions (♀)

Open question:	*How are you doing?*
Closed question:	*Are there times when you feel tearful?*
Leading question:	*You're feeling low, aren't you?*

Closed questions are sometimes necessary, but leading questions should always be avoided.

- Record the patient's principal problems verbatim. For example, "*I have a feeling of unreality, that people are conspiring to make life seem normal when in actual fact it is unreal*" is far more vivid and descriptive than, 'The patient complains of derealization.'
- Establish the precise nature of the symptoms, including:
  - onset and progression
  - possible precipitating and perpetuating factors
  - effect on everyday life
  - exacerbating and relieving factors, including any treatments
- Use the logico-deductive approach rather than the exhaustive approach to history taking: instead of asking about everything under the sun, form a diagnostic hypothesis and try to validate or falsify it by asking discriminating questions. For example, if you think that a patient might be depressed because he lost his job three months ago and complains of feeling tired all the time, ask about other symptoms of depression such as low mood, loss of interest, sleep disturbance, and so on.

Past psychiatric history

- Previous episodes of mental disorder.
- Previous psychiatric admissions, formal (under a Section) and informal.
- Previous physical and psychological treatments and their outcomes.
- History of self-harm or attempted suicide.

Past medical history

- Current illness:
  - acute illness

- chronic illness
- vascular risk factors
- Past and childhood illnesses, including head injury.
- Past hospital admissions and surgery.

Drug history/current treatments

- Psychological treatments such as counselling and CBT.
- Prescribed medication: route, dosage, regimen, adverse effects and longer term complications, compliance.
- Recent changes in prescribed medication which could account for a relapse.
- Over-the-counter and alternative remedies such as St John's Wort (depression), Kava (anxiety), Valerian (insomnia), and Ginkgo (memory).
- Allergic and adverse reactions.

Substance use

- Alcohol.
- Tobacco.
- Illicit drugs such as cannabis, LSD, ecstasy, amphetamines, cocaine, and heroin.

Further questioning to elicit the features of dependence syndrome is required if alcohol or drug use is substantial (Chapter 11).

Family history

- Determine if anyone in the family suffers, or has suffered, from mental disorder. Did they respond to treatment? Start with a question such as:

  Has anyone in the family ever had problems similar to the ones you've been having?
  Has anyone in the family ever had a nervous breakdown?

- Partner: Age, occupation, health.
- Children: Age, schooling, health. Where do they normally live? Who is caring for them?
- Quality of relationships and atmosphere in the home.
- Recent events in the family.

Sketch an annotated genogram if the family history is complex and relevant (Figure 2.2).

Social history

- Self-care.
- Family and social support.

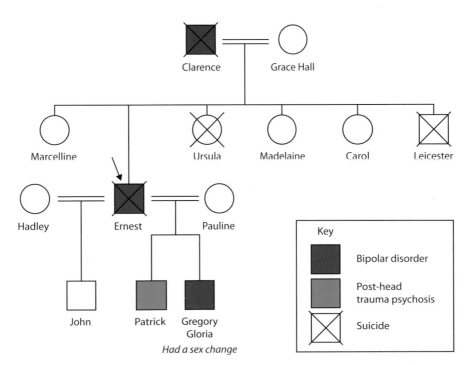

Figure 2.2. Genogram for Ernest Hemingway.

- Housing.
- Finances.
- Typical day.
- Interests and hobbies.
- Predominant mood and premorbid personality.

Clinical skills: Assessment of premorbid personality

Premorbid personality can be assessed through:
- General questions about personality:
    How would you describe your normal self?
    How would others describe you?
    Do you prefer being alone or surrounded by other people?
- 'Situational' questions:
    How did you cope when…?
- Social and personal histories.
- Informant histories.

It is important to focus on the patient's personality before he became ill, and to tease this apart from his current mental state.

You can test your own personality at www.similarminds.com.

Personal history
- Pregnancy and birth.
- Developmental milestones.
- Childhood: Emotional problems, serious illnesses, prolonged separation from parents, bullying.
- Educational achievement: Favourite subjects, academic record, learning difficulties. Did the patient like school?
- Occupational history: Jobs in chronological order, reasons for changes, current job satisfaction.
- Psychosexual history: Past and present partners, quality of relationships, frequency of sexual intercourse, sexual problems, contraception, physical and sexual abuse.
- Forensic history: Arrests, charges, convictions, imprisonment. A good question to ask is:
    Have you ever had problems with the police?
- Spiritual orientation. Good questions are:
    Do you generally believe that there is something beyond us, like God?
    Is religion important to you?

Before closing, use an enjoinder such as:
You've told me a lot about yourself, thank you. Is there anything else that you'd like to mention?

Informant history

If possible, you should check the patient's records and corroborate the history by interviewing an informant such as a relative, friend, carer, police officer, GP, or other healthcare professional (seek the patient's consent first). Informant histories are particularly useful if, owing to his or her mental state, the patient is unable to provide a clear, complete, or reliable history. They are also opportunities for assessing the attitudes and dispositions of relatives and carers, and for involving them in the management plan.

The mental state examination

This section also integrates the descriptive psycho-pathology required for the MSE. Common and important signs and symptoms are in *italics*. The rest are included mainly for interest.

Recall that the MSE can be carried out under seven main headings:
1. Appearance and behaviour
2. Speech
3. Mood, plus anxiety and risk assessment
4. Thoughts
5. Perceptions
6. Cognition
7. Insight

Appearance and behaviour

Note the following:
- Level of consciousness, e.g. hyperalert, vigilant, alert, somnolent.
- Appearance: Body build, posture, general physical condition, grooming and hygiene, dress, physical stigmata such as scars, piercing, and tattoos. Remember that scars result not only from accidents and operations, but also—and importantly—from self-harm.
- Behaviour and attitude to the examiner. In particular, note: Facial expression, degree of eye contact, and quality of rapport.
- Motor activity/abnormalities of movement, e.g. agitation, retardation, tremor, dystonia (Table 2.2). Abnormalities of movement affecting induced movements and posture tend to be associated with catatonic schizophrenia, which, over the past decades, has become rare (Chapter 4).

Table 2.2: Abnormalities of movement

Amount of movement

Agitation	Excessive motor activity and restlessness, e.g. fidgeting or pacing.
Retardation	Lack of motor activity; the opposite of agitation.
Stupor	An extreme form of retardation such that the patient is immobile and mute.

Abnormalities of movement

Spontaneous movements

Mannerism	Odd, repetitive, goal-directed movement, e.g. flicking hair, pulling up socks (cf. stereotypy).
Stereotypy	Odd, repetitive, non-goal-directed movement, e.g. body rocking, head banging.
Tic	Movement or vocalization that is involuntary, sudden, rapid, recurrent, non-rhythmic, and stereotyped.
Static tremor	Resting tremor that is usually attenuated by deliberate movement.
Dystonia	Spasm of muscle groups that most commonly affects the neck, eyes, and trunk, e.g. tongue protrusion, grimacing, torticollis.
Akathisia	Subjective feeling of inner restlessness manifested by fidgety leg movements, shuffling of feet, pacing, etc.
Dyskinesia	Involuntary, repetitive, purposeless movements that may be generalized or affect only certain muscles groups, typically the orofacial muscles ('rabbit syndrome').
Athetosis	Slow semi-rotatory and writhing movements of the limbs.
Myoclonus	Sudden, jerky, and involuntary movement of a muscle or group of muscles.
Chorea	Sudden, jerky, and involuntary movements of several muscle groups that resemble fragments of goal-directed behaviour.

Induced movements

Advertence/aversion	Turning towards/away from the examiner in an exaggerated way when engaged with him or her.
Forced grasping	Repetitive grasping and shaking of the examiner's proffered hand despite requests to desist.
Echopraxia	Imitation of the examiner's body movements despite requests to desist.
Perseveration	Repetition of a movement or behaviour requested by the examiner even though it is no longer appropriate.
Automatic obedience	Indiscriminate obedience of the examiner's commands regardless of their consequences.
Blocking	Interruption of a movement before it can be completed.
Obstruction	Irregular blocking of movements.
Ambitendence	Alternation of opposite movements, e.g. putting out a hand and then pulling it back again before the action can be fully completed.
Mitmachen	In mitmachen the limbs can be placed in any posture, after which they return to their resting position (cf. mitgehen, catalepsy).
Mitgehen	An extreme form of mitmachen: the limbs can be placed in any posture even at a slight touch.

Posture

Posturing	Voluntary assumption and maintenance of unusual and normally uncomfortable body postures, often for hours on end. Includes 'psychological pillow' in which the patient lies prone with his or her head raised by a few centimetres.
Catalepsy (waxy flexibility)	In catalepsy the limbs can be placed in any posture, to be maintained in that posture for unusually long periods of time.
Rigidity	Maintenance of a rigid posture against attempts to be moved.
Gegenhalten	Involuntary resistance to passive movement.
Negativism	Extreme form of gegenhalten involving resistance to instructions or attempts to be moved, or movement in the opposite direction.

> **Clinical skills: Distinguishing between catatonia, catalepsy, and cataplexy** 💡

Catatonia A motor syndrome diagnosable in the presence of two or more of:
- motor immobility
- motor excitement
- negativism or mutism
- posturing, stereotypies, or mannerisms
- echolalia or echopraxia

Catalepsy An occasional feature of catatonia in which the limbs can be placed in any posture, and are maintained in that posture for unusually long periods. Also known as waxy flexibility or *cerea flexibilitas*.

Cataplexy A sudden loss of muscle tone leading to collapse. Cataplexy is a feature of the sleep disorder narcolepsy, and is thus completely unrelated to either catatonia or catalepsy.

Speech

Guard your roving thoughts with a jealous care, for speech is but the dealer of thoughts, and every fool can plainly read in your words what is the hour of your thoughts.

—Alfred, Lord Tennyson

Our speech mirrors our thoughts, but under 'speech' you should limit yourself to recording the technical aspects of speech. The *content* of speech is more appropriately described under 'thoughts'.

Note the following:
- Amount, rate, volume, and tone of speech (Table 2.3).
- *Form* of speech (Table 2.3).

Table 2.3: Abnormalities of speech

Ability for speech

Dysphonia	Impairment of ability to vocalize speech.
Dysarthria	Impairment of ability to articulate speech.
Dysphasia	Impairment of ability to comprehend or express language.

Amount of speech

Logorrhoea	Increased quantity (but not rate) of speech.
Poverty of speech	Decreased quantity (but not rate) of speech.

Rate of speech

Pressure of speech	Increased quantity and rate of speech. Speech is hard to interrupt.
Speech retardation	Decreased quantity and rate of speech.
Mutism	Failure to speak despite the physical ability to do so.

Form of speech

Circumstantiality	Speech is organized and goal-oriented but cramped by excessive or irrelevant detail and parenthetical remarks (Figure 2.3).
Tangentiality	Speech is organized but not goal-oriented in that it is only very indirectly related to the questions being asked (Figure 2.3).
Neologism	Use of a new word or condensed combination of words.
Metonym	Use of an existing word with a new meaning.
Clang association	Linkage of words based on sound rather than meaning.
Word salad (schizophasia)	Loss of associations between words, speech is experienced as an incoherent jumble of words.
Paragrammatism	Incorrect grammatical construction, e.g. *I eaten have apples four*.
Paraphasia	Incorrect selection of words: the production of one word when another is meant.
Logoclonia	Repetition of the last syllable of every word.
Palilalia	Repetition of a word after it is no longer appropriate.
Verbigeration	Senseless repetition of sounds, words, or phrases.
Echolalia	Senseless and parrot-like imitation of the examiner's speech (cf. echopraxia).
Coprolalia	Vocal tic involving the shouting of obscenities.
Glossolalia	Use of non-speech sounds as a substitute for speech.
Cryptolalia	Use of an entire private idiom or language.
Pseudologia fantastica	Fluent and plausible lying.
Vorbeigehen (Ganser symptom)	Approximate answers to the questions being asked, e.g. —*How many legs does a chair have?* —*Three*, thereby demonstrating that the question has been understood.

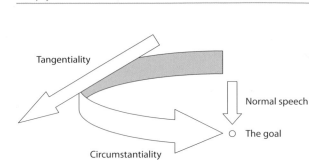

Figure 2.3. Normal speech, circumstantiality, and tangentiality.

Mood

Note the following:

- Current mood and severity. Good screening questions for low mood are:

  Have you been keeping reasonably cheerful?

  Are there times when you feel low-spirited or tearful?

  How would you rate your mood out of 10, where 10 is normal and 1 is the worst you've ever felt?

  Good screening questions for elevated mood are:

  Have you been feeling particularly cheerful?

  Have you been feeling on top of the world?

  If there is the suggestion of a mood disorder, this should be explored further (Chapter 5). It is customary to report both 'subjective mood' (the patient's report of his or her mood) and 'objective mood' (the examiner's impression of the patient's mood).

- Affect, e.g. normal, expansive, constricted, blunted, flattened, labile. In particular, does the patient's affect seem inappropriate?

- Ideas of self-harm and suicide. Asking about these topics can feel uncomfortable. Begin with a formulation such as:

  People with problems similar to yours sometimes feel that life is no longer worth living. Have you ever felt that way?

  If yes, this must be explored further (Chapter 6).

- Ideas of harm to others, especially dependent children.

- Anxiety and its symptoms, e.g. butterflies, palpitations, clamminess. A good screening question for anxiety is:

  Are there times when you become very anxious or frightened?

  If yes, this should be explored further (Chapter 7).

Disorders of mood are listed in Table 2.4.

Table 2.4: Abnormalities of mood

Mood	A pervasive and sustained emotional state such as anxiety, depression, or euphoria.
Affect	Observable *behaviour* associated with changing emotions such as fear, sadness, or joy.
	NB: Affect is to mood as weather is to climate.
Emotional predispositions	
Euthymia	Normal mood.
Dysthymia	A predominantly depressive temperament.
Hyperthymia	A predominantly euphoric temperament.
Cyclothymia	Alternating periods of mild depression and mild euphoria.
Emotional reactions	
Anxiety	A sense of apprehension at a perceived threat.
Irritability	A state of reduced control over aggressive impulses.
Depression	Depressed mood and other symptoms.
Anhedonia	The inability to experience pleasure from previously pleasurable activities.
Euphoria	Undue cheerfulness and elation.
Ecstasy	A pantheistic experience that the subject and the universe are one.
Apathy	A lack or absence of emotion, interest, or concern.
Expressions of emotion	
Blunting/flattening of affect	Dulling of normal emotional responses.
Emotional lability	Sudden, rapid, and often marked shifts in affect.
Emotional incontinence	Complete loss of control over affect, an extreme form of emotional lability.
Dissociation of affect	Affect is inappropriate to thought content, e.g. laughter upon recounting the death of a loved one.
Incongruity of affect	Affect is inappropriate to magnitude of events: an important event leaves the patient emotionless, whereas a small and insignificant event triggers an emotional outburst.
Perplexity	Anxious or puzzled bewilderment.

> It was the autumn of 1826. I was in a dull state of nerves, such as everybody is occasionally liable to; unsusceptible to enjoyment or pleasurable excitement; one of those moods when what is pleasure at other times, becomes insipid or indifferent... In this frame of mind it occurred to me to put the question directly to myself, 'suppose that all your objects in life were realised; that all the changes in institutions and opinions which you are looking forward to, could be completely effected at this very instant: would this be a great joy and happiness to you?' And an irrepressible self-consciousness distinctly answered, 'No!' At this my heart sank within me: the whole foundation on which my life was constructed fell down.
>
> —JS Mill on anhedonia, *Autobiography*

Thoughts

Record the following:

- Stream of thought.
- Form of thought.
- Content of thought. In particular, screen for delusions and overvalued ideas. For obvious reasons, you cannot ask directly about delusions. Begin with an introductory statement and general questions such as:

I would like to ask you some questions that may seem a little strange. These are questions that we put to all of our patients. Is that OK? Do you have any beliefs that your friends and family do not share?

Then, if necessary, ask specifically about common delusional themes (Table 2.6 and Chapter 4). For example, for delusions of control, ask:

Is anyone or anything trying to control you?
Is anyone or anything trying to interfere with your thoughts?

As well as delusions and overvalued ideas, you should also screen for phobias and preoccupations, ruminations, and obsessions. For example:

Do you have any special fears, like some people are afraid of spiders or snakes?
Is anything bothering or weighing on you?
Do certain things keep coming into your mind, even though you try hard to keep them out?

Disorders of thought are listed in Table 2.5.

Table 2.5: Abnormalities of thought

Stream of thought	
Pressure of thought	Thoughts arise in unusual variety and abundance and pass through the mind quickly. This is evidenced as pressure of speech.
Poverty of thought	The opposite of pressure of thought, evidenced as poverty of speech.
Thought blocking	Sudden loss of the train of thought, often in mid-sentence. There is a subjective experience of the mind just 'going blank'.
Form of thought	
Flight of ideas	Thoughts move quickly from one to another and seem to be only loosely connected (e.g. by clang association, punning, or rhyming).
Loosening of associations	Thoughts move quickly from one to another and seem unconnected. This is evidenced as muddled or illogical speech.
Over-inclusive thinking	An inability to preserve the conceptual boundaries of thought. This is evidenced as circumstantiality.
Concrete thinking	An inability to understand abstract concepts and metaphorical ideas, with, for example, a literal understanding of sayings and proverbs.
Dereistic thinking	Idiosyncratic thinking that is not falsified by reality, e.g. day-dreaming.
Content of thought	
Phobia	Persistent irrational fear leading to conscious avoidance of the feared object, activity, or situation.
Rumination	Repetitive and pointless internal debates often involving pseudo-philosophical issues.
Obsessional thought	A recurrent idea, image, or impulse that (1) is perceived as being senseless, (2) is unsuccessfully resisted, and (3) results in marked anxiety and distress.

Table 2.5: Abnormalities of thought – *contd*

Delusion	An unshakeable (fixed) belief held in the face of evidence to the contrary and that cannot be explained by culture or religion. Although a delusion is not necessarily false, the process by which it arises is bizarre and illogical. A delusion can be primary or secondary:
	Primary delusion (autochthonous delusion, delusional intuition, apophany): fully formed delusion that is unconnected to previous thoughts and events and that is psychologically irreducible.
	Secondary delusion: delusion that arises from, and can be understood in the context of, previous ideas or events.
	Systematized delusions: a group of delusions organized around a common theme, or multiple elaborations of a single delusion.
Delusional perception	The attribution of delusional significance to normal perceptions.
Delusional memory	The attribution of delusional significance to a memory or false memory.
Delusional mood or atmosphere	A period in which the world seems subtly altered, uncanny, portentous, or sinister, and which is conducive to the formation of delusions.
Overvalued idea	An idiosyncratic and firmly held belief which is in itself acceptable and comprehensible but which comes to dominate thinking and behaviour. It differs from a delusion in that the belief is not fixed, and from an obsessional thought in that it is not perceived as being senseless.
Idea of reference	The sense that events and happenings refer directly to oneself, for example, the sense that people on the radio are talking to or about oneself. If this sense becomes a fixed belief, it is then called a delusion of reference.
Magical thinking	An irrational (although not delusional) belief that certain outcomes are connected to certain thoughts, words, or actions, e.g. if I hold my nose, someone will die.
Folie à deux	Shared psychotic disorder: one person communicates his delusion to another so that he too becomes psychotic.

Table 2.6: Delusional themes

Delusional theme	Notes
Delusions of persecution	Delusions that one is being persecuted, for example, being spied upon by secret services or poisoned by aliens.
Delusions of control	Delusions that one's thoughts, feelings, or actions are being interfered with by an external agency. Subtypes are: • thought insertion • thought withdrawal • thought broadcasting • passivity of affect, volition, or actions • somatic passivity
Delusions of reference	Delusions that objects, events, or other people have a special significance pertaining to oneself.
Delusions of misidentification	• Capgras syndrome: The delusion that a familiar individual has been replaced by an identical-looking imposter. • Fregoli syndrome: The delusion that a familiar individual is disguising as various strangers. • Intermetamorphosis: The delusion that a familiar person has been transformed into someone else. • Reverse intermetamorphosis: The delusion that one has been transformed into someone else. • Subjective doubles or *Doppelganger*: The delusion that there is a double of oneself. In 'clonal pluralization', there are several doubles. • Reduplicative paramnesia: The delusion that an object, place, or person has been multiplied. • Delusional companions: The delusion that objects are sentient beings, as in children's cartoons.
Delusions of grandeur	Delusions of being invested with special status, a special purpose, or special powers and abilities, for example, being the most intelligent person in Oxford, specially commissioned to save the world from climate change.

Table 2.6: Delusional themes– *contd*

Religious delusions	Delusions of having a special relationship with God or a supernatural force, for example, of being the next messiah, or being pursued by the devil.
Delusions of guilt	Delusions that one has committed a serious crime or sinned greatly, for example, being personally responsible for an earthquake or terrorist attack.
Nihilistic delusions	Delusions that one no longer exists, or that one is about to die or suffer a great catastrophe. Nihilistic delusions may feature the belief that other people or objects no longer exist or that the world is coming to an end. The combination of nihilistic and somatic delusions in depressive psychosis is sometimes referred to as *délire de négation* or Cotard syndrome.
Somatic delusions	Delusions about the body, for example, of having a medical condition or deformity. Cf. somatoform disorder, factitious disorder, malingering (Chapter 7).
Delusions of infestation	Delusion that one's skin is infested by parasites. In the context of a monosymptomatic delusional disorder, this is referred to as Ekbom syndrome.
Delusions of jealousy	Delusions that one's partner is being unfaithful. In the context of a monosymptomatic delusional disorder, this is referred to as Othello syndrome.
Delusions of love (Amorous delusions)	Delusions of being loved by someone who is distant or inaccessible. Erotomania or De Clérambault syndrome (named after French psychiatrist Gaëtan Gatian de Clérambault, author of *Les Psychoses Passionelles*) is the delusion of being secretly loved, usually by someone of a higher social status. Delusions of love are more common in women while delusions of jealousy are more common in men, hinting that delusional themes may have some basis in evolution.

There are fictions when the society supports you, there are fictions where nobody supports you. That is the difference between a sane and an insane person; a sane person is one whose fiction is supported by the society. He has manipulated the society to support his fiction. An insane man is one whose fiction is supported by nobody; he is alone so you have to put him in the madhouse.

—Rajneesh, *The Mustard Seed*

A delusion is defined as 'a strongly held belief that is not amenable to logic or persuasion and that is out of keeping with its holder's background or culture'. But for a strongly held belief to be a delusion, exactly how strongly must it be held? To whose logic must it not be amenable? And at what precise point is it out of keeping with its holder's background?

In the early 1970s, Prof David Rosenhan (1929-2012) of Stanford University and seven colleagues briefly feigned auditory hallucinations in an attempt to gain admission to various psychiatric hospitals. All eight pseudo-patients were admitted and diagnosed with schizophrenia or, in one case, bipolar disorder. Once admitted, the pseudo-patients acted normally, telling staff that the voices had stopped and that they felt fine. Despite this, staff interpreted much of their behaviour in terms of mental disorder. For example, a nurse labelled the note-taking of one pseudo-patient as pathological 'writing behaviour'. The pseudo-patients spent from 7 to 52 days (average 19 days) in hospital, and only secured their release after admitting to mental illness and agreeing to take antipsychotic medication.

In a secondary study, the staff at one hospital was informed that, over the next three months, one or more pseudo-patients would attempt to be admitted into their hospital. Out of 193 new patients, the staff confidently picked out 41 imposters. But Rosenhan had sent no one.

Perceptions

Record the following:

- Sensory distortions. A good screening question is:
  Have you noticed anything unusual about the way things look or sound, or smell, or taste?
- Depersonalization and derealization. Good screening questions are:
  Have you ever felt distant or unreal?
  Have you ever felt that things around you are unreal?
- Illusions and, especially, hallucinations. Begin by an introductory statement and general questions such as:
  I gather that you have been under quite some pressure recently. When people are under pressure they can sometimes find that their imagination plays tricks on them. Have you had any such experiences?
  Have you heard/seen anything unusual?
  Have you heard voices when there was no one around?
  Have you seen things that other people do not see?

For any hallucinations, record their modality, content, and mood congruency. Distinguish true hallucinations from pseudo-hallucinations, which tend to be a feature of personality disorder. Exclude hypnopompic and hynogogic hallucinations, which are very unlikely to be pathological. For voices, determine the number of voices, and if the voices talk *to* the patient (second person) or *about* the patient (third person). Do the voices command the patient to do dangerous things (command or imperative hallucinations), and, importantly, is the patient able to resist these orders? If the voices talk about the patient, do they comment on his or her every thought or action (running commentary)? Disorders of perception are listed in Table 2.7.

Clinical skills: Discussing psychotic symptoms

You should not overtly challenge a patient's delusions and hallucinations, but neither should you validate them. This difficult balance is best achieved by explicitly recognizing that the patient's delusions and hallucinations are important to him or her, while making it clear that you yourself do not experience or share in them. For example:

Patient: The aliens are saying they're going to abduct me.

Doctor: That sounds terrifying.

P: I've never been so frightened in all my life.

D: Gosh, yes, I can understand that, although I myself cannot hear the aliens you speak of.

P: You mean, you can't hear them?

D: No, not at all. Have you tried ignoring them?

P: When I listen to music they don't seem so loud.

D: What about when we chat together, like now?

P: Yes, that's very helpful too.

Table 2.7: Descriptive psychopathology: Disorders of perception

Sensory distortions	Sensory distortions include distortions of intensity, colour, form, and proportions.
Depersonalization	An alteration in the perception or experience of the self, leading to a sense of detachment from one's mental processes or body.
Derealization	An alteration in the perception or experience of the environment, leading to a sense that it is strange or unreal.
Illusion	A percept that arises as a misinterpretation of a stimulus (Figure 2.4), e.g. hearing voices in rustling leaves.
Affect illusion	Illusions that arise during periods of heightened emotion.
Completion illusion	Illusions that arise during periods of inattention.
Pareidolic illusion	Illusions that arise from poorly defined stimuli, e.g. seeing 'shapes' in the clouds.
Hallucination	A percept that arises in the absence of a stimulus. A true hallucination is experienced as arising from the sense organs (outer space) and not from within the mind, and shares the quality of a real perception.
Auditory hallucinations	
Simple	Simple sounds.
Complex	Complex sounds e.g. voices, music. Voices may be in the second person (you, addressing the patient directly) or the third person (he/she, talking about the patient).
Gedankenlautwerden	German for 'thoughts becoming loud': thoughts are 'heard' as they are being formulated (cf. thought broadcasting and *echo de la pensée*.)
Echo de la pensée	French for 'thought echo': thoughts are 'heard' shortly after they are formulated.

Table 2.7: Descriptive psychopathology: Disorders of perception – *contd*

Visual hallucinations

Simple	Flashes of light.
Complex	Images of objects, animals, people.
Panoramic	Images of objects, animals, people—plus the background.
Lilliputian	Images of objects, animals, people that are smaller than in reality (In *Gulliver's Travels*, the inhabitants of Lilliput are six inches tall).
Autoscopic	Image of the self is projected into external space. Differs from a near-death experience in that it does not involve a feeling of being outside the body.
Negative autoscopy	Image of the self cannot be seen in mirrors.
Eidetic image	Unusually vivid mental image of an object e.g. flashbacks, 'photographic memory'.
Charles Bonnet syndrome	Isolated, complex visual hallucinations, usually secondary to sudden loss of vision.
Olfactory & gustatory hallucinations	Olfactory and gustatory hallucinations may be difficult to differentiate from each another. They are usually of unpleasant odours/flavours.

Specific types

Hypnopompic	Visual or auditory hallucinations upon awaking.
Hypnagogic	Visual or auditory hallucinations upon falling asleep.
Extracampine	Hallucinations from outside the limits of the sensory field, e.g. hearing voices from Antarctica.
Functional	Hallucinations triggered by environmental stimuli in the same modality, e.g. voices triggered by the sound of a running tap.
Reflex	Hallucination triggered by environmental stimuli in a different modality, e.g. voices triggered by the sight of a photograph.
Pseudo-hallucinations	A pseudo-hallucination may differ from a true hallucination in that:

- It is perceived to arise from within the mind rather than from the sense organs.
- It is less vivid.
- It is less distressing.
- The patient has some degree of control over it.

Palinopsia	The persistence or recurrence of an image long after its stimulus has been removed.
Synaesthesia	In synaesthesia, sensations in one modality produce sensations in another. For example, a piece of music is experienced as a concert of colours. Arthur Rimbaud's *Voyelles* is a synaesthetic poem. Other artists to experiment with synaesthesia include Charles Baudelaire, Wassily Kandinsky, and Alexander Scriabin.

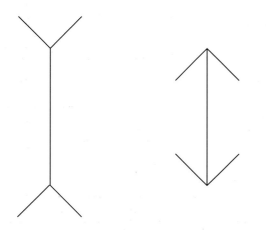

Figure 2.4. The Müller-Lyer illusion arises from the misinterpretation of a stimulus: both lines are in fact the same length. In contrast to an illusion, a hallucination arises in the absence of a stimulus.

Cognition

Record the following:
- Orientation in time, place, and person.
- Attention and concentration, e.g. ask the patient to subtract 7 from 100 and keep on going (serial sevens test).
- Memory: Short-term memory, recent memory, and remote memory.
- Grasp, e.g. ask the patient to name the current prime minister.

If cognition appears to be impaired, consider carrying out a more formal assessment such as the 30-point Folstein Mini-Mental State Examination (MMSE) or the freely available Montreal Cognitive Assessment (MoCA, Figure 2.5). For the MMSE, scores of less than 22 suggest

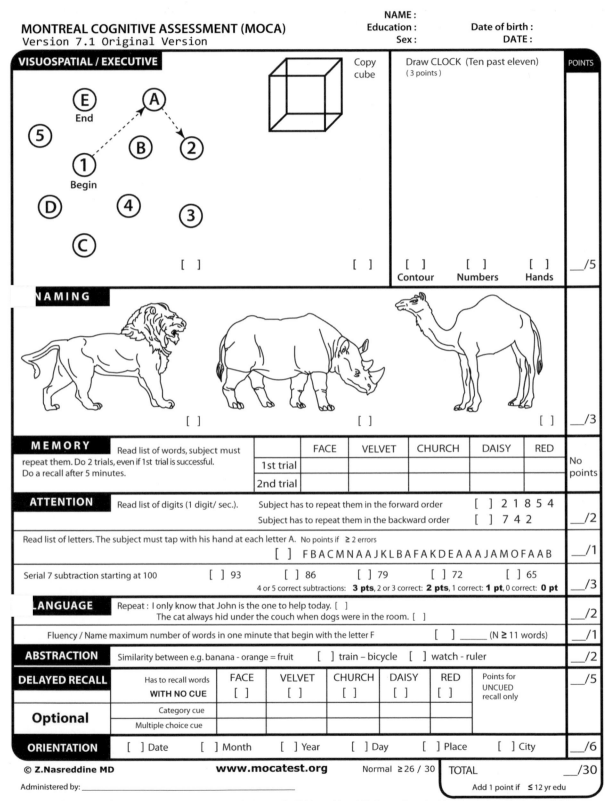

Figure 2.5. The Montreal Cognitive Assessment (MoCA). Copyright Z. Nasreddine MD. Reproduced with permission. Copies available at www.mocatest.org.

2

significant cognitive impairment, and scores of 22 to 25 suggest moderate cognitive impairment. The test cannot be interpreted if the patient is delirious or suffering from a mood disorder, or simply not co-operating!

Insight

To determine insight, ask the patient:

Do you think there's anything wrong with you?

If no:

Why did you come to hospital?

If yes:

What do you think is wrong with you?

What's caused it?

Do you think you need treatment?

What do you think treatment will achieve?

Note that insight is not synonymous with agreeing with the medical team!

The formulation

The formulation is not merely a synopsis of the psychiatric history and MSE, but also an assessment of the case.

Like the MSE, it can be carried out under seven headings:

1. Case summary
2. Further information
3. Differential diagnosis
4. Risk assessment
5. Aetiology
6. Management
7. Prognosis

Case summary

This ought to consist of a short paragraph summarizing the salient features of the history and MSE.

Further information required

Consider:

- Fuller psychiatric history and MSE.
- Informant histories from relatives, friends, carers, the police, and/or other healthcare professionals, including the patient's GP.
- Old records, e.g. medical records, school reports, police record.

- Physical examination. Required:
    - to exclude organic causes of the presentation, e.g. endocrine disorder, space-occupying lesion
    - to exclude complications of the presentation, e.g. malnutrition, burns, injuries from falls
    - as a baseline for starting psychotropic drugs
- Brain imaging (CT or MRI head), particularly if the presentation is atypical or suggestive of an organic, neurological aetiology.
- Psychological tests and inventories.

Clinical skills: The physical examination in psychiatry

Psychiatrists take responsibility for the physical health of their day- and in-patients, and an integral physical examination (vital signs and cardiovascular, respiratory, abdominal, and neurological examination) should be carried out on all aforesaid patients.

Medical disorders are commoner in psychiatric patients and may arise from a shared aetiology, as a direct or indirect consequence of mental disorder, or from psychotropic drugs.

In some cases, medical disorders actually underlie psychiatric signs and symptoms. For instance, depressive symptoms can result from endocrine disorders such as hypothyroidism and Cushing's syndrome, metabolic disorders such as hypercalcaemia and vitamin B12 deficiency, infective disorders such as hepatitis and HIV/AIDS, neurological disorders such as stroke and Parkinson's disease, and alcohol and drug misuse.

Differential diagnosis

List likely diagnoses in order of probability, and make a brief note of the evidence for and against each diagnosis.

This simple sieve should prevent you from overlooking the most important diagnostic possibilities:

Psychiatric differential

- Psychotic disorder
- Mood disorder
- Anxiety disorder
- Personality disorder

Organic differential

- Substance misuse
- Dementia and delirium
- Medical disorder e.g. endocrine disorder, space-occupying lesion...

Diagnoses that are higher up in the 'diagnostic hierarchy' (Figure 2.6) should take precedence over those that are lower down. For example, if a patient meets the criteria for all of schizophrenia, depression, and an anxiety disorder, the schizophrenia 'trumps' the depression and anxiety disorder because affective symptoms and anxiety symptoms are common in schizophrenia and often remit if the schizophrenia is treated.

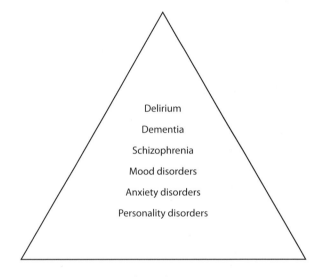

Figure 2.6. The diagnostic hierarchy.

Table 2.8: Factors that increase risk
(See also Chapter 6)

Personal factors	Previous violence to self or to others (best predictor)
	Male sex
	Young or elderly
	Recent life crisis
	Unemployed
	Divorced
	Socially isolated
	Socially unstable
	Victim of physical or sexual abuse
	Access to means
	Access to victims
Illness-related factors	Depressive symptoms
	Psychotic symptoms
	Substance misuse
	Treatment resistance
	Treatment non-compliance
Factors in the mental state	Suicidal ideation
	Anger
	Hostility
	Paranoia
	Expressed intent to harm or take revenge
	Command hallucinations
	Delusions of persecution
	Delusions of control
	Delusions of jealousy
	Delusions of guilt

Risk assessment

Assess the patient's risk:
- To self, through
  - self-harm
  - neglect
  - exploitation
- To others.

Aetiology

Identify predisposing, precipitating, and maintaining factors. For exam purposes, it can help to classify these factors as biological, psychological, or social, as per the biopsychosocial model (Table 2.9). You can also identify strengths or positive prognostic factors, e.g. first episode, good premorbid functioning, in a supportive relationship.

Table 2.9: Common aetiological factors for mental disorder

	Biological	**Psychological**	**Social**
Predisposing Factors	Family history	Cognitive distortions	Childhood abuse
	Substance misuse	Maladaptive behaviours	Bullying
	Organic conditions	Psychodynamic factors	Poor social support
			Poor housing
			Unemployment
Precipitating Factors	Substance misuse	Stress	Life events
	Organic conditions	Bereavement or loss	
	Non-compliance		
	Pattern of sleep		

Table 2.9: Common aetiological factors for mental disorder – *contd*

	Biological	Psychological	Social
Maintaining Factors	Substance misuse	Poor insight	Stigma
	Organic conditions	Cognitive distortions	Poor coping skills
	Non-compliance	Maladaptive behaviours	Poor social support
	Treatment-resistance	Psychodynamic factors	Poor housing
	Pattern of sleep	High expressed emotion	Unemployment
		Lack of confiding relationships	
Strengths	No family history	Good insight	Good premorbid
	No substance misuse	Strong motivation	functioning
	Responsive to medication	Confiding relationships	Good social support
	Compliant with medication		Employment

Management

The management plan should not omit psychological and social dimensions, which, especially in the longer term, may be far more important than the biological dimension.

Identify short-term and medium-term interventions. As with aetiological factors, it can help to classify interventions as biological, psychological, or social.

Table 2.10: Some possible interventions for mental disorder

	Biological	Psychological	Social
Short-term	Drugs	Counselling	Family education
	Detoxification	Psychoeducation	Carer support
	ECT		
Medium/long-term	Maintenance treatment	Self-help guides	Patient groups
	Depot antipsychotic	Meditation	Charities
	Mood stabilizer	Cognitive behavioural therapy	Benefits
	Family planning	Psychodynamic psychotherapy	Housing
		Family therapy	Rehabilitation
		Addictions counselling	Power of
			attorney

Prognosis

Make a clear prognosis both for the current episode and for the long-term, and explain your reasoning. You can also list any relevant positive and negative prognostic factors. Examples of important positive prognostic factors are first episode, good premorbid functioning, good social support, and good response to medication. Examples of important negative prognostic factors are strong family history, non-compliance with medication, and substance misuse.

Classification of Mental Disorders

If any man were bold enough to write a history of psychiatric classifications he would find when he had completed his task that in the process he had written a history of psychiatry as well.

—Robert Kendell, *The Role of Diagnosis in Psychiatry*

The majority of medical disorders are defined by their cause (aetiology) or by the bodily damage that they result in or from (pathology) and so are relatively easy to define and recognize. For instance, if someone is suspected of having malaria, a blood sample can be taken and examined under a microscope for malarial parasites of the genus *Plasmodium*; and if someone appears to have suffered a stroke, a brain scan can be taken to look for evidence of obstruction of an artery in the brain. In contrast, mental disorders cannot (as yet?) be defined according to their aetiology or pathology, but only according to their manifestations or symptoms. This means that they are more difficult to describe and diagnose, and more open to misunderstanding and misuse.

Psychiatric classifications represent an attempt to address these problems with clearly defined concepts and reliable operational criteria by which to diagnose them. One of the disadvantages of psychiatric classifications is that, by adopting a 'menu of symptoms' approach to diagnosis, they encourage health professionals to focus too closely on validating and treating an abstract diagnosis, and not enough on the person's distress, its context, and its significance or meaning.

The World Health Organization (WHO) classification

The ICD-10 classification of mental and behavioural disorders: clinical descriptions and diagnostic guidelines is chapter V of the *Tenth Revision of the International Classification of Diseases* (ICD-10). ICD-10 dates back to 1992, and the next edition, ICD-11, is due by 2018. Other than simply listing and coding the names of diseases and disorders like other chapters in ICD-10, Chapter V provides clinical descriptions, diagnostic criteria, and diagnostic criteria for research. These are based on the scientific literature and on international consultation and consensus. The principal aims of Chapter V are to serve as a reference for national classifications and to facilitate international comparisons of morbidity and mortality statistics. It comes in four different versions: (1) clinical descriptions and diagnostic guidelines, (2) diagnostic criteria for research, (3) primary care version, and (4) multiaspect (axial) systems.

The broad categories of mental and behavioural disorders listed in Chapter V are:

F0-F9	Organic, including symptomatic, mental disorders
F10-F19	Mental and behavioural disorders due to psychoactive substance use
F20-F29	Schizophrenia, schizotypal and delusional disorders
F30-F39	Mood (affective) disorders
F40-48	Neurotic, stress-related and somatoform disorders
F50-F59	Behavioural syndromes associated with physiological disturbances and physical factors
F60-F69	Disorders of adult personality and behaviour
F70-F79	Mental retardation
F80-F89	Disorders of psychological development
F90-F98	Behavioural and emotional disorders with onset usually occurring in childhood and adolescence
F99	Unspecified mental disorder

Note that these are organized in a loose diagnostic hierarchy (see previous section).

The American classification

The first classification of mental and behavioural disorders appeared in ICD-6, published in 1948. The American Psychiatric Association (APA) lost little time in publishing an alternative classification, the Diagnostic and Statistical Manual of Mental Disorders (DSM), for use in the USA. The fifth revision of the DSM, published in 2013, is broadly similar to the ICD-10 classification. Although it introduced some small improvements, it attracted criticism for further narrowing the realm of normality, for instance, by dropping the 'bereavement exclusion' for depressive disorders, lowering the threshold for 'gambling disorder', and introducing such constructs as 'minor neurocognitive disorder', 'disruptive mood dysregulation disorder' (temper tantrums), 'premenstrual dysphoric disorder', and 'binge-eating disorder'.

Although some psychiatrists prefer ICD-10 to DSM-5 and *vice versa*, the classifications should be seen as complementary, not competing. Both are used throughout this book.

If homosexuality is a disease, let's all call in queer to work.

'Hello. Can't work today, still queer.'

—Robin Tyler

In the 1950s and 1960s, some therapists employed aversion therapy of the kind featured in *A Clockwork Orange* to 'cure' male homosexuality. This typically involved showing patients pictures of naked men while giving them electric shocks or drugs to make them vomit, and, once they could no longer bear it, showing them pictures of naked women or sending them out on a 'date' with a young nurse. Needless to say, these cruel and degrading methods proved entirely ineffective.

First published in 1968, DSM-II listed homosexuality as a mental disorder. In this, the DSM followed in a long tradition in medicine, which in the 19th century appropriated homosexuality from the Church and transformed it from sin to mental disorder.

In 1973, the American Psychiatric Association (APA) asked all members attending its convention to vote on whether they believed homosexuality to be a mental disorder. 5,854 psychiatrists voted to remove homosexuality from the DSM, and 3,810 to retain it. The APA then compromised, removing homosexuality from the DSM but replacing it, in effect, with 'sexual orientation disturbance' for people 'in conflict with' their sexual orientation. Not until 1987 did homosexuality completely fall out of the DSM.

Meanwhile, the World Health Organization (WHO) only removed homosexuality from the ICD classification with the publication of ICD-10 in 1992, although ICD-10 still carries the construct of 'ego-dystonic sexual orientation'. In this condition, the person is in no doubt about his or her sexual preference, but 'wishes it were different because of associated psychological and behavioural disorders'.

The evolution of the status of homosexuality in the classifications of mental disorders highlights that concepts of mental disorder can be social constructs that change as society changes. Today, the standard of psychotherapy in the U.S. and Europe is gay affirmative psychotherapy, which encourages gay people to accept their sexual orientation.

Case study: Psychiatric Assessment

LD, 22 year old Caucasian male referred by his GP for hearing voices. Currently a student in architectural engineering at Y University.

Presenting problem

LD is hearing critical voices for about half an hour every evening.

- The voices belong to his three best friends.
- They speak both to him and about him, telling him, for example, that his parents are going to die because of his poor exam performance.
- Although he experiences them as coming from outside his head, he does not believe that they are real and tries to ignore them as much as possible.
- They do not tell him to harm himself or anyone else.
- They do not stop him from leading his life, but he finds it difficult to talk about them and worries that he may spiral into a florid psychosis similar to the one he suffered some 16 months ago.
- On further questioning, LD revealed that he sometimes feels that people in public places are talking about him, even though he recognizes that this is a product of his mind.

- LD goes to bed in the early hours of the morning to accommodate his busy social life. Despite this, he enjoys a full complement of seven or eight hours of uninterrupted sleep every night.

History of presenting problem

The voices started about one month ago, while LD was revising for his end-of-year exams. Since then, they have been becoming more prominent.

Past psychiatric history

- First episode of (? Cannabis-induced) psychosis some 16 months ago: involved prominent auditory hallucinations and delusions of persecution.
- Informally admitted under Dr X for ten days.
- Diagnosed with drug-induced psychotic episode and started on risperidone.
- Made a good recovery.
- No other psychiatric history.

Past medical history

- Mild asthma.
- Hay fever.

- Uncomplicated appendicectomy at 16 years old.
- No history of epilepsy or head injury.

Current treatments

- History of patchy compliance on oral medication. Started on risperidone depot.
- Risperidone depot recently increased to 37.5mg once every two weeks by his GP, Dr Z. On this dose he is suffering from troublesome adverse effects, including sedation and ejaculatory failure.
- Salbutamol inhaler PRN.
- Allergic to penicillin (rash).

Substance use

- LD used to be a heavy cannabis user, but denies having used drugs since his first psychotic episode 16 months ago.
- He smokes 10 cigarettes a day.
- He drinks 2-3 pints of craft beer a day in the pub with his friends, although on Friday and Saturday nights he may drink considerably more than this.

Family history

- LD's maternal grandfather died from complications of catatonic schizophrenia at the age of 43.
- His mother is on an SSRI antidepressant for panic disorder.
- His parents separated a year ago and since then he has been spending his holidays with his father. Mum is supportive but dad is a 'constant nag' and finds it difficult to accept that he is mentally ill.
- He is the youngest of three. His brother and sister both live abroad.

Social history

- During term-time LD lives in university halls.
- His parents are both accountants and are funding him through university.
- He has a busy social life and often goes to bed in the early hours of the morning. As a result, he can sometimes miss 2pm lectures. He finds it difficult to talk to friends about his voices for fear of being mocked or rejected.

- He describes himself as socially outgoing despite a natural shyness. He regrets not having achieved his full potential at school and university, and at one point asked me which novels I thought he should be reading.

Personal history

- LD has no history of birth complications or of developmental delay.
- He got on well with his parents but was bullied by his brother, who once gave him a black eye.
- He enjoyed school, did moderately well, and had a fair few friends.
- He left school with three good A-levels and spent a year in the Australian outback, where he was attacked by a koala. He then began a course in architectural engineering at X University but dropped out after his first episode of psychosis. Last October, he re-started a similar course at Y University.
- He has never had a girlfriend, which he regrets. He says he is not confident around girls.
- When I asked him whether he believes in God, he replied, 'I sometimes go to church, but only for the bells and smells.'
- He has never been in trouble with the police.

Informant history (with consent from LD)

LD's mother corroborated LD's history. As far as she is aware, LD has not smoked cannabis since his first episode of illness. She is concerned that he is unable to concentrate on his studies and likely to fail his exams.

MENTAL STATE EXAMINATION

Appearance and behaviour

- Tall, slightly stooped.
- Well kempt.
- Shy but co-operative. Good eye contact. Good rapport.
- No motor abnormalities.

Speech

No abnormalities of speech.

Mood

- Affect is normal.
- Mood is objectively and subjectively euthymic.
- No thoughts of self-harm or harming others.
- No anxiety symptoms.

Thoughts

- Normal stream and form of thought.
- Sometimes feels that people in public places are talking about him, but is able to recognize that this is a product of his mind.
- Worried that he may spiral into a florid psychosis similar to the one he suffered some 16 months ago.
- Preoccupied about failing his exams.
- Preoccupied about never having been in a relationship.
- No obsessions or phobias.

Perceptions

- Although he is not currently hearing voices, he describes hearing voices for about half an hour every evening.
- No sensory distortions, illusions, or depersonalization or derealization.

Cognition

Fully oriented in time and place. Cognition not formally tested.

Insight

He believes that he is suffering a second psychotic episode and is asking for support.

FORMULATION

Synopsis

- 22-year-old Caucasian male with ideas of reference and second and third person auditory hallucinations for half an hour every evening since starting exam revision one month ago.
- First episode of drug-induced psychosis with prominent auditory hallucinations and delusions of persecution 16 months ago. Informally admitted under Dr X for 10 days and started on risperidone. Made a good recovery and has stopped using drugs.
- Switched to depot risperidone owing to poor compliance. Dose recently increased to 37.5 every two weeks, leading to multiple adverse effects.

Further information required

- Physical examination unremarkable.
- Urine drug screen negative.
- Blood tests normal.
- Waiting to speak to GP.

Differential diagnosis

- F20.0 Paranoid schizophrenia (ICD-10). Has one first rank symptoms of schizophrenia (third person auditory hallucinations) and fulfils the duration criteria. Also, there is a family history of schizophrenia.
- Drug-induced psychotic disorder—but he claims not to have been taking drugs and the urine drug screen was negative.

Risk assessment

Symptoms remain mild and contained. Risk to self and others is currently low.

Aetiology

	Biological	Psychological	Social
Precipitating Factors	? cannabis Irregular sleep pattern	Exam stress	Parental separation Going to university
Predisposing Factors	Family history	High expressed emotion Lack of a confiding relationship	Childhood bullying
Perpetuating Factors	? cannabis Irregular sleep pattern	High expressed emotion Lack of a confiding relationship	Stigma of mental illness

Management

	Biological	Psychological	Social
Short-term	Change antipsychotic to amisulpride (less sedating)	Support and educate patient and family In particular, advise on importance of sleeping, staying off drugs, and complying with medication	
Medium-term	Monitor symptoms Monitor response to amisulpride	Schizophrenia support group Consider family therapy for high expressed emotion	Schizophrenia support group
Long-term		Find a confiding relationship (hopefully)	

Next steps

1. Appointment made with Dr A (SHO) next Monday at 3pm to monitor symptoms, monitor response to amisulpride, and support and educate the patient and family.
2. Weekly home visits by CPN to monitor progress and support and educate the patient and family.
3. CPN to provide the patient with contact details of local schizophrenia support group.

Prognosis

In the short-term he is likely to respond to amilsulpiride and make a good recovery. In the longer term, he is likely to suffer further relapses, particularly if he comes under stress, uses drugs, or suddenly stops taking his medication.

Positive prognostic factors, at least initially, include acute onset, presence of precipitating factors, florid symptoms, good premorbid functioning, good social support, early treatment, and good response to treatment.

Negative prognostic factors include family history, history of drug use, history of poor compliance with medication, lack of a confiding relationship, and male sex.

Patient assessment: Checklist and summary

Psychiatric history

1. Introductory information.
2. Presenting problem and history of presenting problem.
3. Past psychiatric history, including previous episodes of mental disorder, treatments, admissions, and history of self-harm and harm to others.
4. Past medical history.
5. Current treatments including psychological treatments, recent changes in medication, adverse reactions, and compliance.
6. Substance use.
7. Family history, including quality of relationships and recent events.
8. Social history: Self-care, support, housing, finances, typical day, interests and hobbies, premorbid personality.
9. Personal history: Pregnancy and birth, developmental milestones, childhood problems and setbacks, educational achievement, occupational history, psychosexual history, forensic history, spiritual orientation.
10. Informant history.

Mental state examination

1. Appearance and behaviour: Level of consciousness, appearance, behaviour, motor activity, abnormalities of movement.
2. Speech, especially amount, rate, and form.
3. Mood: Subjective and objective mood, affect, ideas of self-harm and suicide, ideas of harm to others, anxiety.
4. Thoughts: Stream, form, and content, including delusions, overvalued ideas, preoccupations, ruminations, obsessions, and phobias.
5. Perception, especially hallucinations, depersonalization, and derealization.
6. Cognition: Orientation, attention and concentration, memory, grasp.
7. Insight.

Formulation

1. Case summary
2. Further information required: Consider fuller psychiatric history and MSE, informant histories, old records, physical examination, laboratory investigations, brain imaging, and psychological tests and inventories.
3. Differential diagnosis: Psychiatric and organic differentials, including substance misuse.
4. Risk assessment: Risk to self through self-harm, neglect, or exploitation; and risk to others.
5. Aetiology: Predisposing, precipitating, and perpetuating factors; biological, psychological, and social.
6. Management: Short-, medium-, and long-term; biological, psychological, and social.
7. Prognosis: Current episode and long-term.

Self-assessment

Answer by true or false:

1. The MSE is a snapshot of the patient's mental state at, or around, that time.
2. The MSE can be compared to both a physical examination and a functional enquiry.
3. One of the most important principles of descriptive psychopathology is to make assumptions about the causes of signs and symptoms of mental disorder.
4. Asking about suicide often suggests it to the patient.
5. Before interviewing an informant, consent from the patient is generally required.
6. On the Folstein Mini-Mental State Examination, scores of 22 to 25 are indicative of moderate cognitive impairment, while scores of less than 22 are indicative of significant cognitive impairment.
7. A stereotypy is an odd, repetitive movement with a functional significance.
8. Apraxia describes a reduced ability to carry out purposive movements in spite of intact comprehension and motor function.
9. *Mitmachen* is an extreme form of *mitgehen*.
10. *Gegenhalten* denotes involuntary resistance to passive movement.
11. Dysphasia denotes an impairment of the ability to vocalize speech.
12. Echolalia denotes parrot-like imitation of another's speech.
13. In incongruity of affect, affect does not reflect content of thought.
14. In circumstantial thinking, the normal structure of thought is preserved, but thoughts are cramped by irrelevant material.
15. A secondary delusion is a delusion that arises from, and is understandable in context of, previous ideas or events.
16. Delusional perception is the attribution of delusional significance to normal percepts.
17. An overvalued idea differs from a delusion in part because the person accepts that the belief may be false.
18. Fregoli syndrome is the delusion that a familiar person has been replaced by an identical-looking imposter.
19. A pseudo-hallucination differs from a true hallucination in that it is perceived to arise from the sense organs.
20. A reflex hallucination is a hallucination triggered by an environmental stimulus in the same modality.
21. Insight can be assessed independently of the assessor's values.
22. In the diagnostic hierarchy, delirium is higher than dementia, which is itself higher than schizophrenia.
23. DSM-5 is based on international consultation and consensus.
24. DSM-5 comes in four different versions: clinical descriptions and diagnostic guidelines, diagnostic criteria for research, primary care version, and multiaspect (axial) systems.

Answers

1. True.
2. True. The MSE elicits both the signs and the symptoms of mental disorder.
3. False. One of the most important principles of descriptive psychopathology is *not* to make any such assumptions.
4. False. Suicide should be asked about.
5. True.
6. True.
7. False. This describes a mannerism: a stereotypy does not have a functional significance.
8. False. This describes dyspraxia. Apraxia is an *inability* to carry out purposive movements in spite of intact comprehension and motor function.
9. False. *Mitgehen* is an extreme form of *mitmachen*.
10. True.
11. False. This denotes dysphonia, not dysphasia, which is impairment of the ability to comprehend or express language.
12. True.
13. False. This denotes dissociation of affect. In incongruity of affect, affect is inappropriate to circumstances.
14. True.
15. True.
16. True.
17. True
18. False. This is Capgras syndrome. Fregoli is the delusion that a familiar individual is disguising as various strangers.
19. False. Pseudo-hallucinations are generally perceived to come from the mind.
20. False. This denotes a functional hallucination. A reflex hallucination is a hallucination triggered by an environmental stimulus in another modality.
21. False.
22. True.
23. False. This describes ICD-10.
24. False. This describes ICD-10.

3

Mental healthcare

The development of community care

The push for community care in the 1950s and 1960s owed to:

- Important social changes and heavy criticism of the institutional model of psychiatric care, as epitomized by the anti-psychiatry movement.
- The advent of drugs such as the antipsychotic chlorpromazine.
- The perceived cost benefits of community care.

By removing patients from the isolation of the old Victorian asylums and integrating them into the community under the care of community mental health teams, policy-makers hoped to improve their social functioning and reduce the stigma of mental illness.

The expansion in community care carried on through the 1970s and 1980s, but came under heavy criticism in the 1980s after a series of headline-grabbing killings by mentally ill people in the community. (Such killings, though very rare, are often sensationally reported in the press. For instance, the author once spotted an article headed: *Beast freed from prison psycho ward chopped my mum into 16 little pieces.*) This prompted a government inquiry that culminated in the Community Care Act 1990, a major piece of legislation that is at the origin of the present, more 'fail-safe', model of community care.

The advantages of community care are clear. By shifting the emphasis from a person's mental illness to his or her strengths and life aspirations, community care promotes independence and self-reliance, while discouraging isolation and institutionalization and reducing stigma. On the other hand, lack of staff and resources can shift the burden of care onto informal carers and leave some of the most vulnerable people, such as the isolated and homeless, without adequate support.

The pros and cons of community care are summarized in Table 3.1.

Table 3.1: Pros and cons of community care

Pros	Cons
• Promotes independence and self-reliance. • Discourages isolation and institutionalization. • Diminishes stigma. • Emphasizes relapse prevention. • Originally thought to be cheaper.	• Poses a (mostly perceived) threat to the safety of the patient and community. • Places a heavy burden on carers. • Makes it harder to care for people without a solid support network. • Places a heavy burden on staff and resources. • Has resulted in a shortage of hospital beds as resources are diverted to community services.

3

One Flew Over the Cuckoo's Nest, adapted from Ken Kasey's popular 1962 novel by the same name, stars Jack Nicholson as the spirited Mac and Louise Fletcher as the chilly but softly spoken Nurse Ratched. When Mac arrives at the Oregon state mental hospital, he challenges the stultifying routine and bureaucratic authoritarianism personified by Nurse Ratched, and pays the price by being drugged, electroshocked, and, ultimately, lobotomized. Nominated for nine Academy Awards, the film is a (belated and contentious) critique of the institutional model of psychiatric care, as well as a metaphor for total institutions, that is, institutions that repress individuality to create a compliant society. This sort of critique paved the way for community care.

Organization of mental health services

Mental health services are currently undergoing a great deal of change. In many areas, the traditional Community Mental Health Team (CMHT) is being re-structured into new specialist teams. Teams in different areas may differ quite significantly, or, more often than not, just carry different names. Figure 3.1 offers no more than a notional template.

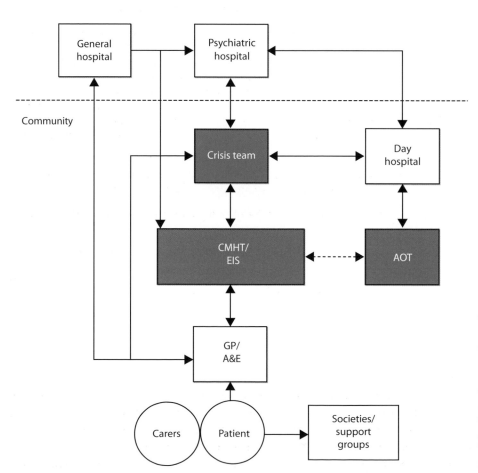

Figure 3.1. Example of organization of mental healthcare services (local services may differ, not least in their nomenclature). Mental healthcare services are organized so as to avoid unnecessary hospital admissions. CMHT, Community Mental Health Team; AOT or AORT, Assertive Outreach Team; EIS, Early Intervention Service.

GP and A&E

Most mental disorder that presents to medical attention is treated in general practice. If a referral to secondary care is required, this is usually to the CMHT, or, in an emergency or at night, to the crisis team. A minority of patients first present to Accident & Emergency rather than to the GP, in which case they are screened by a casualty doctor and, if appropriate, referred for further assessment by mental health services.

Community Mental Health Team (CMHT)

The CMHT is at the centre of mental healthcare provision. It is a multidisciplinary team led by a consultant psychiatrist and operating from a team base in the geographical sector that it covers. Community psychiatric nurses and social workers often play key roles within the CMHT, co-ordinating patient care, monitoring patients in the community, and taking urgent referrals. Other important members of the team include more junior psychiatrists, clinical psychologists, occupational therapists, and administrative staff (Table 3.2). A new referral to the CMHT usually undergoes an initial assessment by a psychiatrist, sometimes in the presence of another member of the team such as a CPN or social worker. The skill mix of the multidisciplinary team means that different aspects of the patient's life can be understood, and addressed, from multiple angles.

Table 3.2: Key non-medical members of the CMHT

Community psychiatric nurse	The CPN is the team member with whom the patient is likely to come into contact most often. The CPN usually visits the patient's home to facilitate the treatment plan and monitor progress.
Social worker	Sometimes a patient may be allocated a social worker instead of a CPN, in which case the social worker fulfils a role similar to that of the CPN. The social worker can also help to sort out housing and benefits.
Clinical psychologist	The clinical psychologist may spend a lot of time hearing and making sense of a patient and his or her carers, and also deliver talking treatments such as cognitive behavioural therapy or family therapy. People often confuse psychiatrist, psychologist, psychotherapist, and psychoanalyst. A psychiatrist is a medical doctor specialized in the diagnosis and treatment of mental disorders such as schizophrenia and depression. A clinical psychologist is an expert in human experience and behaviour. A psychotherapist is any person trained in delivering specialized talking treatments, commonly a clinical psychologist or psychiatrist. Finally, a psychoanalyst is a type of psychotherapist trained in delivering specialized talking treatments based on the psychoanalytic principles pioneered by Sigmund Freud and others, including Alfred Adler, Carl Jung, and Melanie Klein.
Occupational therapist	The role of the occupational therapist is to help the patient maintain skills and develop new ones. This keeps the patient engaged and motivated, and, in the longer term, helps him or her back into work.
Pharmacist	Patients with a physical illness or who are pregnant or breastfeeding may find it particularly helpful to engage with a pharmacist, who might be able to help with their medication.
Administrative staff	Administrative staff work at the interface between patients and team members. They are responsible for arranging appointments and are often the first port of call in an emergency.

NB: Other forms of support which are available but which do not form part of the CMHT include support groups, telephone helplines, hobby groups, and the Citizen's Advice Bureau.

Crisis team

The crisis team is a 24-hours-a-day, 365-days-a-year multidisciplinary team that acts as a gatekeeper to a variety of mental health services, including admission to a psychiatric hospital. Patients in a crisis are referred to the crisis team from a variety of places, most commonly GPs, A&E, and CMHTs. A member of the team, most often a CPN, promptly assesses the patient in conjunction with a psychiatrist to determine if hospital admission can be prevented by short-term intensive home care. If so, the crisis team arranges for a team member to visit the patient's home up to thrice a day, gradually decreasing the frequency of visits as the patient recovers. Other than simply providing support, the crisis team can assist in implementing a care and treatment plan and in monitoring progress. It can also expedite and ease the discharge of in-patients. The key features of the crisis team are summarized in Table 3.3.

Table 3.3: Crisis team key features

- Gatekeeper to psychiatric services, including hospital admission.
- Prompt assessment of patients in a crisis.
- Intensive, round-the-clock community support in the early stages of the crisis.
- Continued involvement until the crisis has resolved.
- Action to prevent similar crises from re-occurring.
- Partnership with the patient and his or her relatives and carers.

Assertive Outreach Team (AOT)

Some people with severe mental disorder are reluctant to seek help and treatment, and as a consequence only appear in times of crisis. These so-called 'revolving door' patients, who often have the most complex mental health needs and social problems, are best dealt with by the AOT, a multidisciplinary team which specializes in engaging them in treatment and supporting them in the community.

Early Intervention Service (EIS)

Like the AOT, the EIS may also operate from the CMHT base. Its role is specifically to improve short- and long-term outcomes of psychotic disorders through a three-pronged approach involving preventative measures, earlier detection of untreated cases, and intensive treatment and support in the early stages of illness.

Hospital and day hospital

If a patient requires admission, this is usually because care in the community is no longer an option. Commonly this is because:

- The patient is a danger to himself or others, or is very vulnerable.
- The patient requires specialized care or supervised treatment.
- The patient is lacking a social structure.
- Carers can no longer cope and need respite.

Some patients are admitted on an informal, that is, voluntary, basis, but many are admitted under a Section of the Mental Health Act (see later). Another option may be to attend a day hospital, which only operates within office hours. Day hospitals can provide suitable patients with a less restrictive and more tolerable (and less expensive) alternative to conventional hospital admission.

Rehabilitation

Some patients, especially those suffering from prominent negative symptoms of schizophrenia, may need a period of long-term rehabilitation either in in-patient units or in the community. Areas that are considered during rehabilitation include accommodation, activities of daily living, occupational activities, leisure activities, and social skills (Chapter 4).

General hospital (liaison psychiatry)

'Liaison psychiatry' (sometimes also 'psychological medicine') refers to psychiatric services within the general hospital. Since the 1970s, liaison psychiatry has evolved into a recognized sub-specialism of psychiatry, devoted to the overlap between psychiatry and the rest of medicine and surgery. At its core, it involves providing expert advice and treatment to in-patients and out-patients referred by physicians and surgeons, and assessing patients with suspected psychological or psychiatric complaints in A&E. Cases vary greatly, for example, self-harm, somatization disorder, and depression following a mastectomy.

Societies and support groups

Selected societies and support groups relevant to psychiatric practice in the UK include MIND, Rethink, SANE, The Mental Health Foundation, MDF the Bipolar Organisation, Depression Alliance, Cruse Bereavement Care, Relate (support with relationships), Anxiety UK, No Panic, OCD Action, Beat (support with eating disorders), Alzheimer's Society, The Sleep Council, Drinkline, Alcoholics Anonymous, Al Anon, QUIT (support with smoking cessation), Cocaine Anonymous, Narcotics Anonymous, The Samaritans, CRISIS (support with homelessness), Carers UK, and the Royal College of Psychiatrists.

The Care-Programme Approach (CPA)

The management of patients accepted into specialist mental health services is planned at one or more CPA meetings attended by the patient and his or her carers. These meetings are useful in establishing the context of the patient's problems, evaluating his circumstances, assessing his medical, psychological, and social needs, and formulating a detailed care plan to ensure that these needs can be met.

Other than ensuring that the patient takes his medication and is regularly reviewed by a member of the multidisciplinary team, any care plan is likely to include a number of psychosocial measures such as attendance at self-help groups, carer education and support, and home help.

A care co-ordinator, most often a CPN or social worker, is appointed to ensure that the care plan is implemented and revised in light of changing circumstances.

At the outcome of the CPA meeting, the patient should feel that his needs and concerns have been considered, and that the care plan that he has helped to formulate reflects these in as far as possible.

Ethics and the law

A full discussion of psychiatric ethics is beyond the scope of this book, and this section merely highlights some of the more salient ethical principles involved in daily psychiatric practice, as brought out by the story of AB.

Case study: Mr AB

Mr AB, a 48-year-old bank manager, arrives in A&E complaining of burning pains in the head. He is carrying a letter from his GP in which she opines that he is suffering from severe depression. He has a history of recurrent depressive disorder and once made an impulsive and near-fatal suicide attempt.

Although Mr AB appears to be depressed, he denies feeling suicidal. Oddly, he refuses to let the casualty officer call his wife. The casualty officer tries to call his GP but she is out on a home visit. He obtains Mr AB's telephone number from directory enquiries and calls Mr AB's wife, who is unaware that her husband is in A&E or even that he has been to see their GP.

Mrs AB reports that Mr AB has become increasingly gloomy and preoccupied over the past three or four weeks. She is alarmed to discover that he is complaining of burning pains in the head: the last time he did so was when he tried to kill himself. She is adamant that he should not be allowed to leave the hospital, or, at any rate, not until she can get there.

The casualty officer calls the duty psychiatrist to Mr AB's bedside. Although guarded and suspicious, Mr AB eventually reveals that he has 'advanced brain cancer'. After a careful neurological examination, the psychiatrist finds no evidence of a tumour and carefully explains this to Mr AB. Unfortunately, Mr AB does not believe him, and asks several times to be discharged with a painkiller.

Mrs AB arrives and tells the psychiatrist that her husband is most probably designing to kill himself, as he is behaving just as he did in the run-up to his suicide attempt. As Mr AB insists upon leaving the hospital, he is admitted involuntarily under a Section of the Mental Health Act and started on an antidepressant drug.

Confidentiality

Patient information should not be disclosed and further information collected unless the patient has provided consent. However, in exceptional circumstances, there is an obligation to disclose information if:

- It is in the public interest, for example, to help prevent, detect, or prosecute a serious crime.
- It is in the best interests of the patient, when the patient is legally incapable owing to severe mental or physical disorder.

The casualty officer breached Mr AB's confidentiality by discussing his case with his wife. This could be justified on the grounds of best interest, as Mr AB was deemed to be suffering from a severe mental disorder and lacking in capacity. In our autonomy-dominated ethic, a breach of confidentiality to Mr AB's family must be 'justified' on certain grounds. But in cultures that value families and communities ahead of individuals, it may be considered entirely natural and appropriate to contact Mr AB's family. This reveals that our autonomy-dominated ethic, which we often take for granted, is heavily values-laden.

3

In August 1969, during his ninth session with Dr Lawrence Moore, a psychologist at UC Berkeley's Cowell Memorial Hospital, Prosenjit Poddar revealed that he was going to kill Tatiana Tarasoff, a fellow student who had spurned his romantic advances.

Dr Moore told the campus police that Poddar posed a threat and ought to be hospitalized against his will, but the police released Poddar because they felt that he had 'changed his attitude'. The psychiatric director who had been apprised of the situation instructed his staff not to pursue further attempts to hospitalize Poddar. Meanwhile, Tarasoff and her parents remained unaware of Poddar's threats.

On October 27, Poddar went to Tarasoff's house and stabbed her to death with a kitchen knife. He then called the police and asked to be handcuffed.

When Tarasoff's parents sued Moore and various other members of the university, the California Supreme Court ruled that physicians have a duty to breach confidentiality if maintaining confidentiality might result in harm to the patient or community.

Capacity

Doctors and in particular psychiatrists may be called upon to assess a patient's capacity and competence to give informed consent or enter into another contract. Having deemed Mr AB to be lacking in capacity on the grounds of mental illness, the casualty officer acted in his best interests by breaking confidentiality and speaking to Mrs AB. The information that he received from Mrs AB turned out to be of vital importance to Mr AB's assessment and management. Similarly, the psychiatrist acted in Mr AB's best interests by admitting him involuntarily and starting him on an antidepressant drug.

The Mental Capacity Act 2005 (MCA) is a piece of legislation intended to protect people who lack the ability to make decisions about their health, welfare, and finances. According to the MCA, 'a person lacks capacity in relation to a matter if at the material time he is unable to make a decision for himself in relation to the matter because of an impairment of, or a disturbance in the functioning of, the mind or brain.' Capacity refers to the natural ability to make decisions: a person has a certain degree of capacity in relation to a particular decision at a particular time. Competence on the other hand is the legal right to have one's decision regarding treatment respected. It is a binary concept: one is either 'competent' or not. Competence is informed by capacity: if capacity is beyond a certain threshold, the person is deemed 'competent' to make a decision. This threshold varies according to the seriousness of the decision at hand.

The main principles of the MCA are:
- Presumption of capacity. A person is presumed to have capacity to make a decision unless it is established otherwise.

- Maximizing capacity. Before a person is deemed to lack capacity, all practicable steps must have been taken to help that person make his or her own decisions.
- Right to make unwise decisions. A person must not be treated as unable to make a decision merely because the decision appears unwise to others.
- Best interests. Decisions made on behalf of a person who lacks capacity must be made in their best interests.
- Least restrictive option. Courses of action that are least restrictive to the person's rights and freedom must be considered first.

According to Section 3 of the MCA, a person has capacity to make a particular decision if he:
- Understands the information relevant to decision-making.
- Retains the information for long enough to make a decision.
- Weighs up the information and understands the consequences of a decision.
- Communicates this decision by whatever means necessary.

Note that capacity is contextual and should not simply be inferred from the patient's diagnosis or from previous assessments of his capacity.

Historical case: Re C (1994)

Mr C was a patient in a psychiatric secure hospital who had chronic paranoid schizophrenia with grandiose delusions of being a world famous doctor. When he developed gangrene in his right foot, he refused to consent to a below-knee amputation, and was granted an injunction to prevent such an operation. In granting the injunction, Justice Thorpe held that Mr C sufficiently understood the nature, purpose, and effects of the proposed amputation, and that he retained sufficient capacity to consent to, or refuse, medical treatment. The case of Mr C has helped to establish the 'Re C criteria' or legal criteria for capacity.

Clinical skills: Assessment of capacity in adults

1. Diagnostic test: Assess whether there is a disturbance or impairment of the mind (e.g. intoxication, head injury, intellectual disability, dementia) which may affect decision-making at this moment in time. Your assessment must lean on standardized criteria such as the ICD-10 or DSM-5 diagnostic criteria.
2. Assess by the four criteria in Section 3 of the MCA whether, on the balance of probabilities, this disturbance or impairment renders the person unable to make a decision about the matter in hand. In particular, ensure that the patient understands:
   - What the intervention is.
   - Why the intervention is being proposed.
   - The alternatives to the intervention, including no intervention.
   - The principal benefits and risks of the intervention and its alternatives.
   - The consequences of the intervention and its alternatives.

Efforts to optimize capacity might include:
- Making your explanations easier to understand, for example, by using diagrams.
- Seeing the patient at his best time of day.
- Seeing him with one of his friends or relatives.
- Improving his environment, e.g. finding a quiet side-room.
- Adjusting his medication, e.g. decreasing the dose of sedative drugs.

Remember to ensure that the patient is not subject to coercion or threat.

Clinical skills: Assessment of capacity in minors

As far as possible, minors ought to be involved in decisions about their care, whether or not they are deemed competent.
- Decisions on behalf of a minor can be made by a person with parental responsibility or by a High Court.
- 16- and 17-year olds are deemed competent by the same standards as adults (Family Law Reform Act 1969). However, they cannot refuse treatment if it has been agreed by a person with parental responsibility or the Court and it is in their best interests.
- Under-16s may be deemed competent to accept an intervention if they are mature enough to fully understand what is proposed ('Gillick competency', after Gillick v. West Norfolk and Wisbech Area Health Authority, 1986). Much will depend on the relationship between the clinician and the child and family, and also on what intervention is being proposed.
- Ideally, the consent of a person with parental responsibility should also be sought. However, the decision of a competent minor to accept treatment cannot be overruled by a parent.
- A court order may be obtained to overrule the decision of a competent minor or parent if it is considered in the best interests of the minor.

Deprivation of Liberty Safeguards (DoLS)

DoLS is an amendment to the MCA intended to protect vulnerable adults in care from arbitrary or excessive restrictions on their freedom, and also to give them the right to legally challenge their detention. In practice, DoLS is pertinent to most mentally incapacitated adults living in care who, for the sake of their own welfare, are prevented from leaving. In such cases, the hospital or care home must apply for authorization from a DoLS supervisory authority, whether or not the patient (who lacks capacity) is 'agreeing' to the arrangements.

Clinical skills: MHA or MCA DoLS?

The Mental Health Act (MHA) pertains to people with a mental disorder who need to be detained for assessment or treatment in the interests of their own health and safety or the safety of others. DoLS pertains to people with mental disorders such as dementia and intellectual disability who do not require assessment and for whom there is no medical treatment (for the mental disturbance), and who therefore do not meet the MHA criteria, but who nevertheless require deprivation of liberty for their wellbeing, including for the treatment of physical illness. Note that DoLS cannot be applied to people detained under the MHA.

Common law

Common law is law based on previous court rulings (case law, such as Re C), as opposed to law enacted by parliament (statute law, such as the MHA). Under common law, adults have a right to refuse treatment, even when doing so may result in permanent physical injury or death. If a competent adult refuses consent or lacks the capacity to provide consent, no one can provide consent on his behalf, not even his next of kin.

However, treatment without consent can be delivered under common law:

- If serious harm or death is likely and there is doubt about the patient's capacity at the time and no advance directive (or 'living will') has been made; and the clinician is able to justify that he is acting in the patient's best interests and in accordance with established medical practice ('Bolam's test').
- In an emergency to prevent serious harm to the patient or others, or to prevent a crime.

Had Mr AB tried to leave A&E before being detained under a Section of the Mental Health Act, he could have been held back under Common Law.

The Mental Health Act (MHA)

Some people with severe mental disorders pose a risk to themselves or others, but lack insight and refuse the care and treatment that they require. In most countries, there are special legal provisions to protect such people, and society, from the consequences of their mental disorder.

In England and Wales, the Mental Health Act 1983 (amended in 2007) is the principal Act governing not only the compulsory admission and detention of people to a psychiatric hospital, but also their treatment, discharge from hospital, and aftercare. People with a mental disorder as defined by the Act can be detained under the Act in the interests of their health or safety or in the interests of the safety of others. To minimize the potential for abuse, the Act specifically excludes as mental disorder dependence on alcohol or drugs.

Scotland is governed by the Mental Health (Care and Treatment) (Scotland) Act 2003 and Northern Ireland by the Mental Health (Northern Ireland) Order 1986. In the USA, each state produces its own mental health legislation.

Two of the most common Sections of the MHA used to admit people with a mental disorder to a psychiatric hospital are the so-called Sections 2 and 3.

Section 2

Section 2 allows for an admission for assessment and treatment that can last for up to 28 days. An application for a Section 2 is usually made by an Approved Mental Health Professional (AMHP) with special training in mental health, and recommended by two doctors, one of whom must have special experience in the diagnosis and treatment of mental disorders.

Under Section 2, treatment can be given, but only in so far as it aims at treating the mental disorder or conditions directly resulting from the mental disorder (so, for example, treatment for appendicitis cannot be given under the Act).

A Section 2 can be 'discharged' or revoked at any time by the Responsible Clinician (usually the consultant psychiatrist), the hospital managers, or the nearest relative. Moreover, the patient can appeal against the Section, in which case the appeal is heard by a specially constituted tribunal. The patient is represented by a solicitor who helps him to construct a case for discharge. The tribunal is by nature adversarial, and it falls upon members of the patient's care team to argue the case for continued detention. This can be quite trying for both the claimant and his care team, and can at times undermine their relationship.

Section 2 in England and Wales is broadly equivalent to Section 26 in Scotland, except that Section 26 cannot be used to admit a patient to hospital. Instead, Section 26 tags onto Section 24 (Emergency admission to hospital) or Section 25 (Detention of patients already in hospital).

Section 3

A patient can be detained under Section 3 after a conclusive period of assessment under Section 2, or if his diagnosis has already been established by the care team and is not in reasonable doubt. Section 3 corresponds to an admission for treatment and lasts for up to six months. As for Section 2, it is usually applied for by an AMHP and approved by two doctors, one of whom must have special experience in the diagnosis and treatment of mental disorders.

Treatment can be given only in so far as it aims at treating the mental disorder or conditions directly resulting from the mental disorder. After the first three months, any treatment requires either the consent of the patient or the recommendation of a second doctor.

A Section 3 can be discharged at any time by the Responsible Clinician, the hospital managers, or the nearest relative. Moreover, the patient can appeal against the Section, in which case the appeal is heard by a specially constituted tribunal, as above.

If the patient still requires detention after six months, Section 3 can be renewed for further periods.

Section 3 is broadly similar to Section 18 of the Health (Care and Treatment) (Scotland) Act 2003.

Aftercare

A patient under Section 3 is automatically placed under Section 117 at the time of his discharge from the Section 3.

Section 117 corresponds to 'aftercare', and places a duty on services to provide the patient with a care package aimed at rehabilitation and relapse prevention. Although the patient is under no obligation to accept aftercare, in some cases he may also be placed under 'Supervised Community Treatment' or 'Guardianship' to ensure that he receives aftercare. Under Supervised Community Treatment, the patient is made subject to certain conditions, which, if unmet, can result in recall to hospital.

Other civil Sections

Important civil Sections of the MHA are summarized in Table 3.4.

Table 3.4 Commonly used Sections of the Mental Health Act

Section	Description	Duration	Treatment	Application/ recommendation	Discharge/renewal
2	Admission for assessment	28 days	Can be given, but note that the MHA only authorizes treatment of the mental disorder itself or conditions directly resulting from the mental disorder	Application by AMHP or nearest relative. Recommendation by two doctors (at least one must be Section 12 approved)	Patient may appeal to tribunal. Can be discharged by RC, hospital managers, or nearest relative. Usually converted to Section 3 if longer period of detention is required
3	Admission for treatment	6 months	Can be given for first 3 months, then consent or second opinion is needed	Application by AMHP or nearest relative. Recommendation by two doctors (at least one must be Section 12 approved)	Patient may appeal to tribunal. Can be discharged by RC, hospital managers, or nearest relative. Can be renewed if need be
4	Emergency admission for assessment (usually used in lieu of a Section 2)	72 hours	Consent needed unless treatment is being given under common law	Application by AMHP or nearest relative. Recommendation by any doctor	Patient cannot appeal. Can be discharged by RC only
5(2)	Emergency holding order (patient already admitted to hospital on an informal basis)	72 hours	Consent needed unless treatment is being given under common law	Recommendation from the doctor or AC in charge of the patient's care or their nominated deputy	Patient cannot appeal. Can be discharged by RC only
5(4)	Emergency holding order (patient already admitted to hospital on an informal basis)	6 hours	Consent needed unless treatment is being given under common law	Recommendation from a registered mental nurse	Patient cannot appeal
117	Automatically applies if a patient has been detained under Section 3. Under Section 117 it is the duty of the local health authority and the local social services authority to provide aftercare. Unlike under Supervised Community Treatment, there is no obligation for the patient to accept it.				

AC, approved Clinician; AMHP, Approved Mental Health Professional; RC, Responsible Clinician, usually the consultant in charge. Section 12 approval is usually granted to a psychiatrist having obtained Membership of the Royal College of Psychiatrists (MRCPsych) or having more than 3 years of relevant experience.

Police Sections

Section 135 allows the removal of a person from his premises to a 'place of safety' (often a specially designated part of a psychiatric hospital), and lasts for up to 72 hours.

Section 136 allows for the removal of a person from a public place to a 'place of safety', and also lasts for up to 72 hours. The person must appear to the police to be suffering from a mental disorder.

Criminal Sections

The principal criminal Sections are Sections 35 and 36, and Sections 37 and 41.

Sections 35 and 36 mirror Sections 2 and 3 for persons suffering from a mental disorder and awaiting trial for a serious offence. Section 35 can be enacted by a Crown Court or Magistrates' Court on the evidence of a Section 12 approved doctor. Section 36 can only be enacted by a Crown Court on the evidence of two doctors, one of whom must be Section 12 approved. In contrast to Section 36, Section 35 does not permit treatment, and is used solely for remanding a person to hospital for a report on his mental state. Both Sections 35 and 36 have an initial duration of 28 days, but can be extended for up to 28 days at a time, for up to 12 weeks.

Section 37 is used for the detention and treatment of persons suffering from a mental disorder and convicted of a serious offence punishable by imprisonment. It is enacted by a Crown Court or Magistrates' Court on the evidence of two Section 12 approved doctors. Section 37 has an initial duration of six months, and can be either discharged or extended. Sometimes a Section 41 'restriction order' is appended to a Section 37, such that leave and discharge can only be granted with the approval of the Ministry of Justice.

Consent to treatment

Patients on a long-term treatment order can be treated with psychiatric drugs with or without consent for up to three months, after which an additional order, Section 58, is required for their continued treatment. If the patient does not consent to the Section 58, a second opinion must be obtained.

Clinical skills: Mental disorders and driving

The following advice applies to mania, schizophrenia, and other schizophrenia-like psychotic disorders, and more severe forms of anxiety and depression.

Patients should stop driving during a first episode or relapse of their illness, because driving while ill can endanger lives. In the UK, the patient must notify the Driver and Vehicle Licensing Authority (DVLA). Failure to do so makes it illegal for him to drive and invalidates his insurance. The DVLA then sends the patient a medical questionnaire to fill in, together with a form asking for permission to contact his psychiatrist.

The patient's driving licence can generally be reinstated when the psychiatrist can confirm that:
- The illness has been successfully treated with medication for a certain amount of time, typically at least three months.
- The patient is conscientious about taking his medication.
- The adverse effects of the medication are not likely to impair the patient's driving.
- The patient is not misusing drugs.

People with substance misuse or dependence should also stop driving, as should some people with other mental disorders such as dementia, intellectual disability, or personality disorder. Further information can be obtained from the DVLA website at www.dvla.gov.uk.

Note that the rules for professional driving are stricter than those outlined above.

Psychological treatments

He said the soul was treated with certain charms, my dear Charmides, and that these charms were beautiful words.

—Plato, *Charmides*

In the *Charmides*, one of Plato's early dialogues, Socrates tells the young Charmides, who is suffering with headaches, about a charm for headaches which he learnt from one of the mystical physicians to the king of Thrace. However, this great physician taught that it is best to cure the soul before curing the body, since health and happiness ultimately depend on the state of the soul.

He said all things, both good and bad, in the body and in the whole man, originated in the soul and spread from there… One ought, then, to treat the soul first and foremost, if the head and the rest of the body were to be well. He said the soul was treated with certain charms, my dear Charmides, and that these charms were beautiful words. As a result of such words self-control came into being in souls. When it came into being and was present in them, it was then easy to secure health both for the head and for the rest of the body.

Drugs are the most available treatment option for mental disorders such as anxiety and depression, but, very often, psychological treatments can offer a safer, more effective, and more empowering alternative. Many people prefer psychological treatments on the grounds that they address underlying problems, rather than merely masking superficial symptoms.

Of course, psychological treatments and drugs are not mutually exclusive, and in some cases, such as severe psychosis, drugs can be hard to avoid.

The type of psychological treatment that is chosen depends not only on the patient's diagnosis, but also on his personal circumstances, his preferences, and, all too often, on available funding and human resources.

Supportive therapy

At its most basic, psychological treatment involves little more than explanation, reassurance, and encouragement. Such 'supportive therapy' is often sorely lacking, but ought to be offered to all people diagnosed with mental disorder.

In people diagnosed with milder forms of mental disorder, supportive therapy is often the only intervention that is either necessary or appropriate.

Counselling

Counselling is similar to supportive therapy in that it involves explanation, reassurance, and encouragement.

However, counselling also aims at identifying and resolving life problems, and so is more problem-focused and goal-oriented than supportive therapy.

Psychodynamic psychotherapy

In contrast to supportive therapy and counselling, exploratory psychotherapy endeavours to examine the person's thoughts and feelings. Two important, yet very different, forms of exploratory psychotherapy are psychodynamic psychotherapy and cognitive behavioural therapy (CBT).

Psychodynamic psychotherapy is founded on psychoanalytic theory. It is similar to psychoanalysis, but less

intensive and more limited in duration. Like psychoanalysis, psychodynamic therapy aims to bring unconscious feelings to the surface so that they can be experienced and understood, and so 'dealt with'.

In contrast to CBT, which is based on learning and cognitive theories, psychodynamic psychotherapy can, and usually does, delve into past and childhood experiences, which can be particularly helpful if the person's problems are deep-rooted.

Cognitive behavioural therapy (CBT)

Developed by psychiatrist Aaron Beck (born 1921) in the 1960s, CBT has become a mainstream treatment for non-severe anxiety and depression and a number of other mental disorders. In the short-term, it is at least as effective as antidepressants, and in the longer term may be more effective at preventing relapses.

CBT is most often carried out on a one-to-one basis, but can also be delivered in small groups. It involves a defined number of sessions, typically between ten and twenty, but principally takes place outside of sessions through 'homework'. The patient and a trained therapist (who may be a doctor, psychologist, nurse, or counsellor) develop a shared perspective of the patient's current problems, and try to understand them in terms of his thoughts (cognitions), emotions, and behaviours, and of how these are likely to relate to one another. This leads to the identification of realistic, time-limited goals, and of cognitive and behavioural strategies for achieving them.

For instance, in panic disorder, cognitive and behavioural strategies may involve cognitive restructuring (examining, testing, and modifying unhelpful thoughts and beliefs), relaxation training, and graded exposure to anxiety-provoking situations. In depression, the principal focus of CBT is on modifying automatic and self-perpetuating negative thoughts. These 'thinking errors' are considered to be hypotheses which, through gentle questioning and guided discovery, can be examined, tested, and modified. Behavioural tasks might include self-monitoring, activity scheduling, graded task assignments, and assertiveness training.

3

How effective is CBT?

CBT for depression in particular has garnered a great deal of institutional support on the basis that it is cheap and effective. However, critics question the robustness of the research into CBT for depression, and claim that it is in fact no more effective than other psychological treatments.

Curiously, one study published in 2015* found that the effectiveness of CBT for depression has been declining ever since the seminal CBT trials of the 1970s, with the steepest decline in the period from 1995. One explanation might be that, as CBT for depression has become ever more common, the quality of training, or the quality of trained therapists, has declined.

More fundamentally, by leaning so heavily on patterns of cognition, CBT may be mistaking the symptoms of depression for its causes, while implying to the patient that depression has little or nothing to do with life circumstances.

Furthermore, in assuming that people are entirely determined by involuntary or unreflective cognitive processes, CBT undermines the possibility of free will or agency.

This confused and reductive approach may frustrate and even alienate the patient, and contribute to the relatively high drop-out rates observed in CBT for depression.

* Johnsen TJ & Friborg O (2015): The effects of cognitive behavioural therapy as an anti-depressive treatment is falling: A meta-analysis. *Psychological Bulletin* 141(4):747-68.

Mindfulness

Some of the concerns with CBT are addressed by mindfulness-based cognitive therapy (MBCT), which combines traditional CBT methods with 'newer' psychological strategies such as mindfulness and mindfulness meditation.

In essence, mindfulness, which derives from Buddhist spiritual practice, aims at increasing our awareness and acceptance of incoming thoughts and feelings, and so the flexibility or fluidity of our responses, which become less like unconscious reactions and more like conscious reflections.

Mindfulness can be harnessed for the treatment of recurrent depression, stress, anxiety, and addiction, among others; but it can also be used to broadly improve our quality of life by decentering us and shifting our focus from doing to being.

Family therapy

Family therapy involves the identification and resolution of negative aspects of couple or family dynamics that may be contributing to mental disorder, such as deeply rooted conflict or high expressed emotion (Chapter 4). It usually requires the direct participation of each of the parties.

Other psychological treatments

Other types of psychological treatment include interpersonal therapy (IPT) and dialectical behavioural therapy (DBT). IPT involves a systematic and standardized treatment approach to personal relationships and life problems contributing to depression. DBT is a psychological method based on Buddhist teachings for the treatment of borderline personality disorder and recurrent self-harm.

Clinical skills: Selection criteria for psychological treatments

Selection criteria for CBT and other forms of psychological treatment are:
- 'Psychological-mindedness'.
- Adequate ego strength.
- Ability to form and maintain relationships.
- Motivation for insight and change.
- Ability to tolerate change and a degree of frustration.

Self-assessment

Answer by true or false:

1. Community care was originally thought to be cheaper than in-patient care.
2. If a GP refers a patient to specialist care, this is usually to the CMHT or AOT.
3. The crisis team is a 24-hours-a-day, 365-days-a-year multidisciplinary team dedicated to engaging 'revolving door' patients in treatment and supporting them in their daily activities.
4. The case of Re C (1994) helped to establish the legal criteria for capacity.
5. A child can be competent to consent to treatment if he or she at least partially understands the treatment proposed.
6. Simple measures such as ensuring that an elderly person has access to his spectacles or hearing aid can have a significant impact on level of capacity.
7. Common law can be invoked to restrain and medicate a patient if there are doubts as to his capacity.
8. According to the MHA, immoral conduct can be tantamount to mental disorder.
9. Section 2, admission for assessment, lasts 28 days, and Section 3, admission for treatment, lasts six months.
10. An application for Section 2 must be recommended by two doctors, both of whom must have special experience in the diagnosis and treatment of mental disorders.
11. Under Section 2, treatment cannot be given unless under common law.
12. A patient with a severe mental disorder can be treated for life-threatening diabetic ketoacidosis under the Mental Health Act.
13. Only a psychiatrist can make a recommendation for Section 5(2).
14. A patient in A&E can be detained under Section 5(2).
15. A patient in A&E can be detained under Section 2, 3, or 4.
16. Under Section 117, there is an obligation for the patient to accept aftercare.
17. If a person in a public place appears to the police to be suffering from a mental disorder, the police can remove him to a place of safety under Section 135.
18. Supportive therapy is more problem-focused and goal-oriented than counselling.
19. Psychodynamic psychotherapy and cognitive behavioural therapy are both forms of exploratory psychotherapy.
20. Several psychological treatments have been inspired by Buddhist teachings.

Answers

1. True.
2. False. Psychiatric referrals are usually to the CMHT or, in an emergency or at night, to the crisis team.
3. False. This best describes the AOT.
4. True.
5. False—*fully* understands.
6. True.
7. True.
8. False.
9. False. *Up to* 28 days, and *up to* six months.
10. False. Only one of the doctors must have special experience in the diagnosis and treatment of mental disorders.
11. False. Under Section 2, treatment can be given, but only in so far as it aims at treating the mental disorder or conditions directly resulting from the mental disorder.
12. False. Under common law perhaps.
13. False. Any fully registered doctor.
14. False. A patient can only be detained under Section 5(2) if he has already been admitted to hospital. Technically, patients in A&E have not yet been admitted to hospital.
15. True.
16. False.
17. False. Section 136.
18. False. The other way round.
19. True.
20. True.

Part 2

'That he's mad, 'tis true, 'tis true 'tis pity,
And pity 'tis 'tis true—a foolish figure,
But farewell it, for I will use no art.
Mad let us grant him then, and now remains
That we find out the cause of this effect,
Or rather say, the cause of this defect,
For this effect defective comes by cause:
Thus it remains, and the remainder thus.

—Shakespeare, *Hamlet*

4

Schizophrenia and other psychoses

A brief history of schizophrenia

The term 'schizophrenia' was coined in 1910 by psychiatrist Paul Eugen Bleuler (1857-1939), and derives from the Greek *schizo* ('split') and *phren* ('mind'). Although people often mistakenly think of schizophrenia as a 'split personality', Bleuler had intended the term to reflect the 'loosening' of thoughts and feelings which he had found to be a prominent feature of the illness.

Unfortunately, the term 'schizophrenia' has led to much confusion about the nature of the illness. Ironically, Bleuler had intended it to clarify matters by replacing the older, even more misleading term of *dementia praecox* ('dementia of early life'). This older term had been championed by Emil Kraepelin (1856-1926), who wrongly believed that the syndrome only occurred in young people and inevitably led to mental deterioration. Bleuler disagreed on both counts, and so renamed it 'schizophrenia'.

Bleuler held that, contrary to mental deterioration, schizophrenia led to a sharpening of the senses and to a heightened consciousness of memories and experiences. Compared to Kraepelin, he put more emphasis on thought disorder and negative symptoms than on the more florid positive, or psychotic, symptoms. He described the primary symptoms of schizophrenia as ambivalence, autistic behaviour, abnormal associations, and abnormal affect (the so-called 'four A's').

Although Kraepelin had some misguided beliefs about schizophrenia, he was the first person to distinguish it from other forms of psychosis, and in particular from the 'affective psychoses' that occur in mood disorders such as depression and bipolar disorder. He further distinguished three clinical presentations of schizophrenia: (1) paranoia, dominated by delusions and hallucinations; (2) hebephrenia, dominated by inappropriate reactions and behaviours; and (3) catatonia, dominated by extreme agitation or immobility and odd mannerisms and posturing.

Kraepelin first isolated schizophrenia from other forms of psychosis in 1887, but that is not to say that schizophrenia—or *dementia praecox*, as he called it—had not existed in some form or other long before his day. The oldest available description of an illness closely resembling schizophrenia can be found in the Ebers papyrus, which dates back to the Egypt of 1550 BC. And archaeological discoveries of Stone Age skulls with burr holes—drilled, one presumes, to release evil spirits—have led to speculation that schizophrenia is as old as mankind itself.

Symptoms of schizophrenia

ICD-10: F20 Schizophrenia

The schizophrenic disorders are characterized in general by fundamental and characteristic distortions of thinking and perception, and by inappropriate or blunted affect. Clear consciousness and intellectual capacity are usually maintained, although certain cognitive deficits may evolve in the course of time. The disturbance involves the most basic functions that give the normal person a feeling of individuality, uniqueness, and self-direction. The most intimate thoughts, feelings, and acts are often felt to be known to or shared by others, and explanatory delusions may develop, to the effect that natural or supernatural forces are at work to influence the afflicted individual's thoughts and actions in ways that are often bizarre. The individual may see himself or herself as the pivot of all that happens. Hallucinations, especially auditory, are common and may comment on the individual's behaviour or thoughts. Perception is frequently disturbed in other ways: colours or sounds may seem unduly vivid or altered in quality, and irrelevant features of ordinary things may appear more important than the whole object or situation. Perplexity is also common early on and frequently leads to a belief that everyday situations possess a special, usually sinister, meaning intended uniquely for the individual. In the characteristic schizophrenic disturbance of thinking, peripheral and irrelevant features of a total concept, which are inhibited in normal directed mental activity, are brought to the fore and utilized in place of those that are relevant and appropriate to the situation. Thus thinking becomes vague, elliptical, and obscure, and its expression in speech sometimes incomprehensible. Breaks and interpolations in the train of thought are frequent, and thoughts may seem to be withdrawn by some outside agency. Mood is characteristically shallow, capricious, or incongruous. Ambivalence and disturbance of volition may appear as inertia, negativism, or stupor. Catatonia may be present…

In 1959, psychiatrist Kurt Schneider (1887-1967) defined the 'first rank' symptoms of schizophrenia, symptoms supposed to be specific to, and therefore pathognomic of, schizophrenia (Table 4.1). Schneider's first rank symptoms largely consisted of florid psychotic symptoms such as thought insertion, thought broadcasting, and third person auditory hallucinations—symptoms held together by a common theme of loss of control over thoughts, feelings, and the body. Unfortunately, these symptoms are common to many psychotic disorders, and therefore not as useful as originally thought at distinguishing schizophrenia from other psychotic disorders. They are also absent in about 20% of schizophrenia sufferers.

Table 4.1: Schneider's First Rank Symptoms

Auditory hallucinations	
Third person	Voices discuss or argue about the patient.
Running commentary	Voices comment on the patient's thoughts and actions.
Gedankenlautwerden and *écho de la pensée*	The patient's thoughts are heard as, or shortly after, they are formulated.
Delusions of thought control	
Thought insertion	Alien thoughts are inserted into the patient's mind by an external agency.
Thought withdrawal	The opposite; thoughts are withdrawn from the patient's mind by an external agency.
Thought broadcasting	The patient's thoughts are overheard by, or otherwise accessible to, others.
Delusions of control (passivity phenomena)	
Passivity of affect, volition, and impulses	The patient's affect, volition, and impulses are under the control of an external agency.
Somatic passivity	The patient's bodily sensations are under the control of an external agency.
Delusional perception	The patient attributes delusional significance to normal percepts.

Reminder of some important definitions:

Delusion: An unshakeable (fixed) belief held in the face of evidence to the contrary and that cannot be explained by culture or religion.

Hallucination: A percept that arises in the absence of a stimulus, and that is not subject to conscious manipulation.

Case studies: Schneider's first rank symptoms

Echo de la pensée

A 32-year-old housewife complained of a man's voice, speaking in an intense whisper from a point about two feet above her head. The voice would repeat almost all the patient's goal-directed thinking—even the most banal thoughts. The patient would think, 'I must put the kettle on,' and after a pause of not more than one second the voice would say, 'I must put the kettle on.' It would often say the opposite, 'Don't put the kettle on.'

Thought insertion

A 29-year-old housewife said, 'I look out of the window and I think the garden looks nice and the grass looks cool, but the thoughts of Eamonn Andrews come into my mind. There are no other thoughts there, only his... He treats my mind like a screen and flashes his thoughts onto it like you flash a picture.'

Thought withdrawal

A 22-year-old woman said, 'I am thinking about my mother, and suddenly my thoughts are sucked out of my mind by a phrenological vacuum extractor, and there is nothing in my mind, it is empty...'

Thought broadcasting

A 21-year-old student said, 'As I think, my thoughts leave my head on a type of mental ticker-tape. Everyone around has only to pass the tape through their mind and they know my thoughts.'

Passivity of affect

A 23-year-old woman reported: 'I cry, tears roll down my cheeks and I look unhappy, but inside I have a cold anger because they are using me in this way, and it is not me who is unhappy, but they are projecting unhappiness onto my brain. They project upon me laughter, for no reason, and you have no idea how terrible it is to laugh and look happy and know it is not you, but their emotions.'

Passivity of volition

A 29-year-old shorthand typist described her actions as follows: 'When I reach my hand for the comb it is my hand and arm which move, and my fingers pick up the pen, but I don't control them... I sit there watching them move, and they are quite independent, what they do is nothing to do with me... I am just a puppet who is manipulated by cosmic strings. When the strings are pulled my body moves and I cannot prevent it.'

Passivity of impulse

A 26-year-old engineer emptied the contents of a urine bottle over the ward dinner trolley. He said, 'The sudden impulse came over me that I must do it. It was not my feeling, it came into me from the X-ray department, that was why I was sent there for implants yesterday. It was nothing to do with me, they wanted it done. So I picked up the bottle and poured it in. It seemed all I could do.'

Somatic passivity

A 38-year-old man had jumped from a bedroom window, injuring his right knee which was very painful. He described his physical experience thus: 'The sun-rays are directed by U.S. army satellite in an intense beam which I can feel entering the centre of my knee and then radiating outwards causing the pain.'

Delusional perception

A young Irishman was at breakfast with two fellow-lodgers. He felt a sense of unease, that something frightening was going to happen. One of the lodgers pushed the salt cellar towards him (he appreciated at the time that this was an ordinary salt cellar and his friend's intention was innocent). Almost before the salt cellar reached him he knew that he must return home 'to greet the Pope, who is visiting Ireland to see his family and to reward them... because our Lord is going to be born again to one of the women... And because of this they [the women] are born different with their private parts back to front.'

C. S. Mellor (1970): First rank symptoms in schizophrenia. *Brit. J. Psychiat.* 117, 15-23.

Today, the symptoms of schizophrenia are divided into three groups: positive symptoms, disorganized symptoms, and negative symptoms, as detailed in Table 4.2.

Table 4.2: Symptoms of schizophrenia

Positive symptoms	Disorganized symptoms	Negative symptoms
Delusions	Disorganized thinking/speech	Affective flattening
Hallucinations	Disorganized behaviour	Apathy
	Inappropriate affect	Avolition
		Anergia
		Anhedonia
		Alogia
		Asociality
		Attentional impairment

Positive symptoms consist of psychotic symptoms (hallucinations and delusions), which are usually as real to the sufferer as they are unreal to everybody else. Positive symptoms are often considered to be the hallmark of schizophrenia, and tend to be most prominent in its early stages.

Disorganized symptoms (sometimes also referred to as cognitive symptoms or 'thought disorder') involve problems with concentration and memory that can make it difficult to register and recall information, and to formulate and communicate thoughts. Although less manifest than positive symptoms, disorganized symptoms can be just as distressing and disabling.

Whereas positive symptoms can be thought of as an excess or distortion of normal functions, negative symptoms can be thought of as a diminution or loss of normal functions. In some cases, negative symptoms dominate the clinical picture; in others, they are altogether absent. Compared with positive symptoms, negative symptoms tend to be more subtle and less noticeable, but also more persistent, and can perdure right through periods of remission, long after any positive symptoms have burnt out. Negative symptoms are often misconstrued by the public, and sometimes also by relatives and carers, as indolence or obstinacy, rather than the manifestations of a mental disorder. For health professionals, they can be difficult to distinguish from symptoms of depression, or from the adverse effects of antipsychotics (see later).

Case study: Valerie

Valerie is a 23-year-old anthropology student who shares a house with three other students on her course. According to her housemates, she has been behaving oddly for the past six months, and since the beginning of term four weeks ago has not attended a single lecture. One month ago, she found out that her close childhood friend, Chloe, had died in a motorbike accident. Since then, she has been secluding herself in her room for hours on end, banging on the furniture, and, it seems, shouting to herself. Her housemates eventually persuaded her to see a doctor.

When Valerie arrived in A&E, she was so agitated and distressed that she could not reply to most of the junior psychiatrist's questions. However, he was able to make out that she was hearing three or four male voices coming from outside her head, and that the voices were talking together about her, disparaging her, and blaming her for her family's financial problems. She said the voices belonged to SAS paratroopers engaged by her parents to destroy her by putting certain thoughts, such as the thought of cutting her wrists, into her head.

Towards the end of the consultation, Valerie screamed at the psychiatrist, "I've seen your belt! They've sent you to distract me! I can't... I can't fight them anymore!" and ran out into the waiting area.

Having ascertained that Valerie does not have a psychiatric or medical history and does not take drugs, the psychiatrist made a provisional diagnosis of acute schizophrenia-like psychosis and called for a Mental Health Act assessment.

Clinical skills: Asking about delusions

Begin with an introductory statement and general questions, such as: *I would like to ask you some questions that may seem a little strange. These are questions that we ask to everyone who comes to see us. Is that all right with you? Do you have any thoughts or beliefs that your friends and family do not share?*

Then ask specifically about common delusions, tailoring your questioning to the particular patient—for instance, you do not need to ask a manic patient about nihilistic delusions.

- Delusions of persecution: *How are you getting on with other people? Do you fear for your safety? Is anyone trying to harm you?*
- Delusions of reference: *Do people talk about you behind your back? Do you receive messages from the newspapers, radio, or television?*
- Delusional perception: *Do things happening around you carry a special meaning?*

- Delusions of control and passivity phenomena: *Is someone or something controlling you? Is someone or something forcing you to think or say or do certain things?*
- Delusions of thought control, including thought insertion, thought withdrawal, and thought broadcasting: *Are your thoughts being interfered with? Are someone else's thoughts being put into your head? Are your own thoughts being removed from your head? Can your thoughts be heard or otherwise accessed by others?*
- Delusions of misidentification: *Do you feel that people are not who they seem to be?*
- Delusions of grandeur: *How do you compare yourself to others? Do you have a special calling in life? Do you have any special abilities or powers?*

- Religious delusions: *Are you a very religious person? Are you especially close to God?*
- Delusions of guilt: *Do you have any regrets? Is there anything for which you blame yourself?*
- Nihilistic delusions: *Do you feel that something terrible has happened or is about to happen? Do you feel that a part of your body is dead or missing? Do you feel dead inside?*
- Somatic delusions: *Are you worried that you may be suffering from a serious physical illness?*
- Delusions of jealousy: *How are you getting on with your partner? Does she reciprocate your loyalty?*

Explore any possible delusions. In particular, ask about their onset, their effect on the patient's life, and the patient's explanation for them (degree of insight).

Clinical skills: Asking about hallucinations (voices)

Begin with an introductory statement and general questions, such as: *I gather you've been under quite some pressure lately. When people are under pressure they sometimes find their imagination playing tricks on them. Have you had any such experiences? Have you heard unusual things? Have you heard or seen things which others cannot hear or see?*

Then ask more closed questions to determine:

- Content: Whose voices are they? Where are they coming from? What are they saying? Are they ordering the patient to do anything dangerous (command hallucinations)? Can the patient resist these commands?
- Type: Do the voices speak directly to the patient (second person), or about him (third person)? Do they comment on his every thought and action (running commentary), or repeat or echo his thoughts (*Gedankenlautwerden, echo de la pensée*)? If necessary, distinguish between true hallucinations and pseudohallucinations, and exclude hypnagogic and hypnopompic hallucinations (Table 2.7).
- Onset and precipitating factors.
- Frequency and duration.
- Effect on the patient's life.
- The patient's explanation for the voices (degree of insight).

Course

The course of schizophrenia can vary considerably from one person to another, but is often marked by a number of distinct phases. In the acute phase, positive symptoms come to the fore, while any cognitive and negative symptoms that may already be present sink into the background. The sufferer typically reaches a crisis point at which he comes into contact with mental health services. An antipsychotic is started and the acute phase resolves, even though residual positive symptoms may remain.

In some cases, the onset of schizophrenia can be preceded by an insidious prodromal phase lasting for anything from days to years, and consisting of subtle and non-specific abnormalities or oddities in language, cognition, and behaviour that may be mistaken for depression or normal teenage behaviour, and that are associated with a loss of function.

As the acute phase remits, any cognitive and negative symptoms start to dominate the picture. This chronic phase, if it occurs, can last for a period of several months or even several years, and may be punctuated by relapses into a state resembling the acute phase. Such relapses are often caused by a sudden reduction or discontinuation of antipsychotic medication, substance misuse, or a stressful life event, although in many cases there is no identifiable trigger.

Diagnosis and types

ICD-10

A minimum of one very clear symptom (and usually two or more if symptoms are less clear-cut) from groups (a) to (d), or symptoms from at least two of the groups (e) to (h).

These symptoms should have been present for most of the time during a period of **one month or more**. If present for less than one month, a diagnosis of acute schizophrenia-like psychotic disorder should be made.

(a) Thought echo, thought insertion or withdrawal, thought broadcasting.

(b) Delusions of control, influence, passivity; delusional perception.

(c) Hallucinatory voices of running commentary, third-person discussion, or other types of voices coming from some part of the body.

(d) Persistent delusions of other kinds that are culturally inappropriate and completely impossible.

(e) Persistent hallucinations in any modality if accompanied by fleeting or half-formed delusions that are not affective delusions, or by persistent over-valued ideas, or if occurring every day for months on end.

(f) Breaks in the train of thought resulting in incoherence, irrelevant speech, or neologisms.

(g) Catatonic behaviour such as excitement, posturing, waxy flexibility, negativism, mutism, and stupor.

(h) Negative symptoms such as apathy, paucity of speech, blunting or incongruity of emotional responses, social withdrawal not due to depression or neuroleptic (antipsychotic) medication.

(i) Significant and consistent change in overall quality of some aspects of personal behaviour, manifest as loss of interest, aimlessness, idleness, a self-absorbed attitude, and social withdrawal.

ICD-10 subtypes of schizophrenia

F20.0 Paranoid schizophrenia
F20.1 Hebephrenic schizophrenia
F20.2 Catatonic schizophrenia
F20.3 Undifferentiated schizophrenia
F20.4 Post-schizophrenic depression
F20.5 Residual schizophrenia
F20.6 Simple schizophrenia
F20.8 Other schizophrenia
F20.9 Schizophrenia, unspecified

Paranoid schizophrenia

In paranoid schizophrenia, the commonest type of schizophrenia, the clinical picture is dominated by relatively stable, often paranoid, delusions, usually accompanied by hallucinations and perceptual disturbances. Disturbances of affect, volition, and speech, and catatonic symptoms, are not prominent. Onset tends to be later than for hebephrenic or catatonic schizophrenia, and the course may be either episodic or chronic.

Hebephrenic schizophrenia

Hebephrenic schizophrenia is marked by prominent affective changes. Mood is inappropriate and often accompanied by giggling or self-satisfied, self-absorbed smiling, or by a lofty manner, grimaces, mannerisms, pranks, hypochondriacal complaints, and reiterated phrases. Thought is disorganized and speech rambling and incoherent. Behaviour is characteristically aimless and empty of purpose. Compared to paranoid schizophrenia, delusions and hallucinations are fleeting and fragmentary. Hebephrenic schizophrenia is normally diagnosed for the first time only in adolescents or young adults, and has a poor prognosis owing to rapid development of negative symptoms.

Catatonic schizophrenia

Catatonic schizophrenia is diagnosed in the presence of prominent psychomotor disturbances that may alternate between extremes such as hyperkinesis and stupor, and automatic obedience and negativism (See chapter 2 for a full description of catatonia). Catatonic schizophrenia, which several decades ago used to be more common, has become very rare: this could be because the symptoms of schizophrenia are culturally shaped, and there has been a shift in culture.

Undifferentiated schizophrenia

Undifferentiated schizophrenia is a diagnosis reserved for conditions meeting the general diagnostic criteria for schizophrenia but not conforming to any of the above subtypes, or exhibiting features of more than one of them without any one predominating.

Post-schizophrenic depression

A diagnosis of post-schizophrenic depression can only be made if the patient has had a schizophrenic illness in the past 12 months, and if some schizophrenic symptoms are still present although no longer dominating the clinical picture. The depressive symptoms must independently fulfil the diagnostic criteria for a depressive episode.

Residual schizophrenia

For a diagnosis of residual schizophrenia, there must have been a clear progression from an early stage (comprising one or more episodes with psychotic symptoms that meet the general criteria for schizophrenia) to a later stage characterized by long-term, although not necessarily irreversible, negative symptoms. For a confident diagnosis, this later stage should already have lasted for at least one year, and conditions such as dementia, chronic depression, or institutionalization should have been excluded.

Simple schizophrenia

Simple schizophrenia is characterized by the insidious but progressive development of oddities of conduct, an inability to meet the demands of society, and a decline in total performance. The characteristic negative symptoms of residual schizophrenia develop without having been preceded by any overt positive or psychotic symptoms. The diagnosis is difficult to secure.

Although the biological validity of all these subtypes is highly questionable, it is interesting to note that paranoid schizophrenia tends to be dominated by positive symptoms, hebephrenic schizophrenia by disorganized symptoms, and simple schizophrenia by negative symptoms (Table 4.2).

DSM-5

The DSM-5 diagnostic criteria for schizophrenia can be summarized as follows:

The difficulty with diagnosing schizophrenia

The majority of medical disorders are defined by their aetiology or pathology, and so are relatively easy to define and recognize. For instance, if someone is suspected of having malaria, a blood sample can be taken and examined under a microscope for malarial parasites; and if someone appears to have suffered a stroke, a brain scan can be taken to look for evidence of arterial obstruction. In contrast, mental disorders such as schizophrenia cannot (as yet?) be defined according to their aetiology or pathology, but only according to their manifestations or symptoms. This means that they are more difficult to describe and diagnose, and more open to misunderstanding and misuse.

If a person is suspected of having schizophrenia, there are no laboratory or physical tests that can objectively confirm the diagnosis. Instead, the psychiatrist is left to base his diagnosis on nothing but the person's symptoms, without the support of any tests. If the symptoms tally with the diagnostic criteria for schizophrenia, the psychiatrist is justified in making a diagnosis of schizophrenia.

The problem here is one of circularity: the concept of schizophrenia is defined according to the symptoms of schizophrenia, which in turn are defined according to the concept of schizophrenia. Thus, it is impossible to be sure that 'schizophrenia' maps into any real or distinct disease entity. Given the 'menu of symptoms' approach to diagnosis, it is even possible for two people with no symptoms in common to receive the same label of schizophrenia. Perhaps for this reason, a diagnosis of schizophrenia is a poor predictor of either the severity of the condition or its likely outcome or prognosis.

1. The person must have at least two characteristic symptoms from a list of five: delusions, hallucinations, disorganized speech, disorganized behaviour, and negative symptoms. One of these two symptoms must be delusions, hallucinations, or disorganized speech.

2. These symptoms must have been present for at least one month, and signs of disturbance for at least six months.

3. The symptoms must undermine the person's ability to function in his social or occupational setting.

4. Other mental and medical disorders that can present like schizophrenia—such as drug intoxication, mood disorder, and head injury—must have been excluded.

Compared to DSM-IV and indeed ICD-10, DSM-5 accords much less importance to Schneiderian first rank symptoms, and does away with the classic subtypes of schizophrenia owing to their 'limited diagnostic stability, low reliability, and poor validity'.

What's more, psychotic symptoms may form an inadequate basis for diagnosing schizophrenia. Delusions and hallucinations occur in a number of different disorders and states, and therefore represent relatively non-specific indicators of mental disorder. Most of the disability associated with schizophrenia is related to chronic cognitive and negative symptoms, not acute, albeit more florid, positive symptoms. Diagnosing schizophrenia on the basis of psychosis may be akin to diagnosing pneumonia on the basis of nothing more than a fever.

Both clinical practice and research into the causes of mental disorders suggest that many of the concepts delineated in classifications of mental disorders, including schizophrenia, depression, and bipolar disorder, do not in fact map onto any real or distinct entities, as Kraepelin led us to believe, but instead lie at different extremes of a single spectrum of mental disorders or states.

Even assuming that the concept of schizophrenia is valid, the symptoms and clinical manifestations that define it are open to interpretation. Recent studies have found that, in reaching a diagnosis of schizophrenia, the rate of agreement between any two independent assessors, that is, the inter-rater reliability, is 65 per cent *at most*. So the concept of schizophrenia is lacking not only in validity, but also in reliability.

That this is so is a consequence of the empirical challenges of investigating the brain, but also, and above all, of the conceptual challenges of understanding the structure and content of human experience.

Differential diagnosis

Psychiatric differential

- Drug-induced psychotic disorder (common), for example, amphetamines, cocaine, cannabis, alcohol, LSD, phencyclidine, glucocorticoids, L-dopa.
- Schizoaffective disorder.
- Depressive psychosis.
- Manic psychosis.
- Other psychotic disorder such as brief psychotic disorder, persistent delusional disorder, or induced delusional disorder.
- Puerperal psychosis.
- Personality disorder.

Organic differential

- Delirium.
- Dementia.
- Stroke.
- Temporal lobe epilepsy.
- Central nervous system infections such as AIDS, neurosyphilis, herpes encephalitis.
- Other neurological conditions such as head trauma, brain tumour, Huntington's disease, Wilson's disease.
- Endocrine disorders, especially Cushing's syndrome.
- Metabolic disorders, especially vitamin B12 deficiency and porphyria.
- Autoimmune disorders, especially systemic lupus erythematosus (SLE).

Schizophrenia and depression ⊙

Chronic or residual schizophrenia ought to be distinguished from the symptoms of depression and from the motor side-effects of antipsychotics. About a quarter of patients with schizophrenia develop depression once their psychotic symptoms have resolved.

Epidemiology

Prevalence

Figures for the lifetime prevalence of schizophrenia vary according to diagnostic criteria, but are usually quoted at around 1%. Point prevalence is about 0.4%.

Sex ratio

Unlike many other mental disorders such as depression and anxiety disorders, which are more common in women, schizophrenia affects men and women in more or less equal numbers. However, it tends to present earlier in men, and also to affect them more severely. Why this is so remains unclear.

Age of onset

Onset can be at any age, but the syndrome is rare in childhood and early adolescence and uncommon after the age of 45. Mean age of onset in males is about 28 years, and in females about 32 years. If symptoms first present in middle or old age, it is particularly important to exclude organic conditions that may masquerade as schizophrenia.

Geography

Generally speaking, lifetime prevalence is similar across populations and stable over time, despite the reduced reproductive fitness of affected individuals. Prevalence and severity tend to be greater in urban areas, maybe because schizophrenia sufferers drift into urban areas as a consequence of their illness or its prodromal symptoms (the drift hypothesis), or else because the stress of urban living actually plays a part in the aetiology of the syndrome (the breeder hypothesis).

Migration

The prevalence of schizophrenia seems to be higher in immigrants, especially second-generation Afro-Caribbean immigrants to the UK (about a 10-fold increase). This may reflect such factors as poor integration, socioeconomic deprivation, or diagnostic bias among doctors.

Seasonality of births

The lifetime prevalence of schizophrenia is increased by about 5-10% if born from January to April in the northern hemisphere or July to September in the southern hemisphere. This may reflect a viral contribution to aetiology.

Socioeconomic status

As the socioeconomic backgrounds of the fathers of schizophrenia sufferers are normally distributed, observed socioeconomic differences most probably result from social drifting. For instance, schizophrenia sufferers are much more likely to be unemployed.

Schizophrenia and creativity

Genes for potentially debilitating illnesses usually become less common over time: the fact that this has not happened for schizophrenia suggests that the responsible genes are being selected despite their potentially debilitating effects on a significant proportion of the population. This could be because the genes confer important adaptive advantages, such as the abilities for language and creativity. Our abilities for language and creativity not only set us apart from other animals, but also make us highly adept at the game of survival.

Some highly creative people have suffered from schizophrenia, including Syd Barrett, the early driving force behind the rock band Pink Floyd; John Nash, the father of game theory and Nobel Prize winner; and Vaslav Nijinsky, the legendary choreographer and dancer. However, these cases are exceptional, and many people with schizophrenia are intensely disabled by their symptoms. Even highly creative people with schizophrenia tend to be incapacitated during active phases of the illness, while being much more productive before its onset and during later phases of remission.

Many more highly creative people, while not themselves suffering from schizophrenia, have close relatives who do or did. Albert Einstein's son suffered from schizophrenia, as did Bertrand Russell's son and James Joyce's daughter. Several studies suggest that this may not be simple coincidence, and that the relatives of schizophrenia sufferers enjoy above average creative intelligence.

According to one theory, both people with schizophrenia and their non-affected relatives lack lateralization of function in the brain. While this tends to handicap the former, it tends to benefit the latter, who gain in creativity from increased use of the right hemisphere and increased communication between the right and left hemispheres. This increased inter-hemispheric communication also occurs in schizophrenia sufferers, but their cognitive processes tend to be too disorganized for them to make productive use of it.

Some healthy relatives of schizophrenia sufferers may be so close to schizophrenia on the spectrum of normality as to meet the diagnostic criteria for schizotypal personality disorder (Chapter 7). Many more relatives who do not meet the threshold for schizotypal disorder may nonetheless have mild schizotypal traits, such as divergent or idiosyncratic thinking, which are associated with creativity.

Aetiology

The stress-vulnerability model

Any given individual has a certain complement of genetic variations that make him more or less vulnerable to developing schizophrenia. A person who is highly vulnerable to developing schizophrenia but who is never subjected to severe stress may be less likely to develop or express the syndrome than a person who is only moderately vulnerable but who comes under severe stress. (Figure 4.1). Examples of severe stress include losing a friend or relative in an accident, being badly bullied at school, or smoking cannabis (a form of physical, as opposed to emotional, stress).

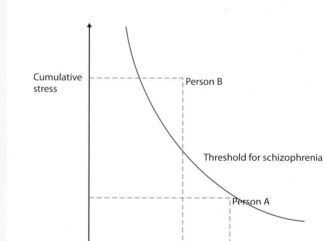

Figure 4.1. The stress-vulnerability model of schizophrenia. A person develops schizophrenia when the stress that he faces becomes greater than his ability to cope with it. Person A is highly vulnerable to developing schizophrenia but suffers only moderate stress and so does not cross the threshold for the illness. In contrast, Person B, though only moderately vulnerable, is subjected to unusually high stress and so does cross the threshold.

Genetic factors

A concordance rate of about 50% in monozygotic twins suggests that genetic and environmental factors are more or less equally involved in the expression of the disorder. In adoption studies, biological offspring of schizophrenic parents adopted by non-schizophrenic parents maintain their increased risk, whereas biological offspring of non-schizophrenic parents adopted by schizophrenic parents do not suffer any increased risk. Figure 4.2 conveys the approximate lifetime risk of schizophrenia according to relative(s) affected.

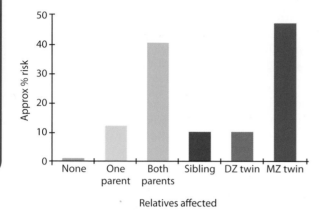

Figure 4.2. Approximate lifetime risk of schizophrenia according to relative(s) affected.

Environmental factors

Developmental factors

Cytoarchitectural abnormalities and a lack of gliosis in certain parts of the brains of schizophrenia sufferers point to a neurodevelopmental rather than a neurodegenerative pathological process. Further support for a neurodevelopmental aetiology comes from the season of birth effect (see above), which may owe to prenatal exposure to influenza or other viruses. Interestingly, a season of birth effect has also been reported for autism, depression, and bipolar disorder. Obstetric complications, childhood head injury, and childhood encephalitis have also been proposed as aetiological factors.

Life events and background stressors

Schizophrenia sufferers experience more adverse life events in the month prior to the onset of acute symptoms. This suggests that schizophrenia is precipitated by adverse life events, but the converse may also hold (adverse life events are precipitated by schizophrenia), and even the prodromal phase may predispose to life events such as failing exams or dropping out of school.

It is also important to remember that most of our daily stress comes not from life events, but from seemingly smaller 'background' stressors such as strained relationships, painful memories, loneliness, discrimination, poor housing, and unpaid bills.

Expressed emotion

High expressed emotion (EE) can increase the risk of relapse in schizophrenia by up to fourfold. EE can be thought of as a specific type of stress. It refers to the amount of critical, hostile, or emotionally over-involved attitudes directed to the schizophrenia sufferer by his relatives and carers. Such attitudes often originate in a misunderstanding that the schizophrenia sufferer is actually in control of his illness and merely 'choosing' to be ill. In some cases, it owes to an unjustified sense of guilt, or a desire to 'share out' the burden of the illness. As with life events, the relationship between high EE and schizophrenia is far from simple: in some cases, high EE may simply reflect legitimate feelings of anxiety and distress at the illness of a loved one.

Cannabis and other drugs

People who smoke cannabis are up to six times more likely to develop schizophrenia, and people with schizophrenia who smoke cannabis suffer more frequent and severe relapses. Other drugs that have been associated with schizophrenia include stimulant drugs such as amphetamines, ecstasy, and cocaine. It could be that cannabis causes schizophrenia, but it could also be that people who are predisposed to schizophrenia are also predisposed to smoking cannabis as a means of relieving their distress.

Neurochemical abnormalities

According to the original dopamine hypothesis of schizophrenia, which dates back to 1976, positive symptoms are produced by an increase in dopamine in the mesolimbic tract (Figure 4.3). Support for the dopamine hypothesis comes, in the main, from two observations: (1) drugs such as amphetamines and cannabis that increase dopamine in the mesolimbic tract can exacerbate positive symptoms or even induce a schizophrenia-like psychosis; and (2) antipsychotics that are effective in the treatment of positive symptoms block the effects of increased dopamine in the mesolimbic tract.

The revised dopamine hypothesis, which dates back to 1991, adds that the negative symptoms of schizophrenia result from a *decrease* in dopamine in the mesocortical tract (Figure 4.3).

The dopamine hypothesis has supplied researchers with a basic model of schizophrenia, but says little about the actual cause of the changes in dopamine lev-

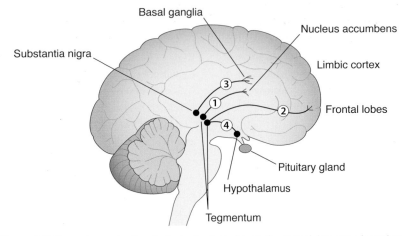

Figure 4.3. Dopamine projections in the brain. According to the revised dopamine hypothesis of schizophrenia, positive symptoms result from hyperdopaminergia in the mesolimbic tract (1), whereas negative symptoms result from hypodopaminergia in the mesocortical tract (2). The other dopamine projections are the nigrostriatal tract (3) and the tuberoinfundibular tract (4).

els, and can by no means account for all the subtleties and complexities of the syndrome or its treatment. More recent research has implicated a number of other neurotransmitters such as glutamate and serotonin, and it is notable that NMDA antagonists such as phencyclidine hydrochloride (PCP, 'angel dust') and ketamine, and the 5-HT receptor agonist lysergic acid diethylamide (LSD), can all induce a schizophrenia-like psychosis. It may be that altered levels of dopamine and other neurotransmitters are interrelated, once more raising the age-old problem of the chicken and the egg.

Other neurological differences

Structural differences, which are only present in some cases, include a reduction in brain volume principally affecting the frontal and temporal lobes and medial temporal lobe structures such as the hippocampus, parahippocampus, and amygdala, ventricular enlargement, and cytoarchitectural abnormalities. The reduction in brain volume seems to owe to decrease in neuronal size rather than to a neurodegenerative process. It remains unclear whether structural differences preexist prior to the onset of illness, or whether they result from the illness or from its treatment with antipsychotics. Functional abnormalities include hypofrontality, that is, poor performance on tests of frontal lobe function, and soft neurological signs such as abnormalities of stereognosis and proprioception.

Investigations

In as far as practicable, investigations for a first psychotic episode should include a full physical (including neurological) examination; a serum or urine drug screen; liver, renal and thyroid function tests; full blood count; fasting blood glucose (or HbA1c); and lipids. The purposes of these investigations are chiefly to uncover possible organic causes of psychosis, and to establish baselines for the administration of antipsychotics. Other, more specific investigations should be considered on a case-by-case basis, and might for example include brain imaging if there is a suggestion of a space-occupying lesion.

Management

Introduction

Febrile illnesses such as malaria had been observed to temper psychotic symptoms, and in the early 20th century 'fever therapy' became a standard treatment for schizophrenia. Psychiatrists attempted to induce fevers in their patients, sometimes by means of injections of sulphur or oil. Other common but objectionable treatments included sleep therapy, gas therapy, electroconvulsive therapy, and prefrontal leucotomy (lobotomy), which involved severing the part of the brain that processes emotions. Sadly, many such 'treatments' aimed more at controlling disturbed behaviour than at curing illness or alleviating suffering. In some countries and periods, such as Germany during the Nazi era, the belief that schizophrenia resulted from a 'hereditary defect' led to atrocious acts of forced sterilization and genocide. The first antipsychotic drug, chlorpromazine, first became available in the 1950s. Although far from perfect, it opened up an era of hope and promise for people with schizophrenia.

The dopamine hypothesis submits that antipsychotics are effective in the treatment of positive symptoms because they block the action of dopamine in the mesolimbic tract. Unfortunately, they also block the action of dopamine in other brain tracts, commonly leading to a number of unpleasant adverse effects such as negative symptoms (mesocortical tract), disturbances of voluntary muscle function (nigrostriatal tract), and loss of libido, amenorrhoea, and erectile dysfunction (tuberoinfundibular tract). They also interfere with neurotransmitters other than dopamine, which can result in further adverse effects, first among which sedation and weight gain.

Still, antipsychotics remain the primary treatment for schizophrenia, although psychosocial interventions can also play an important role in reducing symptoms and preventing relapse and re-hospitalization.

Antipsychotics

The following are guidelines to treatment with antipsychotics:

- Prior to starting an antipsychotic, it is good practice to carry out a physical examination and to check, at the very least, urea and electrolytes, liver function tests, fasting plasma glucose, blood lipids, and prolactin. Clozapine additionally requires registration with a monitoring service, baseline full blood count and ECG, and weekly full blood counts for the first 18 weeks. It also requires close monitoring of pulse rate, blood pressure, and temperature during the titration period.

- Patients are more likely to respond if treatment is started early. It is claimed that antipsychotics are effective against positive symptoms in about 70-85% of cases, but it can be several days before they take effect and a benzodiazepine such as lorazepam may have to be prescribed in the interim if the patient is particularly distressed or agitated.

- In the first instance, the patient should be started on an antipsychotic other than clozapine. Choice of antipsychotic should be guided by the patient on the basis of adverse effect profiles (Tables 4.4, 4.5) and, if applicable, previous response to antipsychotic treatment.

- The starting dose should be small to minimize adverse effects, and then increased according to clinical response to no more than the minimum effective dose.

- If the patient fails to respond to the chosen drug or cannot tolerate it, an alternative from a different class should be tried.

- If the patient fails to respond to two or more antipsychotics after an adequate trial of each (6-8 weeks), clozapine should be considered. Clozapine is effective in about half of treatment-resistant patients.

- If the patient has improved on a particular drug, he or she should continue taking it at same dose for at least the next six months.

- Where necessary, depot preparations can be used to improve long-term compliance. The principal pros and cons of oral versus depot preparations are listed in Table 4.3. Upon converting a patient to a depot antipsychotic, it is usual to first administer

Table 4.3: Principle pros and cons of oral versus depot preparations

	Pros	Cons
Oral	• Short duration of action • Flexibility	• Variable absorption/first-pass effect • Potential for poor compliance • Potential for misuse and overdose
Depot	• Better bioavailability • Less potential for poor compliance • Less potential for misuse and overdose • Ensures regular contact with healthcare team	• Potential damage to therapeutic alliance • Needle injections may involve pain and local complications such as abscess • Adverse effects may be delayed and/or prolonged

a small test dose. The first treatment dose can be administered after about seven days if the patient has not suffered from any unacceptable adverse effects. The treatment dose can then be increased at regular intervals as the oral antipsychotic is tapered off.

The old so-called typical antipsychotics include chlorpromazine, fluphenazine, flupenthixol, zuclopenthixol, and haloperidol. The clinical efficacy of typical antipsychotics seems related to their antagonism of the dopamine D2 receptor. Their common adverse effects are listed in Table 4.4. Extra-pyramidal side-effects (EPSEs) include acute dystonias, akathisia, Parkinson-like symptoms, and tardive dyskinesia (Table 4.5).

Managing EPSEs (!)

Drugs can be used to treat EPSEs. However, in the first instance it is usually preferable to reduce the dose of the antipsychotic or switch to another (usually atypical) antipsychotic. The prophylactic use of anticholinergics to prevent EPSEs is to be avoided.

Strictly speaking, the definition of an atypical or second generation antipsychotic is 'a drug which does not produce catalepsy in rats despite having an antipsychotic profile in behavioural tests'—that is, a drug which has a high therapeutic index in relation to EPSEs. This may owe to 'fast dissociation' at the dopamine D2 receptor, or simply to lower equivalent doses than with typical antipsychotics. The group of atypical antipsychotics is considered to include clozapine, risperidone, olanzapine, quetiapine, amisulpride, sertindole, ziprasidone, zotepine, paliperidone, and aripiprazole. Clozapine is associated with a 1% risk of agranulocytosis, and patients on clozapine must have their differential leucocyte counts monitored. Despite this inconvenience, clozapine is the drug of choice in treatment-resistant schizophrenia.

In recent years, critics have argued that the distinction between typical and atypical antipsychotics is little more than a marketing ploy by the pharmaceutical industry: atypical antipsychotics are in fact a disparate mix of compounds with significant differences in potency and adverse effects (Table 4.6), and nothing in common to distinguish them from typical antipsychotics, which are more cost-effective.

Table 4.4: Adverse effects of antipsychotics according to receptor action
NB. Individual drugs differ somewhat in their actions and adverse effects.

Receptor action	Potential therapeutic effect	Potential adverse effects
Antidopaminergic	Improvement in positive symptoms	Extrapyramidal symptoms (Table 4.5), negative symptoms, hyperprolactinaemia*, neuroleptic malignant syndrome, weight gain
Serotonergic	Unknown, possibly a small improvement in affective symptoms and negative symptoms	Anxiety, insomnia, change in appetite leading to weight gain, hypercholesterolaemia, diabetes§
Antihistaminergic	Unknown	Sedation (can be a benefit), weight gain
Anti-adrenergic	Unknown	Postural hypotension, tachycardia, ejaculatory failure
Anticholinergic	Unknown	Dry mouth, blurred vision, glaucoma, constipation, urinary retention...

* Symptoms of hyperprolactinaemia include loss of libido, amenorrhoea, erectile dysfunction, galactorrhoea, gynaecomastia, and reduced bone density.

§ Type II diabetes may be related to weight gain or insulin resistance. Interestingly, the prevalence of type II diabetes is also increased in the non-affected relatives of schizophrenia sufferers.

NB. Other adverse effects of antipsychotics include hypo- or hyper-thermia, convulsions, cardiotoxicity (increased QTc, myocarditis, cardiomyopathy), hepatotoxicity, blood dyscrasias, photosensitivity, and allergic reactions.

4

Table 4.5: Extrapyramidal side-effects of antipsychotics

Acute dystonias	Often painful spastic contraction of certain muscles or muscle groups most commonly affecting the neck, eyes, and trunk, for instance, tongue protrusion, grimacing, torticollis. Acute dystonias may respond to anticholinergics.
Akathisia (Greek, *not to sit*)	Distressing feeling of inner restlessness manifested by fidgety leg movements, shuffling of feet, pacing, and so on. Akathisia may respond to anticholinergics, propanolol, the antihistamine cyproheptadine, benzodiazepines, or clonidine.
Parkinson-like symptoms	Triad of parkinsonian tremor, muscular rigidity, and bradykinesia. Parkinson-like symptoms may respond to anticholinergics.
Tardive dyskinesia (TD)	Involuntary, repetitive, purposeless movements of the tongue, lips, face, trunk, and extremities that may be generalized or affect only certain muscle groups, typically orofacial muscle groups ('Rabbit syndrome'). TD occurs after several months or years of antipsychotic treatment and is often irreversible. Risk factors are length and dose of antipsychotic treatment, advanced age, female sex, prominent negative symptoms, head injury/brain damage, and organic brain disease. TD may be *exacerbated* by anticholinergics, and there is no consistently effective treatment. Although TD is typically thought of as an antipsychotic-related EPSE, it may also occur in untreated schizophrenia and in the normal elderly population.

Table 4.6: Adverse effect profiles of four common antipsychotics

Antipsychotic	EPSEs	Hyperprolactinaemia	Sedation	Weight gain	Orthostatic hypotension	Anticholinergic side-effects
Risperidone	+	++	+	+	++	0/+
Olanzapine	0/+	+	++	+++	+	+/++
Quetiapine	0/+	0/+	++	++	++	0/+
Clozapine*	0	0	+++	+++	+++	+++

* Clozapine in particular is also associated with sialorrhoea (hypersalivation), tachycardia, myocarditis, cardiomyopathy, insulin resistance, increased risk of convulsions at higher doses, and agranulocytosis.

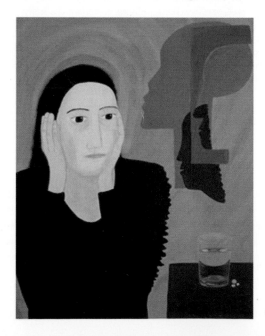

Figure 4.4. 'Medication' by Philippa King. The artist explains: The side-effects I was experiencing on antipsychotic medication were tremors in my arms and hands (illustrated by the wavy line of the sleeve), a dry mouth (another reason for including a glass of water), and weight gain.

Neuroleptic malignant syndrome (NMS) (!)

NMS is a rare but under-diagnosed and potentially fatal idiosyncratic reaction to antipsychotics and some other drugs, including antiparkinsonian drugs, antidepressants, and recreational drugs such as cocaine and ecstasy. It results, among others, from blockade of dopaminergic hypothalamospinal tracts that tonically inhibit preganglionic sympathetic neurones. It is characterized by a tetrad of hyperthermia, muscle rigidity, autonomic instability, and altered mental status. Rhabdomyolysis, as reflected by a high creatinine phosphokinase (CPK) blood level, may lead to renal failure. Other complications include respiratory failure, cardiovascular collapse, seizures, arrhythmias, and disseminated intravascular coagulopathy (DIC).

Differential diagnosis includes infection, catatonia, parkinsonism, and malignant hyperthermia.

The mainstay of treatment involves discontinuing the drug and supportive measures such as oxygen, IV fluids, and cooling blankets. Drugs such as dantrolene and lorazepam can also be used to decrease muscle rigidity. If left untreated, mortality from NMS is as high as 10%.

How effective are antipsychotics?

Critics of antipsychotics claim that there is nothing specifically 'anti-psychotic' about them, and that they are no more than a form of chemical control, or 'chemical straightjacket'. They highlight that, before being rebranded as 'antipsychotics', the drugs used to be referred to as 'neuroleptics' (a portemanteau coined from the Greek for 'nerve seizure') or 'major tranquillizers'. Physician Henri Laborit (1914-1995) who first trialled chlorpromazine himself described its effect as one of 'artificial hibernation'.

Today, antipsychotics are used not only in the treatment of psychosis, but also, in many cases, in the treatment or management of bipolar disorder, depression, dementia, insomnia, obsessive-compulsive disorder, post-traumatic stress disorder, personality disorder, and autism, among others—suggesting that any effect that they exert is far from targeted.

Critics also argue that discontinuation-relapse studies overstate the effectiveness of antipsychotics, not least because the drugs sensitize the brain. This means that their discontinuation, especially if sudden, can leave the brain in 'over-drive' and precipitate a relapse. The critics cite, among others, a 20-year longitudinal study led by psychologist Martin Harrow, which found that longer-term antipsychotic treatment is associated with *lower* rates of recovery.

Last but not least, critics point out the obvious, which is that antipsychotics often lead to unpleasant and disabling adverse effects, and are associated with a significant decrease in life expectancy.

Pioneered in Western Lapland, Finland, the innovative Open Dialogue approach to the management of a mental health crisis, including acute schizophrenia, de-emphasizes antipsychotics and other drugs. Instead, it focuses on immediate intervention to encourage the person and his family and wider network to come together and talk to one another, in part so that the person may find the words with which to express and lend meaning to his distress. Further studies are planned, but early indications are that the Open Dialogue approach can secure much better treatment outcomes while markedly reducing the use of antipsychotics.

In 1949, neurologist Egas Moniz (1874-1955) received a Nobel Prize for his discovery of 'the therapeutic value of leucotomy in certain psychoses'. Today, prefrontal leucotomy is derided as a barbaric treatment from a much darker age, and it is to be hoped that, one day, so too might antipsychotics.

Other drugs

In some cases symptoms do not respond to antipsychotics, perhaps owing to treatment-resistance, non-compliance, ongoing stressors, substance misuse, or an overlooked organic aetiology. If these factors have been excluded or addressed, a benzodiazepine, lithium, or carbamazepine are sometimes added to the antipsychotic. These so-called adjunctive or augmentative drugs are *not* as effective as clozapine, and therefore should only be considered following an adequate trial of clozapine. Clozapine itself is sometimes augmented with sulpiride or risperidone, but never with carbamazepine which is also linked to agranulocytosis. It should be noted that the overall evidence for augmentation or combination (two drugs of the same group) treatment in schizophrenia is very poor. Non-pharmacological strategies for distressing chronic hallucinations include music on earphones, subvocal counting or singing, and earplugs.

Benzodiazepines can be used in the management of ancillary symptom complexes such as anxiety and agitation, and in the emergency treatment of acute psychosis ('rapid tranquillization'). A typical regimen for rapid tranquillization is lorazepam 1mg as required, up to 4mg per 24 hours, delivered either orally or intramuscularly.

Insomnia is common in schizophrenia, and is both an effect and a cause of symptoms. Simple sleeping tablets can help to lengthen sleep and restore a regular sleeping pattern, which can be highly therapeutic.

Antidepressants and electroconvulsive therapy can be used to treat depressive symptoms.

Clinical skills: Coffee and a cigarette

The vast majority of schizophrenia sufferers smoke, often very heavily. Perhaps nicotine functions as a neuroprotective agent, or else alleviates symptoms or improves cognitive performance. Nicotine induces the hepatic microsomal enzyme CYP1A2, which metabolizes olanzapine and clozapine and so reduces their levels. CYP1A2 also metabolizes caffeine, which is why smokers tend to drink more coffee than non-smokers. Caffeine competes with olanzapine and clozapine for CYP1A2, thereby *increasing* their levels. These and other interactions may be clinically significant.

Psychosocial interventions

The management of a patient with schizophrenia is usually planned at one or more Care Programme Approach (CPA) meetings (see Chapter 3). The care plan formulated during these meetings should include a number of psychosocial interventions such as patient and family education, self-help groups, cognitive-behavioural therapy (CBT), family therapy, social and vocational skills training, and sheltered employment. Psychosocial measures are cheap, de-stigmatizing, and empowering, with both short- and very long-term benefits and no adverse effects.

In addition to the support received from the mental health team, the patient and his or her relatives ought to be directed or referred to one or more charitable organizations for further information and support. Charitable organizations also run local self-help groups at which the patient can meet other schizophrenia sufferers and share feelings and experiences. Relatives and carers invariably need explanation and support, not least so as to involve themselves optimally in the patient's care plan. CBT may be indicated if the patient continues to suffer from residual symptoms such as drug-resistant delusions, from negative or depressive symptoms, or from poor insight into the illness. CBT for delusions typically involves exploring the subjective nature of the delusions, gently challenging them, and gradually subjecting them to testing by reality. Family therapy can address high expressed emotion and other complex emotions and stressors arising from the family dynamics.

Some patients, especially those with prominent negative symptoms, may benefit from a period of rehabilitation. Areas considered during rehabilitation include accommodation, activities of daily living, occupational activities, leisure activities, and social skills. Several members of the multidisciplinary team, such as the community psychiatric nurse, occupational therapist, and clinical psychologist, may be co-opted into the patient's rehabilitation. Sheltered employment programmes using the place-and-train vocational model significantly increase the patient's likelihood of re-entering competitive employment. Social skills training involves breaking down complex social activities such as making conversation and taking part in recreational activities into simpler steps that can then be learnt and practised through role-play. Despite best efforts at rehabilitation, some patients may require long-term supported accommodation. This is often found in a sheltered home or group home—a house shared by several schizophrenia sufferers and supported by a group homes organization.

Prognosis

Complete recovery from schizophrenia is possible, but most often the illness runs a protracted course punctuated by episodes of relapse and remission. According to the 'rule of thirds', about one third of sufferers recover and lead normal or almost normal lives, about one third improve but continue to experience significant symptoms, and about one third do not improve significantly and require frequent hospitalization. Positive and negative prognostic factors are listed in Table 4.7.

Table 4.7: Prognostic factors in schizophrenia

Good prognosis	Bad prognosis
Acute onset	Insidious onset
Late onset	Early onset
Precipitating factors	No precipitating factors
Florid symptoms or associated mood disorder	Negative symptoms
Female sex	Male sex
No family history	Family history
No substance misuse	Substance misuse
Good premorbid functioning	Poor premorbid functioning
Good social support and stimulation	Poor social support and stimulation
Married	Unmarried (including separated, etc.)
Early treatment and compliance	Delayed treatment and non-compliance
Good response to treatment	Poor response to treatment

Overall, the life expectancy of schizophrenia sufferers is reduced by about 8-10 years compared to average, but this gap is narrowing owing to better standards of physical care. Perhaps surprisingly, the leading cause of death in schizophrenia is cardiovascular disease. Other important causes of death include accidents, drug overdoses, and suicide. The suicide rate is of the order of 5%, although rates of attempted suicide and self-harm are considerably higher. Risk factors for suicide include being young, being male, being early in the course of the illness, having good insight into the illness, coming from a high status background, being intelligent or ambitious, being unmarried, lacking social support, and having recently been discharged from hospital.

Surprisingly, the outcome of schizophrenia tends to be more favourable in traditional societies. This could be because people living in these tightknit communities see mental disorder more as a part of life than a sign of illness or failure, and enable people with conditions that might otherwise be diagnosed as mental disorder to occupy an honourable place in their very midst.

Schizophrenia and the abuse of psychiatry

While a lack of validity and reliability is a problem for all mental disorders, it is a particular problem for schizophrenia, which has a history of being abused for political purposes. China, for one, has established a system of maximum-security psychiatric hospitals (*Ankang*), in part for confining political dissidents and Falun Gong practitioners who represent a 'social danger'. According to a US Department of State report on human rights in China, still in 2014 'there were widespread reports of activists and petitioners being committed to mental health facilities and involuntarily subjected to psychiatric treatment for political reasons.'

The risks of abuse and mistakes are much higher under authoritarian regimes, not least because institutional safeguards such as a strong professional culture among psychiatrists, an independent judiciary, and an open appeals procedure are lacking. But as the Rosenhan experiment (Chapter 2) makes clear, mistakes can take place, and abuse can be perpetrated, even under the most liberal of regimes, because, ultimately, a diagnosis of schizophrenia rests on nothing more concrete than subjective opinion.

Other psychotic disorders

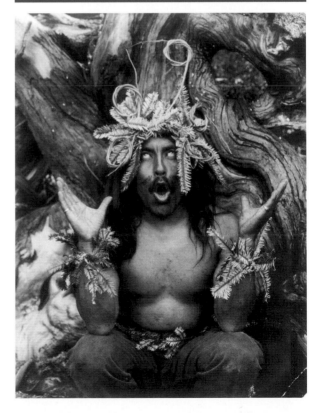

Figure 4.5. Hamatsa shaman possessed by a supernatural power.

Psychosis is a condition or state associated not only with schizophrenia, but also with mood disorders (Chapter 5); other mental disorders such as 'brief psychotic disorder'; medical and neurological disorders such as temporal lobe epilepsy, brain tumour, stroke, and dementia; and drugs such as amphetamines, cocaine, cannabis, LSD, and the entheogens peyote and sage of the diviners. Entheogens ('generating the divine from within') are chemical substances used in a religious, shamanic, or spiritual context. This section covers the other mental disorders with which psychosis is associated, as follows.

Acute or brief psychotic disorder

Brief psychotic disorder looks similar to acute-phase schizophrenia, but is characterized by a rapid, often stress-induced, onset, vivid delusions or hallucinations, a short course of less than one month (by definition), and a complete recovery. In France, psychiatrists refer to this state as *bouffée délirante aiguë*, and are apt to describe it as *un coup de tonnerre dans un ciel serein*—'a thunderclap in a clear sky'.

Schizophreniform disorder (DSM-5)

Schizophreniform disorder is characterized by symptoms identical to those of schizophrenia, that last in total for more than one month but less than six months. It is often a provisional diagnosis, since if the disturbance persists beyond six months, the diagnosis is changed to schizophrenia. Unlike with schizophrenia, impaired functioning, though often present, is not necessary for the diagnosis to be made.

Schizoaffective disorder

Schizoaffective disorder is characterized by prominent affective and schizophrenic symptoms in the same episode of illness. Mood symptoms tend to be episodic rather than continuous. The condition is easily confounded with manic psychosis, depressive psychosis, and post-schizophrenic depression. DSM-5 requires at least two episodes of illness for the diagnosis to be made. Prognosis is generally better than for schizophrenia.

Persistent delusional disorder

Persistent delusional disorder, or delusional disorder, features a single delusion or set of related delusions, often persecutory, hypochondriacal, or grandiose in content. The delusions are of a fixed, elaborate, and systematized kind, and can often be related to the patient's life circumstances. Other psychopathology is characteristically absent, although intermittent depressive symptoms may be present in some cases. There may be occasional or transitory auditory hallucinations, but these form only a small part of the overall clinical picture. Eponymous forms include de Clérambault syndrome (erotomania) and Othello syndrome (Chapter 2). Persistent delusional disorder is generally hard to treat, and poorly responsive to antipsychotics.

Schizotypal disorder

Schizotypal disorder, also called latent schizophrenia, is a personality disorder characterized by eccentric behaviour and anomalies of thinking and affect similar to those seen in schizophrenia. First-degree relatives of schizophrenia sufferers are at increased risk of schizotypal disorder. In DSM-5, schizotypal disorder is also classified under personality disorders (Chapter 8).

Late paraphrenia

'Late paraphrenia', or 'paraphrenia', is a term sometimes used to refer to late-onset schizophrenia, which is either an expression of schizophrenia in the elderly or an entity distinct from schizophrenia. The diagnosis is not coded in ICD-10 or DSM-5. Typically, the condition is characterized by prominent hallucinations and delusions (usually although not invariably paranoid delusions) in the absence of disorganized, negative, or catatonic symptoms. Risk factors include brain disease, family history, female sex, social isolation, and visual or hearing impairment. Prognosis is variable.

Induced delusional disorder

Induced delusional disorder (*folie à deux*, *folie à trois*, or even *folie à plusieurs* and *folie à famille*) is a delusional disorder shared by two or more people in a close and dependent relationship. The delusions are usually chronic and either persecutory or grandiose in content. There are several subtypes of *folie à deux*.

- In *folie imposée*, only A suffers from a primary psychotic disorder such that B's delusions disappear if he is separated from A.

- *Folie communiquée* is similar to *folie imposée*, except that B maintains his delusions even after separation from A.
- In *folie simultanée*, both A and B suffer from a primary psychotic disorder but happen to share the same delusions.
- In *folie induite*, both A and B suffer from a primary psychotic disorder and transfer delusions to each other.

So according to the evidence provided by our ancestors, madness is a nobler thing than sober sense… madness comes from God, whereas sober sense is merely human.

—Plato, *Phaedrus*

Psychosis can be a non-specific marker of a serious underlying disorder. But it can also represent one end of a continuum of normal human experiences. Hallucinations in particular are very common, and are experienced at some time by over one third of the general population. In many cases, psychotic phenomena are nothing more than an expression of severe stress or profound emotion, often underlain by a complex, difficult, or deep-seated life problem. In some cases, they may even be a normal or life-enhancing experience, as in, for instance, hearing the comforting voices of ancestors or guardian angels, or seeing visions that are a source of inspiration and revelation.

There can be no doubt that some people have had unusual experiences of different realities at some point in their lives, and been enriched rather than damaged or impaired by them. In a 2006 interview for the *Observer*, philosopher Robert Pirsig (born 1928), author of *Zen and the Art of Motorcycle Maintenance*, revealed that he refers to his own breakdown both as 'catatonic schizophrenia' and 'hard enlightenment': 'I have never insisted on either, in fact I switch back and forth depending on who I am talking to.'

The idea that psychosis or 'madness' and inspiration and revelation are closely related is an old and recurring one. In *De Tranquillitate Animi*, Seneca the Younger (d. 65 AD) writes that 'there is no great genius without a tincture of madness', a sentence which he attributes to Aristotle, and which is also echoed in Cicero. For Shakespeare (1564-1616), 'the lunatic, the lover, and the poet are of imagination all compact;' and for Dryden (1631-1700), 'great wits are sure to madness near allied, and thin partitions do their bounds divide.'

Self-assessment

Answer by true or false:

1. Kraepelin's description of schizophrenia put more emphasis on thought disorder and negative symptoms than on positive symptoms.
2. Schizophrenia tends to present at an earlier age in women, and also tends to affect women more severely.
3. The season of births effect is not mirrored in the southern hemisphere.
4. The lifetime risk of developing schizophrenia if one parent has been affected by the illness is about 12%.
5. According to the revised dopamine hypothesis, the negative symptoms of schizophrenia result from dopamine overactivity in the mesocortical system.
6. The subtle and non-specific problems in language, cognition, and behaviour that constitute the prodromal phase of schizophrenia do not lead to a loss of function.
7. Over-zealous religious beliefs can be classified as delusions.
8. Pseudo-hallucinations tend to point towards a diagnosis of personality disorder rather than schizophrenia.
9. Pseudo-hallucinations typically differ from true hallucinations in that they are perceived to arise in the mind rather than in the sense organs, and are less vivid and distressing.
10. Second person auditory hallucinations are one of Schneider's first rank symptoms.
11. The ICD-10 criteria for schizophrenia are based on Schneider's first rank symptoms.
12. According to ICD-10, a diagnosis of schizophrenia requires symptoms to have been present for most of the time for a period of one month or more.
13. According to DSM-5, a diagnosis of schizophrenia can only be made if the symptoms undermine the person's ability to function in his social or occupational setting.
14. The anti-adrenergic adverse effects of antipsychotics include postural hypotension and tachycardia, but not ejaculatory failure.
15. Oculogyric crisis and akathisia are side-effects of both typical and atypical antipsychotics.
16. Olanzapine typically causes more hyperprolactinaemia than either risperidone or quetiapine.

17. Risperidone typically causes more weight gain that either olanzapine or quetiapine.

18. Patients on clozapine must have their blood counts monitored because they are at risk of thrombocytosis.

19. Symptoms of neuroleptic malignant syndrome include hyperthermia, muscle rigidity, autonomic instability, and altered mental status.

20. Symptoms of neuroleptic malignant syndrome are often confused with symptoms of mental disorder.

21. Anticholinergics can be used in the treatment of tardive dyskinesia.

22. In schizophrenia, acute onset is a negative prognostic factor.

23. In schizophrenia, florid psychosis and associated mood disorder are positive prognostic factors.

24. Suicide is the most common cause of death in schizophrenia.

25. Psychotic experiences are common in the general population, and, for the most part, do not constitute mental disorder or call for medical attention.

26. Brief psychotic disorder has a short course of less than one week.

27. Brief psychotic disorder is often precipitated by acute stress.

28. Schizophreniform disorder is a condition characterized by the development of a single delusion or set of related delusions. The delusions are of a fixed, elaborate, and systematized kind, and can often be related to the patient's life circumstances.

29. Late paraphrenia is not coded in ICD-10 and DSM-5.

30. *Folie à famille* describes a delusional disorder shared by several members of one same family.

Answers

1. False, Bleuler's.
2. False, men.
3. False. It is, albeit to a lesser extent.
4. True.
5. False, hypodopaminergia.
6. False, loss of function helps to rule out schizotypal disorder.
7. False. The definition of a delusion specifies that it cannot be explained by culture or religion.
8. True.
9. True.
10. False, third person.
11. True.
12. True.
13. True. This is a point of difference with ICD-10.
14. False, all three.
15. True, extrapyramidal side-effects.
16. False.
17. False.
18. False, agranulocytosis.
19. True, the tetrad.
20. True.
21. False, TD can be exacerbated by anticholinergics.
22. False.
23. True.
24. False, cardiovascular disease.
25. True.
26. False, less than one month.
27. True.
28. False, this describes persistent delusional disorder.
29. True.
30. True.

5

Mood disturbances

Case study: Mr GG

I have been high several times over the years, but low only once.

When I was high, I became very enthusiastic about some project or other and would work on it with determination and success. During such highs I wrote the bulk of two books and stood for parliament as an independent. I went to bed very late, if at all, and woke up very early. I didn't feel tired at all. There were times when I lost touch with reality and got carried away. At such times, I would jump from project to project without completing any, and did many things that I later regretted. Once I thought that I was Jesus and that I had a mission to save the world. It was an extremely alarming thought.

When I was low, I was an entirely different person. I felt as though life was pointless, with nothing to live for. Although I would not have tried to end my life, I would not have regretted death. I did not have the wish or energy to take on even the simplest task. Instead I spent my days sleeping or lying awake in bed, worrying about the financial problems that I created for myself during my highs. I also had a feeling of unreality, that people were conspiring to make life seem normal when in actual fact there was nothing there. I kept on asking the doctors and nurses to show me their ID because I just couldn't bring myself to believe that they were real.

—Mr GG

Classification

Primary versus secondary mood disorder

A primary mood disorder is one that does not result from another medical or psychiatric condition. A secondary mood disorder is one that results from another medical or psychiatric condition, such as anaemia, hypothyroidism, or substance misuse.

Secondary mood disorder

Having diagnosed a mood disorder, it is important to consider whether it could be secondary, not least because secondary mood disorder is best treated by treating the primary condition that lies behind it.

Unipolar depression versus bipolar disorder

Broadly speaking, a primary mood disorder is either unipolar (depressive disorder, dysthymia), or bipolar (bipolar disorder, cyclothymia). To meet the criteria for a bipolar mood disorder, the patient must have had one or more episodes of mania or hypomania. The unipolar-bipolar distinction is an important one to make, as the course and treatment of bipolar disorder differs significantly from that of unipolar depression.

Unipolar mood disorders

In ICD-10, depressive disorders are classified according to their severity into mild, moderate, severe, and psychotic depressive disorder. If a patient has had more than one episode of depressive disorder, the term 'recurrent depressive disorder' is used, and the current episode classified as for a single episode, for example, 'recurrent depressive disorder, current episode moderate'. In DSM-

5, the term 'major depressive disorder' is used instead of depressive disorder.

Not all people suffering from depressive symptoms have a depressive disorder. Dysthymia can be described as mild chronic depression, and as such is characterized by depressive symptoms that are not sufficiently severe to meet the criteria for depressive disorder.

Bipolar mood disorders

Bipolar disorder, or manic-depressive illness, involves recurrent episodes of mania or hypomania and depression. In mania and hypomania, mood is markedly elated, expansive, or irritable.

Hypomania can be thought of as a lesser degree of mania, with symptoms similar to those of mania but less severe or extreme. Mood is elated, expansive, or irritable, but, in contrast to mania, there are no psychotic symptoms and no marked impairment of social functioning. Hypomania may or may not herald mania.

In bipolar disorder, the frequency and severity of manic/hypomanic episodes and depressive episodes is very variable, as is the proportion of manic/hypomanic episodes to depressive episodes. Occasionally, episodes can be 'mixed', that is, feature symptoms of both mania and depression.

To meet the ICD-10 criteria for bipolar disorder, a patient must have suffered at least two episodes of mood disturbance, at least one of which must have been mania or hypomania. To meet the DSM-5 criteria for bipolar disorder ('bipolar I disorder'), the patient must have suffered at least one episode of mania. A patient who has only ever suffered depressive episodes cannot be diagnosed with bipolar disorder until and unless he has also suffered a manic or hypomanic episode. In that much, mania/hypomania is the hallmark of bipolar disorder.

In the absence of episodes of depression, the diagnosis is either one of bipolar disorder or hypomania, i.e. recurrent episodes of mania are diagnosed as bipolar disorder. This is because sooner or later a depressive episode is almost certain to supervene, and because recurrent episodes of mania and bipolar disorder share a similar course and prognosis.

Since the publication of DSM-IV in 1994, DSM further distinguishes people who have suffered at least one full-blown manic episode (bipolar I disorder) from those who have only ever had one or several hypomanic episodes (bipolar II disorder). Unlike bipolar I disorder, which can

be diagnosed on the basis of a single manic episode, bipolar II disorder cannot be diagnosed unless the person has also suffered at least one depressive episode.

Finally, cyclothymia can be described as mild chronic bipolar disorder. It is characterized by recurrent episodes of mild elation and mild depressive symptoms that are not sufficiently severe or prolonged to meet the criteria for bipolar disorder or recurrent depressive disorder (cf. dysthymia).

ICD-10 classification of mood disorders		
F30	Manic episode	
	F30.0	Hypomania
	F30.1	Mania without psychotic symptoms
	F30.2	Mania with psychotic symptoms
	F30.8	Other manic episodes
	F30.9	Manic episode, unspecified
F31	Bipolar Affective Disorder (BAD)	
	F31.0	BAD, current episode hypomanic
	F31.1	BAD, current episode manic without psychotic symptoms
	F31.2	BAD, current episode manic with psychotic symptoms
	F31.3	BAD, current episode mild or moderate depression
	F31.4	BAD, current episode severe depression without psychotic symptoms
	F31.5	BAD, current episode severe depression with psychotic symptoms
	F31.6	BAD, current episode mixed
	F31.7	BAD, current episode in remission
	F31.8	Other bipolar affective disorders
	F31.9	Bipolar affective disorder, unspecified
F32	Depressive episode	
	F32.0	Mild depressive episode
	F32.1	Moderate depressive episode
	F32.2	Severe depressive episode without psychotic symptoms
	F32.3	Severe depressive episode with psychotic symptoms
	F32.8	Other depressive episodes
	F32.9	Depressive episode, unspecified
F33	Recurrent depressive disorder	
	F33.0	Recurrent depressive disorder, current episode mild
	F33.1	Recurrent depressive disorder, current episode moderate
	F33.2	Recurrent depressive disorder, current episode severe without psychotic symptoms

F33.3 Recurrent depressive disorder, current episode severe with psychotic symptoms

F33.4 Recurrent depressive disorder, currently in remission

F33.8 Other recurrent depressive disorders

F33.9 Recurrent depressive disorder, unspecified

F34 Persistent mood disorders

F34.0 Cyclothymia

F34.1 Dysthymia

F34.8 Other persistent mood disorder

F34.9 Persistent mood disorder, unspecified

F38 Other mood disorders

F38.0 Other single mood disorders

F38.1 Other recurrent mood disorders

F38.8 Other specified mood disorders

F39 Unspecified mood disorders

DSM-5 classification of mood disorders

Mood episodes
- Major depressive episode
- Manic episode
- Hypomanic episode

Depressive disorders
- Major depressive disorder
- Persistent depressive disorder
- Disruptive mood dysregulation disorder (children's temper tantrums)
- Premenstrual dysphoric disorder
- Depressive disorder due to another medical condition
- Substance/medication-induced mood disorder
- Other specified, or unspecified, depressive disorder

Bipolar and related disorders
- Bipolar I disorder
- Bipolar II disorder
- Cyclothymic disorder
- Substance/medication-induced bipolar disorder
- Bipolar disorder due to another medical condition
- Other specified, or unspecified, bipolar disorder

Depressive disorders: Clinical features

…I have of late—but
Wherefore I know not—lost all my mirth, forgone all
Custom of exercises; and indeed it goes so heavily
With my disposition that this goodly frame, the
Earth, seems to me a sterile promontory, this most
Excellent canopy, the air, look you, this brave
O'erhanging firmament, this majestical roof fretted
With golden fire, why, it appears no other thing to
Me than a foul and pestilent congregation of vapours.
What a piece of work is man! how noble in reason!
How infinite in faculty! in form and moving how
Express and admirable! In action how like an angel!
In apprehension how like a god! the beauty of the
World! the paragon of animals! And yet, to me,
What is this quintessence of dust? man delights not
Me: no, nor woman neither, though by your smiling
You seem to say so.

—Shakespeare, *Hamlet*

People colloquially use the term 'depression' to refer to normal disappointment or sadness, although in severe cases depression can lead to psychotic symptoms and even death through self-neglect or suicide.

The symptoms of depression can be divided into three groups: core symptoms, psychological symptoms, and physical symptoms (Table 5.1).

Table 5.1: Symptoms of depression

Core symptoms	Low mood
	Loss of interest and enjoyment
Psychological symptoms	Poor concentration
	Poor self-esteem
	Inappropriate guilt
	Pessimism
	Recurring thoughts of death or suicide
Physical or somatic symptoms	Sleep disturbance, often with early morning waking
	Fatigability
	Loss of appetite and weight loss
	Loss of libido
	Anhedonia*
	Agitation or retardation

* The inability to derive pleasure from previously pleasurable activities.

In contrast to mere disappointment or sadness, the symptoms of depression vary little from day to day and barely respond to changing circumstances. For instance, a depressed person who is normally passionate about his work will not brighten up even upon learning that his efforts and achievements have been recognized with a major award.

Although the most common symptom of depression is low mood, many patients never complain of this and present instead with cognitive, behavioural, or somatic symptoms such as feeling tired all the time or being unable to concentrate at work.

Mild depression is the commonest form of depression and tends to present, if at all, to GPs. The patient often complains of feeling low or tired, and sometimes also stressed or anxious (so-called 'mixed anxiety-depression'). Somatic features are absent, and, although suicidal thoughts can occur, self-harm is uncommon.

Moderate depression is often treated in primary care but can be severe enough to warrant a specialist referral. Many if not most of the clinical features of depression are present to such an intense degree that the patient finds it difficult to discharge his social obligations. Somatic features are present and anhedonia is characteristic. Suicidal ideation is common and may be acted upon.

Severe depression is an exaggerated form of moderate depression defined by intense negative feelings and psychomotor agitation or retardation. Depressive stupor may supervene upon psychomotor retardation, and in such cases urgent electroconvulsive therapy (ECT) may be instigated (see later). Psychotic symptoms are present in a significant minority of cases, and are usually mood-congruent. Common delusional themes are guilt, poverty, and nihilism. Suicide risk is high, and in the retarded patient may actually increase once treatment is started and the patient develops the motivation and energy to act on his or her suicidal thoughts.

Depressive realism

When the shadow of the sash appeared on the curtains it was between seven and eight o'clock and then I was in time again, hearing the watch. It was Grandfather's and when Father gave it to me he said I give you the mausoleum of all hope and desire; it's rather excruciatingly apt that you will use it to gain the reducto absurdum of all human experience which can fit your individual needs no better than it fitted his or his father's. I give it to you not that you may remember time, but that you might forget it now and then for a moment and not spend all your breath trying to conquer it. Because no battle is ever won he said. They are not even fought. The field only reveals to man his own folly and despair, and victory is an illusion of philosophers and fools.

—William Faulkner (1897-1962), *The Sound and the Fury*

Clinical skills: Physical signs of depression

There are few physical signs in psychiatry, but the omega sign and Veraguth's fold are two of them. The omega sign is a fold that looks like the Greek letter Ω in the forehead just above the root of the nose. It is sometimes produced in depression through the action of the corrugator supercilii, the muscle of frowning, activated by grief and suffering, and also bright sunlight. Veraguth's fold is an oblique skin fold in the upper eyelid running medially and superiorly.

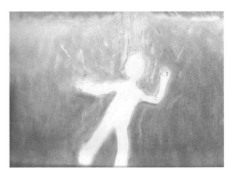

Figure 5.1. Drawing by an in-patient with severe depression. She is drowning: and each time she struggles up near the surface, she is pushed back down.

Case study: William Styron

In depression this faith in deliverance, in ultimate restoration, is absent. The pain is unrelenting, and what makes the condition intolerable is the foreknowledge that no remedy will come—not in a day, an hour, a month, or a minute. If there is mild relief, one knows that it is only temporary; more pain will follow. It is hopelessness even more than pain that crushes the soul. So the decision-making of daily life involves not, as in normal affairs, shifting from one annoying situation to another less annoying—or from discomfort to relative comfort, or from boredom to activity—but moving from pain to pain. One does not abandon, even briefly, one's bed of nails, but is attached to it wherever one goes.

—William Styron (1925-2006), *Darkness Visible: A Memoir of Madness*

Depressive disorders: Diagnosis

ICD-10 Depressive episode

In typical depressive episodes of all three varieties described in ICD-10 (mild, moderate, and severe), the individual usually suffers from depressed mood, loss of interest and enjoyment, and reduced energy leading to increased fatigability and diminished activity. Marked tiredness after only slight effort is common. Other common symptoms are:

(a) reduced concentration and attention;
(b) reduced self-esteem and self-confidence;
(c) ideas of guilt;
(d) pessimism;
(e) ideas of self-harm or suicide;
(f) disturbed sleep;
(g) poor appetite.

Mood varies little from day to day and is often unresponsive to circumstances. In some cases, anxiety, distress, and motor agitation may be more prominent than depressed mood. For depressive episodes of all three grades of severity a duration of at least two weeks is usually required for diagnosis, but shorter periods may be reasonable if symptoms are unusually severe and of rapid onset. The categories of mild, moderate, and severe depressive episode should only be used for a single (first) depressive episode; further episodes should be classified under one of the subdivisions of recurrent depressive disorder.

Mild depressive episode

At least two of depressed mood, loss of interest and enjoyment, and increased fatigability should be present, plus at least two of the other symptoms described above, for a minimum period of two weeks. None of the symptoms should be present to an intense degree.

Moderate depressive episode

At least two of the three most typical symptoms noted for mild depressive episode should be present, plus at least three (and preferably four) of the other symptoms for a minimum of two weeks. Several symptoms are likely to be present to an intense degree. An individual with a moderately severe depressive episode will usually have considerable difficulty in continuing with social, work, or domestic activities.

Severe depressive episode

There is considerable distress or agitation, unless retardation is a marked feature. Loss of self-esteem and feelings of uselessness or guilt are likely to be prominent, and suicide is a distinct danger in particularly severe cases. Psychotic symptoms may be present and are usually mood-congruent.

DSM-5 Major depressive episode

According to DSM-5, for a diagnosis of major depressive episode to be made, five or more symptoms from a list similar to the one in Table 5.1 must have been present for a period of two weeks or more. At least one of the symptoms must be either depressed mood or loss of interest or pleasure, and the symptoms must be associated with significant distress or impairment. The diagnostician must also exclude physical states that can masquerade as depression, such as hypothyroidism, anaemia, and drug adverse effects.

A diagnosis of major depressive disorder, either single episode or recurrent, can only be made in the absence of manic or hypomanic episodes.

Depressive disorders: Differential diagnosis

- Normal reaction to life event or circumstances, or to fresh insight. Not all sustained sadness equates to depression!

> *And I gave my heart to know wisdom, and to know madness and folly: I perceived that this also is vexation of spirit. For in much wisdom is much grief: and he that increaseth knowledge increaseth sorrow.*
>
> —Bible, Ecclesiastes 1:17-18 (KJV)

Psychiatric differential

- Depression.
- Dysthymia.
- Cyclothymia.
- Bipolar disorder.
- Mixed affective states.
- Schizoaffective disorder.
- Schizophrenia and other psychotic disorders, including:

- depression superimposed upon schizophrenia
- negative symptoms of schizophrenia
- adverse effects of antipsychotics
• Adjustment disorder.
• Seasonal affective disorder (SAD).

• Post-traumatic stress disorder (PTSD).
• Generalized anxiety disorder.
• Obsessive-compulsive disorder.
• Eating disorder.

Organic differential

Important organic causes of depression are listed in Table 5.2.

Table 5.2: Important organic causes of depression

Neurological	Stroke, Alzheimer's disease and other dementias, Parkinson's disease, Huntington's disease, multiple sclerosis, epilepsy, intracranial tumours
Endocrine	Cushing's syndrome, Addison's disease, hypothyroidism, hyperparathyroidism
Metabolic	Iron deficiency, B12 or folate deficiency, hypercalcaemia, hypomagnesaemia
Infective	Influenza, infectious mononucleosis, hepatitis, HIV/AIDS
Neoplastic	Non-metastatic effects of carcinoma
Drugs	L-dopa, steroids, beta blockers, digoxin, cocaine, amphetamines, opioids, alcohol

Clinical skills: Assess a patient with low mood

• Introduce yourself to the patient.
• Explain that you are going to ask some questions to uncover exactly how he is feeling, and obtain consent.
• Ensure that he is comfortable.
• First ask open questions about his current mood and feelings, listening attentively and gently encouraging him to open up.
• Aim to cover:
  The core symptoms of depression
  - low mood
  - loss of interest and enjoyment
  The psychological symptoms of depression
  - poor concentration
  - poor self-esteem
  - inappropriate guilt
  - pessimism
  - recurrent thoughts of death or suicide
  The physical or somatic symptoms of depression
  - sleep disturbance and early morning waking

  - fatigability
  - loss of appetite and weight loss
  - loss of libido
  - anhedonia
  - agitation or retardation
• Screen for anxiety, hallucinations, delusions, and mania, to exclude other possible psychiatric diagnoses.
• Ask about the onset of the illness, and possible triggers.
• Assess the severity and impact of the illness.
• Ask about suicidal intent. If there is so much as a hint of suicidality, carry out a full risk assessment (Chapter 6).
• Gather brief psychiatric, medical, drug, and family histories. Remember that drugs and alcohol are commonly associated with depression.
• Ask the patient if there is anything else that he might add that you have forgotten to ask about.
• Thank him and, if appropriate, offer a further course of action (see later).

Depressive disorders: Epidemiology

Figures for the lifetime incidence of depressive disorders depend on the criteria used to define 'depressive disorders'. Using the criteria for major depressive disorder (DSM-5), the lifetime incidence of depressive disorders is about 15%, and the point prevalence about 5%. So common is depression that the costs of treating it exceed the combined costs of treating hypertension and diabetes.

Although depressive disorders can occur at any age, their peak prevalence in males is in old age, and in females in middle age. They are relatively uncommon in children, or present differently (Chapter 13).

Women are twice as likely to be diagnosed with depression than men. The reasons for this asymmetry are unclear, and are thought to be in parts biological, psychological, and sociocultural.

- Possible biological explanations: Compared to men, women are subjected to fluctuating hormone levels, particularly around the times of childbirth and the menopause. Beyond this, they might also have a stronger genetic predisposition to developing depression.

- Possible psychological explanations: Women are more ruminative than men, that is, they tend to think through things more. Men, in contrast, are likelier to respond to life problems with stoicism, anger, or substance misuse. Women also tend to be more invested in relationships, and so more affected and afflicted by relationship problems.

- Possible sociocultural explanations: Women come under greater stress than men. In addition to going to work just like men, they are often expected to bear most of the burden of maintaining the family home, raising the children, and caring for older relatives—and, after all that, they still have to put up with the sexism! Women also live longer than men, and extreme old age is often associated with bereavement, loneliness, poor health, and precarity. Finally, women are more likely to seek out a diagnosis of depression than men. They are more likely to consult a doctor and more likely to discuss their feelings with the doctor. Conversely, doctors, whether themselves men or women, may be more inclined to diagnose them with depression.

There are also important geographical variations in the prevalence of depression, and these can in large part be accounted for by sociocultural rather than biological factors. In traditional societies, emotional distress is more likely to be interpreted as an indicator of the need to address important life problems rather than as a mental disorder requiring professional treatment, and so a diagnosis of depression is correspondingly less common. Some linguistic communities do not even have a word for 'depression', and many people from traditional societies with what may be construed as depression present instead with physical complaints such as fatigue, headache, or chest pain. Being much more exposed to the concept of depression, people in modern societies such as ours are more likely to interpret their distress in terms of depression and to seek out a diagnosis of the illness. At the same time, groups with vested interests actively promote the notion of saccharine happiness as a natural, default state, and of human distress as a mental disorder. The concept of depression as a mental disorder may be useful for the more severe and intractable cases treated by hospital psychiatrists, but perhaps not for the majority of cases, which, for the most part, are mild and short-lived and easily interpreted in terms of life circumstances, human nature, or the human condition.

Another non-mutually exclusive explanation for the important geographical variations in the prevalence of depression may lie in the nature of modern societies, which have become increasingly individualistic and divorced from traditional values. For many people living in our society, life can seem both suffocating and far removed, lonely even and especially among the multitudes, and not only meaningless but absurd. By encoding their distress in terms of a mental disorder, our society is subtly implying that the problem lies not with itself but with them, fragile and failing individuals that they are. Of course, many people prefer to buy into this reductive explanation than to confront their existential angst. But thinking of their unhappiness in terms of an illness or chemical imbalance can prevent them from identifying and addressing the important psychological or life problems that are at the root of their distress.

Depression and creativity

Many of the most creative and insightful people in our society suffered from depression or a state that could have met the DSM-5 criteria for major depressive disorder. They include the politicians Winston Churchill and Abraham Lincoln; the poets Charles Baudelaire, Elizabeth Bishop, Hart Crane, Emily Dickinson, Sylvia Plath, and Rainer Maria Rilke; the thinkers Michel Foucault, William James, John Stuart Mill, Isaac Newton, Friedrich Nietzsche, and Arthur Schopenhauer; and the writers Agatha Christie, Charles Dickens, William Faulkner, Graham Greene, Leo Tolstoy, Evelyn Waugh, and Tennessee Williams—to name but a few. To quote Marcel Proust, who himself suffered from depression, 'Happiness is good for the body, but it is grief which develops the strengths of the mind.'

Depressive disorders: Aetiology

Genetics

First-degree relatives of depression sufferers are at an increased risk of depression (prevalence ~15%, versus ~5% in the general population), but not of bipolar disorder or schizoaffective disorder. The concordance rate for major depressive disorder in monozygotic twins is 46%, compared to 20% in dizygotic twins. Although genes clearly do play a part in the aetiology of depression, with heritability highest in cases of early-onset, recurrent, severe, or chronic depression, the above figures cannot be attributed solely to genetic factors since depression sufferers and their relatives are likely to share much more in common than just their genes.

Environmental factors

A depressive episode can be triggered by one or several adverse life events. Early adverse life events such as the loss of a parent, neglect, or abuse predispose to depression in later life.

In 1978, Brown and Harris studied working class women in inner London boroughs, and found that certain circumstances acted as 'vulnerability factors' for depression. These included:

- Loss of mother by death or separation before age 11.
- Excess of life events or major difficulties prior to onset of depression.
- Lack of a supportive relationship.
- Three or more children under age 14 at home.
- Not working outside the home.

Seasonal affective disorder (SAD)

SAD is a depressive disorder that recurs at the same time each year, and that is often marked by increased sleep and carbohydrate craving. SAD is thought to result from a shortening of daylight hours, and may respond to bright artificial lights at 2500 lux in the morning and evening. There is usually complete summer remission, and, occasionally, summer hypomania or mania, which, along with Shakespeare, may be at the origin of the expression, 'This is very midsummer madness.'

Psychological theories

According to behavioural theory, depression can result from the removal of positive reinforcement from the environment, or from certain stimuli that have become associated with negative emotional states. Depressive behaviour can be learnt through observation and imitation, and inadvertently reinforced by other people's reactions.

According to cognitive theory, depression can result from cognitive distortions (Table 5.3) rooted in negative schemas acquired in childhood and adolescence, for instance, through the loss of a parent, criticism from parents and teachers, or rejection and bullying by peers. In later life, these negative schemas can be reactivated by any event or circumstance that resembles or recalls the initial trauma. People with depression tend to attribute failure to internal, stable, and global causes, as opposed to external, unstable, and specific causes. However, such negative appraisals may be the result rather than the cause of depression.

Table 5.3: Beck's cognitive distortions

Arbitrary inference	Drawing a conclusion in the absence of evidence. *The whole world hates me.*
Overgeneralization	Drawing a conclusion on the basis of a single incident. *My nephew did not come to visit me—the whole world hates me.*
Selective abstraction	Focusing on a single event to the detriment of others. *She gave me an annoyed look three days ago. (But never mind that she spent an hour talking to me this morning.)*
Personalization	Relating independent events to oneself. *The nurse went on holiday because she was fed up with me.*
Dichotomous thinking	'All-or-nothing' thinking. *If he doesn't come to see me today, he doesn't love me.*
Magnification and minimization	Over- or under-estimating the importance of an event. *Now that my cat is dead, I'll never have anything to look forward to.*
Catastrophic thinking	Exaggerating the consequences of an event or situation. *The pain in my knee is getting worse. When I'm reduced to a wheelchair, I won't be able to go to work and pay the mortgage. So I'll end up losing my house and dying in the street.*

Neurochemical abnormalities

According to the monoamine hypothesis of depression, depression results from a depletion of monoamine neurotransmitters, particularly serotonin and noradrena-line. In its revised forms, the monoamine hypothesis states that the problem may lie not with an actual depletion in monoamines, but with some other abnormality such as fewer or less sensitive monoamine receptors. Support for the monoamine hypothesis principally came from the finding that antidepressants increase levels of monoamine neurotransmitters (see later).

Other neurological differences

Computed tomographic and magnetic resonance imaging findings in major depression include enlarged lateral ventricles and loss of volume in the frontal and temporal lobes, hippocampus, and basal ganglia, but such findings are inconsistent.

Endocrine abnormalities

That depression often occurs in endocrine disorders such as Cushing's syndrome, Addison's disease, hypothyroidism, and hyperparathyroidism suggests that endocrine abnormalities play a role in the aetiology of depressive disorders. It has been found that plasma cortisol levels are increased in about 50% of depression sufferers, and that about 50% of depression sufferers fail to respond to the dexamethasone suppression test. These endocrine abnormalities may owe to disturbances of the hypothalamic-pituitary-adrenal axis, which may in turn owe to changes in immune regulation.

Organic causes

The organic causes of depression are listed in Table 5.2.

Ever more people today have the means to live, but no meaning to live for.

—Viktor Frankl (1905-1997)

In *Man's Search for Meaning*, psychiatrist and neurologist Viktor Frankl wrote about his ordeal as a concentration camp inmate during the Second World War. Interestingly, he found that those who survived longest in concentration camps were not those who were physically strong, but those who retained a sense of control over their environment. He observed:

We who lived in concentration camps can remember the men who walked through the huts comforting others, giving away their last piece of bread. They may have been few in number, but they offer sufficient proof that everything can be taken from a man but one thing: the last of human freedoms—to choose one's own attitude in any given set of circumstances—to choose one's own way.

Frankl's message is ultimately one of hope: even in the most absurd, painful, and dispiriting of circumstances, life can be given a meaning, and so too can suffering. Life in the concentration camp taught Frankl that our main drive or motivation in life is neither pleasure, as Freud had believed, nor power, as Adler had believed, but meaning.

Following his liberation, Frankl founded the school of logotherapy (from the Greek *logos*, meaning 'reason' or 'principle'), which is sometimes referred to as the 'Third Viennese School of Psychotherapy' for coming after those of Freud and Adler. The aim of logotherapy is to carry out an existential analysis of the person, and, in so doing, to help him uncover or discover meaning for his life.

According to Frankl, meaning can be found through:
• Experiencing reality by interacting authentically with the environment and with others,

• Giving something back to the world through creativity and self-expression, and
• Changing our attitude when faced with a situation or circumstance that we cannot change.

Frankl is credited with coining the term 'Sunday neurosis' to refer to the dejection that many people feel at the end of the working week when at last they have the time to realize just how empty and meaningless their life has become. This existential vacuum may open the door on all sorts of excesses and compensations such as neurotic anxiety, avoidance, binge eating, drinking, overworking, and overspending. In the short-term, these excesses and compensations carpet over the existential vacuum, but in the longer term they prevent action from being taken and meaning from being found.

For Frankl, depression results when the gap between what a person is and what he ought to be, or once wished to be, becomes so large that it can no longer be carpeted over. The person's goals seem far out of reach and he can no longer envisage a future. As in Psalm 41, *abyssus abyssum invocat*—'hell brings forth hell', or, in an alternative translation, 'the deep calls unto the deep'.

Thus, depression is our way of telling ourselves that something is seriously wrong and needs working through and changing. Unless change can be made, there will continue to be a mismatch between our lived experience and our desired experience, between the meaninglessness of everyday life and the innate drive to find meaning, to self-actualize, to be all that we can be. From an existential standpoint, the experience of depression obliges us to become aware of our mortality and freedom, and challenges us to exercise the latter within the framework of the former. By meeting this ultimate challenge, we can break out of the cast that had been imposed upon us, discover who we truly are, and, in so doing, begin to give deep meaning to our life.

Depressive disorders: Investigations

Investigations in depression, including physical examination, aim at excluding organic causes and physical complications such as dehydration or malnourishment, and, if necessary, establishing a baseline for drug treatment. Laboratory investigations to consider include full-blood count, urea and electrolytes, liver function tests, thyroid function tests, erythrocyte sedimentation rate, vitamin B12 and folate, toxicology screen, antinuclear antibody, HIV test, and dexamethasone suppression test.

Depressive disorders: Management

Psychological and social treatments

Explanation and reassurance are an important part of treatment in all depressions, and in milder depressions may be the only form of treatment that is either necessary or appropriate. It should be stressed that depression is common and treatable, and that it is not a sign of personal or moral failure.

Although drug treatments are the most readily available treatment option, psychological and social interventions can in many cases be more effective. Common psychological treatments for depression are summarized in Table 5.4. The type of psychological treatment chosen depends not only on the patient and his or her symptoms, but also, deplorably, on the available financial and human resources.

Table 5.4: Common psychological treatments for depression

Counselling	Explanation, reassurance, and support. Identification and resolution of current life difficulties.
Cognitive behavioural therapy	Identification of cognitive distortions and associated behaviours. Cognitive restructuring and behavioural modifications.
Dynamic psychotherapy	Effecting change through a higher level of self-understanding.
Family therapy	Effecting change by addressing the dysfunctional aspects of family relationships that contributed to the depressive episode.
Interpersonal psychotherapy	A systematic and standardized treatment approach to personal relationships and life problems.

Antidepressant drugs

The first antidepressant, iproniazid, appeared in the 1950s, some 20 years after electroconvulsive therapy (see later). Iproniazid was initially trialled in people with tuberculosis, who were subsequently noted to be 'inappropriately happy'. Iproniazid and later drugs in the class of the monoamine oxidase inhibitors (MAOIs) are said to exert their antidepressant effect by preventing the enzymatic breakdown of monoamine neurotransmitters. Back in the 1950s, MAOIs revolutionized the treatment of depression. However, with the exception of moclobemide, the drugs also prevent the breakdown of the amino acid tyramine in the gastrointestinal tract, which, through the accumulation of tyramine, can lead to a potentially fatal hypertensive reaction. As a result, people on MAOIs need to steer clear from a long list of tyramine-containing foods and beverages, including such staples as beer, cheese, and sausage. For this and other reasons, MAOIs are seldom used today.

Imipramine, the first tricyclic antidepressant, appeared soon after iproniazid. Tricyclics are said to exert their antidepressant effect by preventing the neuronal re-uptake of noradrenaline and serotonin, and they also antagonize a number of neurotransmitter receptors. Unlike with MAOIs, people on tricyclics can eat and drink freely. However, they often suffer from a range of troublesome and potentially dangerous adverse effects (Table 5.5). Tertiary amines such as amitriptyline, imipramine, and clomipramine are more sedating and more anticholinergic than secondary amines such as nortriptyline, dothiepin, and lofepramine. Tricyclics are still occasionally prescribed, but, owing to their adverse effects and high

Table 5.5: Principal adverse effects of TCAs

Anticholinergic	Dry mouth, blurred vision, glaucoma, constipation, urinary retention
Antihistaminergic	Sedation, weight gain
α-noradrenergic blockade	Sedation, postural hypotension
5-HT$_2$ blockade	Weight gain, sexual dysfunction
Cardiotoxicity*	Arrhythmias, myocardial depression
Neurotoxicity	Delirium, movement disorders, convulsions

*ECG changes indicative of cardiotoxicity include prolonged PR and QT intervals, and ST segment and T wave changes.

toxicity in overdose, ought to be avoided in the elderly, the physically ill, and those at risk of overdosing. Principal contraindications include cardiovascular disease, severe liver disease, glaucoma, and prostatic hypertrophy. Important drug interactions include MAOIs and dental anaesthetics containing lignocaine.

It took another thirty or so years for the next class of antidepressants to make its entry. Fluoxetine, the first selective serotonin reuptake inhibitor (SSRI), only gained regulatory approval in 1987. SSRIs are said to exert their antidepressant effect by preventing the neuronal reuptake of serotonin. Compared to tricyclics, they have milder adverse effects and are less toxic in overdose. Adverse effects include dry mouth, nausea, vomiting, diarrhoea, dizziness, sedation, sexual dysfunction, agitation, akathisia, parkinsonism (rare), and convulsions (rare). Fluoxetine, fluvoxamine, and paroxetine are particularly potent inhibitors of the cytochrome P450 isoenzymes, and can lead to important pharmacokinetic interactions. Today, SSRIs such as fluoxetine, fluvoxamine, paroxetine, sertraline, and citalopram are the drugs of choice for most cases of moderate to severe depression. Like antipsychotics, SSRIs have become something of a panacea, and are also used in the treatment of a broad range of other mental disorders, particularly anxiety disorders, obsessive-compulsive disorder, and bulimia nervosa, and even in some physical disorders such as premature ejaculation in young men and hot flushes in menopausal women. In the UK, the SSRI fluoxetine is so commonly prescribed that trace quantities have been found in the drinking water.

Clinical skills: SSRI discontinuation syndrome

The SSRI discontinuation syndrome consists of headache, dizziness, shock-like sensations, paraesthesia, gastrointestinal symptoms, lethargy, insomnia, and change in mood (depression, anxiety/agitation), and occurs most frequently after the abrupt discontinuation of paroxetine, which has a comparatively short half-life.

The SSRI discontinuation syndrome has led to the suggestion that SSRIs are 'addictive', but this is not strictly accurate in the sense that people do not experience a buzz from SSRIs, and do not crave them as they might a drug of abuse such as cocaine or heroin.

There are also some reports that SSRIs cause, or are associated with, increased suicidal thoughts and behaviours in children and young people, but the studies looking into this are equivocal and the jury is still out.

Serotonin syndrome

The serotonin syndrome is a rare but potentially fatal acute syndrome resulting from increased serotonin activity. It is most often caused by SSRIs, but can also be caused by other drugs such as tricyclic antidepressants or lithium.

Symptoms include:
- Psychological symptoms: Agitation, confusion.
- Neurological symptoms: Nystagmus, myoclonus, tremor, seizures.
- Other symptoms: Hyperpyrexia, autonomic instability.

The principal differential is from neuroleptic malignant syndrome. Management involves discontinuation of the drug and supportive measures.

People starting on an SSRI are usually told to persist in taking their tablets because improvement in mood may be delayed for 10-20 days (in which time, of course, mood may have improved of its own accord), and because potential adverse effects are likely to be only mild and short-lived.

Since 1987, further classes of antidepressants have been developed, such as noradrenaline reuptake inhibitors (NARI e.g. reboxetine), noradrenergic and specific serotonergic antidepressants (NaSSa e.g. mirtazapine), and serotonin and noradrenaline reuptake inhibitors (SNRI e.g. venlafaxine). Such antidepressants are most often used as second- or third-line treatments if SSRI treatment has failed.

How effective are antidepressants?

Medics often assure people starting on an SSRI that they have a 50-70% chance of responding to their medication. However, in 2008, a study published in the *New England Journal of Medicine* suggested that the effectiveness of SSRIs is greatly exaggerated owing to a bias in the reporting of research studies. Out of 74 studies registered with the US Food and Drug Administration (FDA), 37 out of 38 studies with positive results were published in academic journals, compared to only 14 out of 36 studies with negative results. Moreover, out of the 14 studies with negative results that were published, 11 were published in such a way as to convey a positive outcome. Thus, while 94 per cent (37+11/37+14) of published studies conveyed a positive outcome, only 51 per cent (38/38+36) of all studies, published and unpublished, actually demonstrated one.

Another piece of research published in the *Public Library of Science*, also in 2008, combined 35 studies submitted to the FDA before the licensing of four antidepressants including the SSRIs fluoxetine and paroxetine. The researchers found that, while the antidepressants performed better than a placebo, the effect size was very small for all but very severe cases of depression. What's more, the researchers attributed this increased effect size in very severe cases not to an actual increase in the effect of the antidepressants, but to a decrease in their placebo effect.

If, as these studies suggest, the effectiveness of SSRIs has been greatly exaggerated, their cost-benefit urgently needs to be re-evaluated.

Turner EH et al. (2008): Selective publication of antidepressant trials and its influence on apparent efficacy. *New England Journal of Medicine* 358(3):252-60.

Kirsch I et al. (2008): Initial severity and antidepressant benefits: a meta-analysis of data submitted to the Food and Drug Administration. *PLoS Medicine* 5(2):e45.

Other drugs

If psychotic symptoms are prominent or distressing, an antipsychotic can be used in addition to the antidepressant. Rarely, drugs such as lithium, valproate, carbamazepine, tryptophan, tri-iodothyronine, buspirone, and pindolol are used to augment antidepressant treatment.

Electroconvulsive therapy (ECT)

Owing to suicidal ideation, retardation or stupor, food and drink refusal, or psychotic symptoms such as command hallucinations or nihilistic delusions, people with severe depression are often at high risk to themselves. If their level of risk is particularly high, or if their condition has not responded to several trials of antidepressant drugs, they may be prescribed a course of ECT.

It had long been known that convulsions induced by camphor could temper psychotic symptoms. In 1933, psychiatrist Manfred Sakel (1900-1957) began using insulin injections to induce convulsions, but a period of panic and impending doom prior to convulsing made the treatment difficult to tolerate. Psychiatrist Ladislas Meduna (1896-1964) replaced the insulin with a drug called metrazol, but similar problems persisted. Then in 1938, neuropsychiatrist Ugo Cerletti (1877-1963) began the practice of applying a small electric shock to the head. This method, which people found more tolerable—or, rather, less intolerable—soon superseded the injections. In the 1950s, the advent

of short-acting anaesthetics and muscle relaxants made it possible for people to be put to sleep for the treatment, and dramatically reduced complications such as muscle tears and bone fractures.

Clinical skills: Preparing a patient for ECT

In the UK, informed consent is required for ECT except if being treated under the provision of the Mental Health Act. The 2007 amendment to the Mental Health Act introduced new safeguards for the use of ECT. In short, ECT may not be given to a person with the capacity to refuse to consent to it, and then only if this does not conflict with any advance directive, decision of a deputy or donee, or decision of the Court of Protection.

Relative medical contraindications to ECT include:
- Cardiovascular disease.
- Raised intracranial pressure.
- Dementing illnesses.
- Epilepsy and other neurological disorders.
- Cervical spine disease.

Prior to beginning a course of ECT, the patient should have a physical examination, an electrocardiograph (ECG), and blood tests including FBC and U&Es—and should be 'nil by mouth' from the previous midnight.

During ECT treatment, the person is given a standard anaesthetic such as propofol and a muscle relaxant such as suxamethonium. In the UK, the seizure is induced with a constant current, brief-pulse stimulus at a voltage that is just above the person's seizure threshold. The seizure typically lasts for about 30 seconds, and in many cases can only be witnessed on the monitor of the electroencephalogram (EEG) machine. In the UK, most people who are prescribed ECT are prescribed a course of between six and twelve treatments, usually delivered over three to six weeks. The choice of bilateral or unilateral (usually right-sided) ECT should be made on a case-by-case basis: bilateral ECT is considered more effective, while unilateral ECT produces fewer cognitive side-effects. Common adverse effects of ECT include adverse effects of anaesthesia, headache, muscle aches, nausea, confusion, and memory loss for events that occurred around the time of the treatment. Mortality from ECT is largely imputable to the anaesthetic, and is similar to that for any minor surgical procedure.

How effective is ECT?

Opinion is divided as to the effectiveness and value of ECT. Several studies lend weight to the frequent anecdotal reports that ECT can be considerably more effective than antidepressant treatment.

However, opponents claim that the evidence in support of ECT is weak, and that any benefits are short-lived and outweighed by the risks, including the risk of long-term memory impairment. They also highlight that, despite decades of research, proponents of ECT cannot point, or point with certainty, to a mechanism of action for its supposed antidepressant effect.

In addition to these criticisms, ECT suffers from a poor public image. For decades, the media, including Hollywood, has mostly portrayed it as coercive, punitive, and inhumane.

Interestingly, there is emerging evidence that repetitive transcranial magnetic stimulation (rTMS) could in some cases provide a safer and less off-putting alternative to ECT.

Depressive disorders: Course and prognosis

The average length of a major depressive episode is about six months. After a first episode, about 80% of people go on to experience one or more further episodes, with a median of four episodes in the course of a lifetime. Successive episodes tend to be longer than the last, with shorter inter-episode intervals. About 10% of people eventually experience a manic episode, thereby 'converting' to bipolar disorder. While many people with depression are not suicidal, the vast majority of people who commit suicide are deemed to have been suffering from depression or another mental disorder.

Puerperal (postnatal) disorders

The puerperium is marked by unique hormonal changes and psychological stresses, and associated with a number of distinct mental disorders (Table 5.6).

Table 5.6: Puerperal disorders

Puerperal disorder	Incidence (%)	Time of onset post-partum
Maternity blues	50	3-4 days
Postnatal depression	10-15	< 1 month
Puerperal psychosis	0.2	7-14 days

Maternity blues

Maternity blues or 'baby blues' is a minor mood disturbance occurring in about 50% of mothers (especially primiparous mothers) on the third or fourth day post-partum. It is marked by tearfulness, irritability, and lability of affect. The condition usually resolves in a matter of days.

Postnatal depression

Postnatal depression occurs in about 10-15% of mothers in the first month post-partum, and is more common in mothers with a psychiatric history or who lack social support. Tiredness, irritability, and anxiety are often more prominent than depressed mood, and the baby may be at short-term risk of neglect or harm. Management involves explanation and reassurance, and, in some cases, treatment as for depression. If hospital admission is required, this ought to be to a mother-and-baby unit so as not to compromise bonding between the pair.

Puerperal psychosis

Puerperal psychosis affects about 0.2% of mothers at about 7-14 days post-partum. It is more common in primiparous mothers and mothers with a psychiatric history or family history of mental disorder. It can present in one of three forms: delirious, affective, and schizophreniform. The delirious picture results from puerperal sepsis and is in effect an organic psychosis. It has become relatively rare since the advent of antibiotics. In puerperal psychosis, the mother may harbour delusions about the baby, for example, that it is abnormal or evil. This can put the baby at a high risk of neglect or harm. Hospital admission is often required.

5

Mania and bipolar disorder: Clinical features

Case study: Miss SW

Ten months ago, Sophie, a community psychiatric nurse, started feeling brighter and more energetic. At work she took on many additional roles and extra hours, but, much to her astonishment, one of her colleagues reported her as unsafe. She resigned in a fit of pique, claiming that she needed more time to devote to her other plans and projects.

By then, she couldn't stop her thoughts from racing and was sleeping at most three or four hours a night. She bought three houses to rent out to the poor, and also leased out a launderette with the intention of converting it into a multi-purpose centre. She acted completely out of character, dressing garishly, smoking marijuana, and even getting herself arrested for brawling in the street.

Four months ago, her mood began to drop and she felt dreadful and ashamed. Today she is feeling better but has had to sell her house to pay off her debts. Her psychiatrist suggested that she start on a mood stabilizer, but she is understandably reluctant to accept his advice.

People with mania frequently dress in colourful clothing or in unusual, haphazard combinations of clothing which they complement with inappropriate accessories such as hats and sunglasses and excessive make-up, jewellery, or body art. They are hyperactive, and may come across as entertaining, charming, seductive, vigilant, assertive, irritable, angry, or aggressive, and sometimes all of these in turn. Thoughts race through their mind at high speed, as a consequence of which their speech is pressured and voluble and difficult to interrupt.

Case study: John Ruskin

I roll on like a ball, with this exception, that contrary to the usual laws of motion I have no friction to contend with in my mind, and of course have some difficulty in stopping myself when there is nothing else to stop me… I am almost sick and giddy with the quantity of things in my head—trains of thought beginning and branching to infinity, crossing each other, and all tempting and wanting to be worked out.

—John Ruskin (1819-1900), in a letter to his father.

Sometimes, the thoughts and speech of people with mania are so muddled and rambling that they are unable to stay on topic or even make a point. They may ignore the structures and strictures of grammar, step outside the confines of an English dictionary, and even talk in rhymes and puns. All this can make it very difficult for anyone else to be heard, let alone understood, by the person with mania.

On top of this, mania sufferers are typically full of grandiose or unrealistic plans and projects that they begin to act upon but then quickly abandon. They often engage in impulsive and pleasure-seeking behaviour such as spending vast amounts of money, driving recklessly, taking recreational drugs, and having sexual intercourse with near-strangers. As a result, they can end up harming themselves or others, getting into trouble with the police and other authorities, and being exploited by the less than scrupulous.

Case study: Kay Redfield Jamison

When you're high it's tremendous. The ideas and feelings are fast and frequent like shooting stars and you follow them until you find better and brighter ones. Shyness goes, the right words and gestures are suddenly there, the power to captivate others a felt certainty. There are interests found in uninteresting people. Sensuality is pervasive and desire to seduce and be seduced is irresistible… But, somewhere this changes… Everything previously moving with the grain is now against—you are irritable, angry, frightened, uncontrollable, and immersed totally in the blackest caves of the mind.

—Kay Redfield Jamison, An Unquiet Mind

People with mania (although not, by definition, hypomania) may also experience psychotic symptoms that make their behaviour seem all the more bizarre, irrational, and chaotic. Psychotic symptoms are usually in keeping with elevated mood, and often involve delusions of grandeur, that is, delusions of exaggerated self-importance—of special status, special purpose, or special abilities. For instance, a mania sufferer may nurse the delusion that he is a brilliant scientist on the verge of discovering a cure for cancer, or that he is an exceptionally talented entrepreneur commissioned by his cousin the Queen to rid Africa of poverty.

Mania sufferers almost invariably have poor insight into their mental state and find it difficult to accept that they are ill. This means that they are likely to delay and resist getting the help that they need, and, in the meantime, cause tremendous damage to their health, finances, careers, and relationships.

As mentioned at the beginning of the chapter, a single episode of mania suffices to meet the DSM criteria for bipolar I disorder. The thinking behind this is that a person who has suffered a manic episode is very likely, sooner or later, to suffer one or more depressive episodes, as well as further manic or hypomanic episodes and possibly also mixed episodes.

It is important to underline that depressive episodes in bipolar disorder can be severe, with both psychotic symptoms and suicidal thoughts.

Clinical skills: Mental state examination in mania

Appearance	Flamboyant clothing, unusual combinations of clothing, heavy makeup and jewellery, fresh body art.
Behaviour	Hyperactive, entertaining, disinhibited, flirtatious, hypervigilant, assertive, aggressive.
Speech	Pressured speech, neologisms, clang associations.
Affect and mood	Euphoric, irritable, labile.
Thoughts	Optimistic, self-confident, grandiose, pressure of thought, flight of ideas, loosening of associations, circumstantiality, tangentiality, mood-congruent delusions.
Perceptions	Hallucinations.
Cognition	Poor concentration but intact memory and abstract thinking.
Insight	Very poor insight.

Mania and bipolar disorder: Diagnosis

The history of bipolar disorder

The modern concept of bipolar disorder originated in the 19th century. In 1854, psychiatrists Jules Baillarger (1809-1890) and Jean-Pierre Falret (1794-1870) independently presented descriptions of the illness to the *Académie de Médecine* in Paris. Baillarger called it *folie à double forme* ('dual-form insanity'), whereas Falret called it *folie circulaire* ('circular insanity'). Having observed that the illness clustered in families, Falret postulated a strong genetic basis.

In the early 1900s, Kraepelin studied the natural course of the untreated illness and found it to be punctuated by relatively symptom-free intervals. On this basis, he distinguished the illness from *dementia praecox* (schizophrenia) and named it *manisch-depressives Irresein* ('manic-depressive psychosis'). He emphasized that, in contrast to *dementia praecox*, manic-depressive psychosis had an episodic course and a more benign outcome.

Interestingly, Kraepelin did not distinguish people with both manic and depressive episodes from those with only depressive episodes with psychotic symptoms. It is only in the 1950s that German psychiatrists Karl Kleist (1879-1960) and Karl Leonhard (1904-1988) suggested this divide, from which stems the contemporary emphasis on bipolarity, and hence on mania/hypomania, as the defining feature of the illness.

The term 'bipolar disorder' first appeared in the third, 1980 revision of the DSM (DSM-III). It has gradually replaced the older term 'manic depressive illness', which, although more accurate and descriptive, perpetuated the stigmatization of bipolar sufferers as 'maniacs'.

ICD-10 Manic episode

ICD-10 specifies three degrees of severity for manic episode: hypomania, mania without psychotic symptoms, and mania with psychotic symptoms.

Hypomania

'A lesser degree of mania in which abnormalities of mood and behaviour are too persistent and marked to be included under cyclothymia but are not accompanied by hallucinations and delusions. There is persistent mild elevation of mood (for at least several days on end), increased energy and activity, and usually marked feelings of wellbeing and both physical and mental efficiency. Increased sociability, talkativeness, overfamiliarity, increased sexual energy, and a decreased need for sleep are often present but not to the extent that they lead to severe disruption of work or result in social rejection. Irritability, conceit, and boorish behaviour may take the place of the more usual euphoric sociability.'

Mania without psychotic symptoms

'Mood is elevated out of keeping with the individual's circumstances and may vary from carefree joviality to almost uncontrollable excitement. Elation is accompanied by increased energy, resulting in overactivity, pressure of speech, and a decreased need for sleep. Normal social inhibitions are lost, attention cannot be sustained, and there is often marked distractability. Self-esteem is inflated, and grandiose or over-optimistic ideas are freely expressed.

Perceptual disorders may occur, such as the appreciation of colours as especially vivid (and unusually beautiful), a preoccupation with fine details of surfaces or textures, and subjective hyperacusis. The individual may embark on extravagant and impractical schemes, spend money recklessly, or become aggressive, amorous, or facetious in inappropriate circumstances. In some manic episodes the mood is irritable and suspicious rather than elated.

The episode should last for at least one week and should be severe enough to disrupt ordinary work and social activities more or less completely.'

DSM-5 Manic episode

A. A distinct period of abnormally and persistently elevated, expansive, or irritable mood, lasting at least one week (or any duration if hospitalization is necessary).
B. During the period of mood disturbance, three (or more) of the following symptoms have persisted (four if the mood is only irritable) and have been present to a significant degree:
   • Inflated self-esteem or grandiosity.
   • Decreased need for sleep.
   • More talkative than usual or pressure to keep talking.
   • Flight of ideas or subjective experience that thoughts are racing.
   • Distractibility.
   • Increase in goal-directed activity or psychomotor agitation.
   • Excessive involvement in pleasurable activities with a high potential for painful consequences.
C. The mood disturbance is sufficiently severe to cause marked impairment in occupational functioning or in usual social activities or relationships with others, or to necessitate hospitalization to prevent harm to self or others, or there are psychotic features.
D. The symptoms are not due to the direct physiological effects of a substance or a general medical condition.

DSM-5 Hypomanic episode

The criteria and list of symptoms for hypomanic episode are very similar to those for manic episode. However, in this case, the symptoms, which must have been present for at least four days, are not severe enough to cause marked impairment in functioning, or to require hospitalization, and there are no psychotic symptoms.

The specifier 'with mixed features' can be applied to manic and hypomanic episodes with depressive features, and major depressive episodes (whether in the context of bipolar disorder or major depression) with features of mania/hypomania.

Mania and bipolar disorder: Differential diagnosis

Psychiatric differential

• Schizoaffective disorder.
• Schizophrenia.
• Puerperal psychosis.
• Cyclothymia.
• Attention deficit hyperactivity disorder.

Organic differential

• Drugs such as alcohol, amphetamines, cocaine, hallucinogens, anti-depressants, L-dopa, steroids.
• Sleep deprivation.
• Delirium.
• Brain disease of the frontal lobes such as dementia, stroke, multiple sclerosis, tumour, epilepsy, AIDS, neurosyphilis.
• Endocrine disorders such as hyperthyroidism, Cushing's syndrome.
• Systemic lupus erythematosus.

Mania and bipolar disorder: Epidemiology

The lifetime risk for bipolar disorder is difficult to gauge, but is probably in the order of 0.5-1%. As it is a chronic disorder, prevalence is fairly similar. Broadly speaking, all races and populations and both sexes are equally affected. The mean age of onset is 21 years, and a first episode of mania after the age of 50 ought to prompt an investigation for a primary cause such as organic brain disease or endocrine disorder.

False epidemics in psychiatry

Studies indicate that a large proportion of the normal population can be found to have met the diagnostic criteria for both depression and hypomania. The concept of bipolar II disorder, introduced in DSM-IV, has been criticized, first, for lacking biological validity, even by psychiatric standards; and, second, for contributing to a false epidemic of bipolar disorder (especially in the United States), which had hitherto been regarded as a fairly uncommon condition. This 'false epidemic' (the term is in fact that of Allen Frances, the chairman of the task force that drafted DSM-IV) together with aggressive marketing by pharmaceutical companies led to many more people, especially in North America, being prescribed potentially dangerous antipsychotic and mood stabilizing drugs.

DSM-IV has also been blamed for a number of other false epidemics, particularly in attention deficit hyperactivity disorder and Asperger's syndrome. Data from the US National Health Interview Survey indicate that, in 2012, 13.5% of boys aged 3-17 had been diagnosed with ADHD, up from 8.3% in 1997. These figures, which speak for themselves, are far higher than in the UK, partly because the ICD-10 criteria for ADHD (ICD-10: 'hyperkinetic disorder') are much more stringent. Adult ADHD, once looked upon as a rarity, is also becoming much more common, and in Canada now accounts for more than one third of all prescriptions for ADHD psycho-stimulant drugs.

Unusually among mental or indeed physical disorders, bipolar disorder is more common in higher socioeconomic groups, suggesting that the genes that predispose to bipolar disorder also predispose to greater achievement and success in the relatives of bipolar sufferers and perhaps even in bipolar sufferers themselves. There is mounting evidence that bipolar disorder and schizophrenia share some of the same genetic determinants, and that these overlapping sets of genes both predispose to greater creativity through loosened associations or so-called divergent thinking. As Nietzsche remarked in *Thus Spoke Zarathustra*, 'One must have chaos in one, to give birth to a dancing star.'

In her book *Touched with Fire: Manic-Depressive Illness and the Artistic Temperament*, clinical psychologist Kay Redfield Jamison (born 1946) estimates that bipolar disorder is between 10-40 times more common among artists than in the normal population. Artists who suffered, or are thought to have suffered, from bipolar disorder include authors Hans Christian Andersen, Honoré de Balzac, F. Scott Fitzgerald, Victor Hugo, Edgar Allen Poe, Mary Shelley, Mark Twain, and Virginia Woolf; poets William Blake, John Clare, TS Eliot, Florbela Espanca, John Keats, Robert Lowell, Fernando Pessoa, Alfred Lord Tennyson, and Walt Whitman; and composers Ludwig van Beethoven, Hector Berlioz, Edward Elgar, George Frederic Handel, Gustav Mahler, Sergei Rachmaninoff, Robert Schumann, and Peter Tchaikovsky—to name but a handful.

> I am come of a race noted for vigor of fancy and ardour of passion. Men have called me mad; but the question is not yet settled, whether madness is or is not the loftiest intelligence—whether much that is glorious—whether all that is profound—does not spring from disease of thought—from moods of mind exalted at the expense of the general intellect. They who dream by day are cognizant of many things which escape those who dream only by night. In their gray visions they obtain glimpses of eternity, and thrill, in awakening, to find that they have been upon the verge of the great secret. In snatches, they learn something of the wisdom which is of good, and more of the knowledge which is of evil. They penetrate, however rudderless or compassless, into the vast ocean of the 'light ineffable'...
>
> —Edgar Allen Poe (1809-1849), *Eleonora*

Mania and bipolar disorder: Aetiology

Genetics

First-degree relatives of a bipolar sufferer are at increased risks of bipolar disorder (10% lifetime risk), unipolar depression, and schizoaffective disorder. The concordance rate for bipolar disorder in monozygotic twins is 67%, as compared to only 19% in dizygotic twins. Furthermore, children of bipolar sufferers remain at increased risk of mood disorder even after having been adopted by unaffected foster parents. There is thus a strong genetic component to the aetiology of bipolar disorder, stronger, in fact, than in any other mental disorder.

Environmental factors

Life events, severe stresses, and disruptions in daily routines and circadian rhythms (for example, missing a night's sleep or flying from London to Tokyo) may provoke a first manic or hypomanic episode.

Moreover, there is an excess of manic episodes in late spring and summer, and also in the post-partum period.

Neurochemical abnormalities

The monoamine hypothesis of depression suggests that mania results from increased levels of noradrenaline, serotonin, and dopamine, and it has been observed that drugs such as cocaine and amphetamines can precipitate or exacerbate mania.

Other neurological differences

Neuroimaging studies suggest ventricular enlargement and structural differences in certain brain regions, but these findings are inconsistent and could be an effect rather than a cause of the disorder, or even a result of pharmacological treatment.

Mania and bipolar disorder: Investigations

Investigations in bipolar disorder, including physical examination, aim at excluding organic causes and physical complications such as dehydration or malnourishment, and at establishing a baseline for drug treatment. Laboratory investigations should include a serum or urine drug screen, liver, renal, and thyroid function tests, full blood count, erythyrocyte sedimentation rate, and a urine test (including, if appropriate, a pregnancy test). Other, more specific investigations such as antinuclear antibody should be considered on a case-by-case basis. A pre-treatment ECG is required before starting lithium and some other drugs. If the patient is already on lithium, a lithium level should be taken.

Mania and bipolar disorder: Management

Patients with bipolar disorder can generally be managed in the community with the support of the community mental health team or equivalent, although short periods of hospitalization may be required in a crisis.

Education is an important part of the management of bipolar disorder. In particular, patients should be taught to identify early signs of relapse and avoid triggers for relapse such as stress, sleep deprivation, and substance misuse. They should also be given simple lifestyle advice aimed at optimizing their physical health.

The choice of medication in bipolar disorder is largely determined by the person's symptoms. In a manic episode, the treatment most often prescribed is an antipsychotic; in a depressive episode, it is an antidepressant, sometimes in conjunction with an antipsychotic to avoid 'manic switch' (that is, over-treatment into mania). Rarely, ECT might be prescribed, either for a depressive episode that has become life-threatening or unresponsive, or, even more rarely, for a manic episode that cannot be treated with medication, either because it is unresponsive to medication or because medication is contraindicated. Once symptoms of mania or depression have remitted, the antipsychotic or antidepressant is usually discontinued and replaced with a mood stabilizer such as lithium or the anticonvulsant valproate to reduce the risk of further relapses into mania and depression.

Antipsychotics

If a person with mania is not already on a long-term mood stabilizer, the most prevalent practice is to start an antipsychotic and wait for the person to recover before considering a long-term mood stabilizer. If the person with mania is already on a long-term mood stabilizer, it is common to increase its dose and/or add an antipsychotic. In general, a mood stabilizer should not be started during a manic episode when the patient in unable to consent to treatment because this can compromise his or her long-term compliance, which is critical to the effectiveness of the mood stabilizer. In some cases, particularly in the presence of prominent psychotic symptoms, mixed states, rapid cycling (four or more episodes of mania, hypomania, and/or depression within one year), or treatment resistance, the antipsychotic is continued for the long-term instead of, or in addition to, a mood stabilizer, and acts as a de facto mood stabilizer.

Other drugs used in mania

In the initial stages of treatment of mania, the patient may be highly agitated and difficult to manage, and a very fast-acting sedative such as lorazepam may be prescribed in addition to an antipsychotic or mood stabilizer.

If the patient is sleep-deprived, which is likely, a sleeping tablet such as zopiclone or temazepam may also be prescribed. A sleeping tablet can be especially effective in the early, hypomanic stages, when it might singlehandedly succeed in aborting a full-scale manic episode.

In contrast, any antidepressant medication should be rapidly tapered off and stopped.

Lithium

The Australian psychiatrist and researcher John Cade (1912-1980) serendipitously discovered the mood stabilizing properties of lithium in 1949, but the naturally occurring salt took another two decades to enter into mainstream practice. Lithium is often said to decrease the rate of relapse by about one-third, with greater efficacy against mania than depression. Its mode of action is unclear, but it is held to have a range of effects in the brain, including on certain neurotransmitters and their receptors.

Understandably, many bipolar sufferers are reluctant to start on lithium owing to the complexities and risks involved. In particular, some bipolar sufferers who value or depend upon their creativity fear that the drug may leave them unable to think, feel, enjoy, and work. As poet Rainer Maria Rilke (1875-1926) put it, 'If my devils were to leave me, I am afraid my angels will take flight as well.' The other side of the argument is that, by reducing the risk of relapse, lithium can actually enable bipolar sufferers to work and create much more.

Ideally, lithium should only be started if there is a clear intention to carry on with it for at least three years, as poor compliance and intermittent treatment may precipitate 'rebound' mania or hypomania. The starting dose should be cautious and depends on several factors, including the preparation used (lithium carbonate or lithium citrate). The serum level needs to be contained within a narrow range, or 'therapeutic window', of about 0.5-1.0 millimoles per litre: any less and beneficial effects are limited, any

more and adverse and toxic effects become much more likely. Serum levels should be taken at 12 hours post-dose (usually in the morning) and monitored at five-to-seven day intervals until the patient is stabilized, and at three-to-four month intervals thereafter.

The adverse effects of lithium are summarized in Table 5.7. In addition to the adverse effects listed in the table, lithium appears to be teratogenic in early pregnancy, with a small risk of Ebstein's anomaly and other cardiovascular malformations in the foetus. As lithium is excreted into breast milk, breast-feeding is contraindicated.

Table 5.7: Adverse effects of lithium

Short-term	Long-term
Stuffy nose, metallic taste in the mouth	Weight gain
	Oedema
Confusion	Goitre and hypothyroidism*
Fine tremor	Hyperparathyroidism
Gastrointestinal disturbances	Nephrogenic diabetes insipidus
	Irreversible renal damage**
Muscle weakness	Cardiotoxicity§
Polyuria	Exacerbation of acne and psoriasis
Polydipsia	Raised leucocyte and platelet count

* Check thyroid function before starting therapy and monitor every six months.
** Check renal function before starting therapy and monitor every six months. Lithium is eliminated unchanged by the kidneys and its half-life is related to renal function.
§ Perform electrocardiogram before starting therapy. During therapy, lithium cardiotoxicity is manifest as T wave flattening.

Lithium toxicity (!)

High serum lithium levels (beyond about 1.5 millimoles per litre) give rise to additional toxic effects, among which anorexia, nausea, vomiting, diarrhoea, nystagmus, coarse tremor, dysarthria, ataxia, and, in severe cases, loss of consciousness, seizures, and death.

If lithium is started but not tolerated or found to be ineffective, it can be stopped abruptly. However, following successful long-term treatment, it should only be stopped gradually (say, over two or three months), as stopping abruptly in these circumstances can precipitate an episode of rebound mania or hypomania. People on lithium should be advised to drink plenty of fluids and to keep up their salt intake, as dehydration and salt depletion can increase serum levels and lead to lithium toxicity. Common lithium drug interactions are listed in Table 5.8.

Table 5.8: Common lithium drug interactions

Drug	Explanation
Diuretics, especially thiazides	Sodium depletion increases lithium levels, resulting in lithium toxicity.
Carbamazepine	Can result in neurotoxicity, prefer valproate.
NSAIDs	Most NSAIDs can increase lithium levels, resulting in lithium toxicity.
ACE inhibitors	Lithium toxicity.

NSAIDs, non-steroidal anti-inflammatory drugs; ACE inhibitors, angiotensin-converting enzyme inhibitors.

Given all these hazards and hurdles, many bipolar sufferers delay starting on lithium until they have suffered from one or more further relapses, or else carefully consider other options such as valproate or an antipsychotic, which, of course, have drawbacks of their own.

How effective is lithium?

Although lithium has many supporters, Joanna Moncrieff, a psychiatrist, researcher, and co-chair of the Critical Psychiatry Network, argues that the evidence for the effectiveness of lithium in the treatment of bipolar disorder is 'far too weak to outweigh the harm it can cause'.

According to Moncrieff, the main problem with the evidence for lithium is that the higher rate of relapse in control groups is in fact artificial. In every randomized trial looking at lithium, at least some of the people in the control group withdrew from lithium to start on a placebo, and there is substantial evidence that withdrawing from lithium can precipitate a relapse or 'rebound', especially in mania or hypomania.

Even if lithium could be shown to reduce relapse rates, says Moncrieff, this would owe more to its sedating and slowing effects than to any specific mood stabilizing effects.

Moreover, the sudden removal of this neurological suppression could be responsible for the rebound phenomenon.

Valproate

The use of anticonvulsants—principally valproate and, more recently, lamotrigine—in the prophylaxis of bipolar

disorder has been increasing. Anticonvulsants enhance the action of the inhibitory neurotransmitter gamma aminobutyric acid (GABA), but their precise mode of action in the prophylaxis of bipolar disorder remains to be determined.

Valproate, in the form of semisodium valproate (Depakote), is used alone or as an adjunct to lithium or other drugs in the treatment and prophylaxis of bipolar disorder, and in the USA has become the most frequently prescribed mood-stabilizer. Compared to lithium, it is thought to have a similar efficacy but a quicker onset of action, and to be of particular benefit in rapid cycling bipolar disorder.

Although valproate can have a number of adverse effects, it is often better tolerated than lithium, particularly if lithium levels need to be maintained above about 0.8 millimoles per litre. Adverse effects include nausea, tremor, sedation, weight gain, alopecia, blood dyscrasias, hepatotoxicity, and pancreatitis. Valproate can cause neural tube defects and other malformations in the foetus, and for these reasons is best avoided in women of child-bearing age. It is important to check blood cell counts and liver function before starting valproate, and then to monitor these at six-to-twelve month intervals.

Lamotrigine

Lamotrigine is more effective against relapses of depression than relapses of mania, and can be used both in the treatment of relapses of bipolar depression and in the prophylaxis of bipolar disorder. Compared with lithium and valproate, it has fewer adverse effects and does not usually require long-term monitoring with blood tests. Common adverse effects include nausea and vomiting, headaches, dizziness, clumsiness, and blurred vision and diplopia. Other adverse effects include flu-like symptoms, sedation, insomnia, skin rash, and severe skin reactions.

Carbamazepine

Carbamazepine is generally used as a second- or third-line drug in the prophylaxis of bipolar disorder, and is thought to be of particular value in treatment-resistant cases and in rapid cycling. Adverse effects include nausea, headache, dizziness, sedation, diplopia, ataxia, skin rashes, rare but potentially fatal blood dyscrasias, and hepatotoxicity. Bloods should be monitored regularly for leukopaenia, hyponatraemia, and raised liver function tests. In pregnancy, carbamazepine can lead to spina bifida in the foetus, but it is not excreted in breast milk. As it is a strong inducer of hepatic microsomal enzymes, it increases the metabolism of many other drugs.

Mania and bipolar disorder: Course and prognosis

Left untreated, manic episodes last for an average of about four months, and depressive episodes for an average of about six months. A person with bipolar disorder can expect to suffer a total of between eight and ten episodes of mood disturbance in the course of his life, but the exact number varies a lot from one individual to another.

Bipolar disorder tends to strike in the prime of life, when people are likely to be full of plans for the future. A person who has been freshly diagnosed with bipolar disorder may feel that all his hopes and dreams have been dashed, and that he has disappointed or even betrayed the expectations of those he holds most near and dear. Complex and often unrecognized feelings of loss, hopelessness, and guilt may exacerbate or prolong a depressive episode or give rise to further depressive episodes, and even, in some cases, to thoughts of self-harm or suicide.

It is estimated that half of bipolar sufferers attempt suicide at least once in their lifetime, and, tragically, a small number of these attempts do end up being fatal. One recent Swedish cohort study led by C. Crump found that, compared with the normal population, suicide risk in bipolar disorder is increased ten-fold among women and eight-fold among men. Suicide risk is greatest during relapses of the illness, particularly during depressive episodes, mixed episodes, and manic episodes with psychotic symptoms.

In addition to having a higher suicide rate, bipolar sufferers are more prone to potentially fatal accidents, particularly during manic episodes when their behaviour is rash and reckless. A person in the throes of mania is much more likely than average to be involved in a car crash, street fight, accidental drug overdose, or house fire, among others. He may also suffer from self-neglect, commonly, from forgetting or otherwise omitting to eat or drink or take his medication.

Life expectancy in bipolar disorder depends in large part on the course that the illness takes. Overall, life expectancy is reduced by about eight or nine years compared to average, but the gap is narrowing owing to better management, including better physical care. Perhaps surprisingly, important causes of death in bipolar disorder include physical conditions such as cardiovascular disease, diabetes, and respiratory disease. One of the biggest contributors to poor physical health in bipolar disorder is smoking, so stopping smoking can do much to increase life expectancy, as can addressing any alcohol or drug problems, maintaining physical health through sensible diet and regular exercise, developing good sleep hygiene, avoiding stress, and seeking out early treatment for the bipolar disorder and any supervening physical conditions.

I married, and then my brains went up like a shower of fireworks. As an experience, madness is terrific I can assure you, and not to be sniffed at; and in its lava I still find most of the things I write about. It shoots out of one everything shaped, final, not in mere driblets as sanity does. And the six months… that I lay in bed taught me a good deal about what is called oneself.

—Virginia Woolf (1892-1941), in a letter to her friend Ethel Smyth

Virginia Woolf suffered from bipolar disorder from the age of 13. She committed suicide at the age of 59 by walking into the River Ouse with a large rock in her pocket (as portrayed in *The Hours*, a film based on Woolf's novel *Mrs Dalloway*, and starring Nicole Kidman as Woolf).

This is her suicide note to her husband, Leonard:

Dearest, I feel certain I am going mad again. I feel we can't go through another of those terrible times. And I shan't recover this time. I begin to hear voices, and I can't concentrate. So I am doing what seems the best thing to do. You have given me the greatest possible happiness. You have been in every way all that anyone could be. I don't think two people could have been happier till this terrible disease came. I can't fight any longer. I know that I am spoiling your life, that without me you could work. And you will I know. You see I can't even write this properly. I can't read. What I want to say is I owe all the happiness of my life to you. You have been entirely patient with me and incredibly good. I want to say that—everybody knows it. If anybody could have saved me it would have been you. Everything has gone from me but the certainty of your goodness. I can't go on spoiling your life any longer.

I don't think two people could have been happier than we have been.

V.

Self-assessment

Answer by true or false.

1. Poor self-esteem is a core symptom of depression.
2. Low mood is not strictly required to secure a diagnosis of depression.
3. A diagnosis of bipolar disorder can be made if a person has suffered two manic episodes, but never a depressive episode.
4. In mild depression, the person struggles to fulfil his or her social obligations.
5. Bipolar II disorder consists of episodes of major depression and mania.
6. In some respects, people with depression may have a more accurate perception of reality.
7. Psychotic symptoms are more common in mania than in bipolar depression, and more common in bipolar depression than in unipolar depression.
8. 'Rapid cycling' in bipolar disorder refers to four or more episodes of mania within one year.
9. The peak prevalence of depressive disorders in females is in middle age.
10. According to behavioural theory, depressive behaviour can be learnt through observation and imitation, and inadvertently reinforced by other people's reactions.
11. Selective abstraction involves drawing a conclusion on the basis of a single incident.
12. Alcohol misuse is a common cause of depressive symptoms.
13. Stimulant misuse can lead to both mania and depression.
14. The concordance rate for bipolar disorder in monozygotic twins is higher than for major depression or schizophrenia.
15. Interpersonal psychotherapy involves effecting change through a higher level of self-understanding.
16. The tyramine reaction is a hypertensive crisis that can result in subarachnoid haemorrhage.
17. Tertiary amines such as amitriptyline, imipramine, and clomipramine are less sedating and cause less anticholinergic side-effects than secondary amines such as nortriptyline, dothiepin, and lofepramine.
18. The SSRI discontinuation syndrome occurs most frequently upon discontinuing fluoxetine.
19. Serotonin syndrome should be managed in a general hospital.
20. Toxic effects of lithium are experienced beyond about 1.5 millimoles per litre.
21. Serum levels of valproate should be taken at 12-hours post-dose and monitored at five-to-seven day intervals until the patient is stabilized, and at three-to-four month intervals thereafter. Renal and thyroid function should also be monitored.
22. In contrast to lithium, lamotrigine is more effective against relapses of mania than of depression.
23. Adverse effects of carbamazepine include nausea, headache, dizziness, sedation, diplopia, ataxia, skin rashes, blood dyscrasias, and hepatotoxicity.
24. ECT may not be given under the Mental Health Act to a person with the capacity to refuse to consent it.
25. The average length of a treated manic episode is four months.

Answers

1. False.
2. True.
3. True.
4. False. This describes moderate depression.
5. False. Major depression and *hypomania*.
6. True. The phenomenon is called 'depressive realism'.
7. True.
8. False. Rapid cycling refers to four or more episodes of mania, hypomania, and/or depression within one year.
9. True.
10. True. It can also result from the removal of positive reinforcement from the environment, or from certain stimuli that have become associated with negative emotional states.
11. False. This is over-generalization. Selective abstraction involves focusing on a single event to the detriment of others.
12. True.
13. True.
14. True.
15. False. This describes dynamic psychotherapy. Interpersonal psychotherapy is a systematic and standardized treatment approach to personal relationships and life problems.
16. True.
17. False. The other way round.
18. False. Paroxetine.
19. True.
20. True.
21. False. This applies to lithium, not valproate.
22. False. The other way round.
23. True.
24. True.
25. False. This is the average length of an *untreated* manic episode.

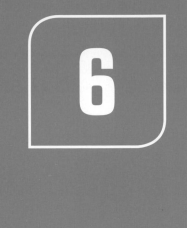

Suicide and deliberate self-harm

6

And so it was I entered the broken world
To trace the visionary company of love, its voice
An instant in the wind (I know not whither hurled)
But not for long to hold each desperate choice.

—Hart Crane (1899-1932), *The Broken Tower*

Definitions

Suicide is a neologism coined from *sui caedes*, Latin for 'murder of oneself', and has been defined by sociologist Emile Durkheim (1858-1917) as applying to 'all cases of death resulting directly or indirectly from a positive or negative act of the victim himself, which he knows will produce this result'.

Suicide can more simply be defined as the act of intentionally bringing about one's own death, although doing so with the primary aim of saving or helping others may be seen more as self-sacrifice than suicide. Thus, a revised and more restrictive definition of suicide is, the act of intentionally bringing about one's own death, *with the primary aim of dying.*

Suicide should be distinguished from assisted suicide, the making available to a person of the information and/or means to end his life; and from voluntary euthanasia (Greek, 'good death'), the deliberate ending of the life of a person who has requested it. A more restrictive definition of euthanasia is, the deliberate ending of the life of an incurably ill person who has requested it, to relieve suffering. Active euthanasia, which in many jurisdictions remains tantamount to murder or manslaughter, involves the use of lethal substances or forces to kill, whereas passive euthanasia merely involves the withholding of common treatments such as antibiotics or surgery.

The act of suicide itself should be distinguished from other acts of self-harm, and particularly from attempted suicide and parasuicide (Figure 6.1). Attempted suicide is the act of trying to kill oneself (with intention), but failing to do so. Parasuicide is any act, or 'suicidal gesture', that resembles suicide but does not result in death. The intention of a parasuicidal act might have been to kill oneself, but it may also have been a means of attracting attention, a 'cry for help', an act of revenge, or an expression of despair, among others. Suicide, attempted suicide, and parasuicide are all forms of deliberate self-harm, which can be defined as the act of intentionally injuring oneself, irrespective of the degree of injury sustained.

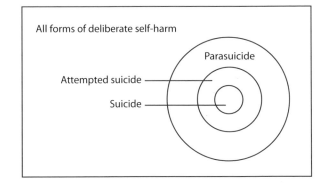

Figure 6.1. Different types of deliberate self-harm.

Suicide: Ethics

The Roman Catholic Church has long argued that one's life is the property of God and thus that to commit suicide is to deride God's prerogatives. The counterargument, by philosopher David Hume (1711-1776) is that, if such is the case, then to save someone's life is also to deride God's prerogatives.

Most religions share the Church's belief in the sanctity of life, although a few have come to regard at least some suicides as honourable. For example, a number of Tibetan monks have killed themselves in protest against the Chinese occupation of Tibet—although this is perhaps more a case of self-sacrifice than suicide proper.

Legal systems have historically been informed by religion, such that in many jurisdictions suicide and attempted suicide are still illegal. The very expression 'commit suicide' implies or at least suggests a crime or sin. In late 2014, the Indian government moved to decriminalize 'attempt to suicide' by deleting Section 209 of the Penal Code from the statute book. Under the said section, a suicide bid could be punished with a prison term of up to one year.

In the UK, the Suicide Act of 1961 decriminalized attempted suicide and suicide, but voluntary euthanasia remains a crime. This may change as the voice of pro-choicers becomes louder than that of pro-lifers. Broadly speaking, pro-choicers argue that a person's life belongs to no one but himself, and that his decision to commit suicide, especially if justified as a rational solution to real problems such as chronic and disabling pain, should be respected and assisted. In contrast, pro-lifers believe that a person's life is not his to take, regardless of circumstances.

Some of the stronger arguments in favour of voluntary euthanasia are that it preserves dignity, prevents suffering, and frees up valuable healthcare resources. On the other side of the argument, a person with a physical or mental disorder may lack the mental capacity to make a rational decision about such an important issue, or may feel pressured into making a decision, and, of course, cannot change his mind once he is dead. Moreover, voluntary euthanasia is difficult to regulate, and could be open to abuse by doctors and relatives keen to unburden themselves and free up or inherit resources.

Unlike most people, some philosophers do not think about suicide in terms of ethics. Existentialist philosophers in particular turn the tables round by arguing that life has no meaning and that there is therefore no reason not to commit suicide. Rather, a person must justify not committing suicide by giving his life a meaning and fulfilling his unique potential through this meaning.

> One is still what one is going to cease to be and already what one is going to become. One lives one's death, one dies one's life.
>
> —Jean-Paul Sartre (1905-1980), *Saint Genet, Actor and Martyr*

Nihilistic (from the Latin *nihil*, 'nothing') philosophers differ from existentialist philosophers in that they believe that a person cannot justify his life even by giving it an individual meaning. For nihilistic philosophers, nothing can have a meaning, not even suicide itself.

Interesting as this may all be, suicide is seldom the product of rational deliberation, the so-called 'rational suicide', but mostly an act of incontrollable anguish and despair.

Around 1755, David Hume, who suffered from melancholy, published *On Suicide* and *On the Immortality of the Soul* in a book of essays entitled *Five Dissertations*. Unfortunately, pre-release copies of *Five Dissertations* stirred up such controversy that both essays had to be removed. In *On Suicide*, Hume argues that, though only 'one step' could put an end to his misery, man dares not commit suicide because of 'a vain fear lest he offend his Maker'. This, combined with his natural fear of death, makes it 'all the more difficult for him to be free'. Hume proposes to 'restore men to their native liberty' by examining all the common arguments against suicide and demonstrating that suicide is 'free from every imputation of guilt or blame'.

According to Hume, God established the laws of nature and enabled all animals, including man, to make use of them by entrusting them with certain bodily and mental powers. Owing to this interaction between the laws of nature and the powers of animals, God has no need to be involved in the world: '...the providence of the Deity appears not immediately in any operation, but governs everything by those general and immutable laws, which have been established from the beginning of time.'

Given this state of affairs, man employs the powers with which he has been invested to provide as best as possible for his 'ease, happiness, or preservation'. If this should bring him to commit suicide, then so be it: the interaction between the laws of nature and the powers of man clearly permit it, so why should it pose an exception?

> *The life of man is of no greater importance to the universe than that of an oyster... I thank Providence, both for the good which I have already enjoyed, and for the power with which I am endowed of escaping the ill that threatens me.*
>
> —David Hume, *On Suicide*

Natural philosopher Pliny the Elder (23-79) goes one step further than Hume in his *Natural History* by regarding the ability to commit suicide as the one advantage that man possesses over God: 'God cannot kill himself if he wishes, but man can do so at any time he chooses.'

Should we be afraid of death?

Regardless of the morality or permissibility of committing suicide, suicide entails death, and so the question naturally arises as to whether death should or should not be feared. In his influential paper of 1970, tersely entitled *Death*, philosopher Thomas Nagel (born 1937) addresses precisely this question: if death is the permanent end of our existence, is it an evil?

Either death is an evil because it deprives us of life, or it is a mere blank because there is no one left to experience this deprivation. Thus, if death is an evil, this is not in virtue of any positive attribute that it has, but in virtue of what it deprives us from, namely, life. For Nagel, the bare experience of life is intrinsically valuable, regardless of the balance of its good and bad elements.

The longer we are alive, the more we 'accumulate' life. In contrast, death cannot be accumulated—it is not 'an evil of which Shakespeare has so far received a larger portion than Proust'. Most people would not consider the temporary suspension of life as an evil, nor would they regard the long period before they were born as an evil. Therefore, if death is an evil this is not because it involves a period of non-existence, but because it deprives us of life.

Nagel draws three objections to this view, but only so as to later counter them. First, it is doubtful whether anything can be an evil unless it actually causes displeasure. Second, in the case of death there is no subject left on whom to impute an evil. As long as we exist, we have not yet died; and once we have died, we no longer exist. So there seems to be no time at which the evil of death might occur. Third, if most people would not

A common argument against suicide is that it is selfish and harms the individuals and society that are left behind. For Hume, a person does no harm in committing suicide, but merely ceases to do good. Assuming that he is under some obligation to do good, this obligation comes to an end with death; and even if it does not, and he is under a perpetual obligation to do good, this should not come at the expense of greater harm to himself, that is, at the expense of prolonging a miserable existence for some 'frivolous advantage that the public may perhaps receive'. In some cases, a person may have become a burden to society, and so may actually do most good by committing suicide. In such cases, says Hume, suicide is better than morally neutral. It is morally good.

regard the long period before they were born as an evil, then why should they regard the period after they are dead any differently?

Nagel counters these three objections by arguing that the good or evil that befalls us depends on our history and possibilities rather than on our momentary state, such that an evil can befall us even if we are not here to experience it. For instance, if an intelligent person receives a head injury that reduces his mental condition to that of a contented infant, this should be considered a serious evil even if the person himself (in his current state) is oblivious to his fate.

Thus, if the three objections are invalid, it is essentially because they ignore the direction of time.

Even though we cannot survive our death, we can still suffer evil; and even though we do not exist during the time before our birth and the time after our death, the time after our death is time of which we have been deprived, time in which we could have carried on enjoying the good of living.

The question remains as to whether the non-realization of further life is an absolute evil, or whether this depends on what can naturally be hoped for: the death of Keats at 24 is commonly regarded as tragic, but that of Tolstoy at 82 (even though he died of pneumonia in a hitherto obscure train station) is not.

'The trouble,' says Nagel, 'is that life familiarizes us with the goods of which death deprives us... Death, no matter how inevitable, is an abrupt cancellation of indefinitely extensive goods.'

Suicide: Epidemiology

Over 4,700 people died by suicide in 2013 in England, just under 78% of whom were men, and suicide remains one of the biggest killers for men under the age of 50. While self-harm is more common in women, completed suicide is more than three times more common in men. This may be because men are more likely to use violent means of suicide, or because men with suicidal thoughts find it harder to obtain and engage with the help and support that they need.

According to the Office for National Statistics (ONS), the highest UK suicide rate in 2013 was among men aged 45 to 59, at 25.1 deaths per 100,000—the highest for that age group since 1981.

An important problem with figures such as these is that they reflect reported suicides, which in turn reflect verdicts reached by coroners' inquests. *Actual* suicide rates may be considerably higher than the statistics suggest, particularly in elderly people in whom suicide is more likely to be mistaken for a natural death.

The most common method of suicide in the UK in 2013, again according to the ONS, was 'hanging, strangulation and suffocation', which accounted for 56.1% of male and 40.2% of female suicides. This is astonishingly high in so far as hanging is both violent and ineffectual, and serves to highlight the important influence of culture and tradition on chosen methods of suicide.

For the first time in 2013, 'hanging, strangulation and suffocation' overtook poisoning as the most common method of suicide in women. In 2013, poisoning accounted for 38% of female suicides, down from 49% in 2002. Drowning, falls, and other methods remained fairly constant over the period.

Methods of suicide are influenced not only by culture but also by availability and accessibility. Thus, the proliferation of barbiturates in the early 1960s led to a marked increase in poisoning as a method of suicide, and gunshot as a method of suicide is far more common in the US than the UK. A small proportion of suicides involve a suicide pact in which two or more people—usually an elderly couple rather than a pair of star-cross'd lovers—agree to commit suicide at or around the same time.

The World Health Organization (WHO) estimates that, each year, there are about 800,000 deaths by suicide throughout the world, which equates to an annual global suicide rate of 11.4 per 100,000. Globally, suicide accounts for 1.4% of deaths, making it the 15th leading cause of death overall and the leading cause of death among people aged 15 to 29. Rates of attempted suicide are, of course, much higher still.

As methods of reporting suicide vary from one country to another, it is difficult to draw robust international comparisons. However, it seems that, in high-income countries, middle-aged men have the highest official sui-cide rates, whereas in low- and middle-income countries it is young adults and elderly women.

In Europe, there is a tendency for suicide rates to increase the more north and the more east one travels. According to the WHO, in 2012, suicide rates in Russia, Lithuania, and Latvia exceeded 30 per 100,000. This compared to 6.3 per 100,000 in Greece, 7.6 in Italy, 8.2 in Spain, 9.8 in the UK, and 19.4 in the US.

Several factors can affect the suicide rate, including the time of year, the state of the economy, and media headlines.

Contrary to popular belief, the suicide rate peaks in the springtime, not the wintertime. This may be because the rebirth that marks springtime accentuates feelings of hopelessness in those already prone to suicide, or because people who are depressed cannot muster the energy to carry through with suicide in the winter.

It comes as no surprise that the suicide rate increases during times of economic depression. More unexpected, however, is that it also increases during times of economic prosperity, presumably because people feel 'left behind' if every Tom, Dick, and Harry seems to be racing ahead. Although economists focus on the absolute size of salaries, several sociological studies have found that the effect of money on happiness results less from the things money can buy (absolute income effect) than from comparing one's income to that of others, especially one's peers (relative income effect). This could help explain the finding that people in developed countries such as the UK and US are no happier than 60 or 70 years ago. Despite being considerably richer, healthier, and more leisured, they have only barely managed to 'keep up with the Joneses'.

On the other hand, the suicide rate decreases during times of national cohesion or coming together, such as during a war or its modern substitute, the international sporting tournament. During such times, there is a feeling of 'being in it together' along with a heady mix of curiosity, suspense, and anticipation. For example, a 2003 study by E Salib looking at England and Wales found that the number of suicides reported for the month of September 2001 was significantly lower than for any other month of that year, and lower than for any month of September in 22 years. According to the author of the study, these findings 'support Durkheim's theory that periods of external threat create group integration within society and lower the suicide rate through the impact of social cohesion'.

Like so much else, suicidal behaviour is culturally shaped. Thus, the suicide rate rises after the depiction or prominent reporting of a suicide in the media. A suicide that is inspired by another suicide, either in the media or in real life, is sometimes referred to as a 'copycat suicide', and the phenomenon itself as the 'Werther effect'. In 1774, JW Goethe (1749-1832) published a novel entitled, *The Sorrows of Young Werther*, in which the fictional Werther shoots himself following an ill-fated romance. Within no time, young men all over Europe began committing suicide using exactly the same method as Werther, prompting the novel to be banned in several places. In some cases, suicide can spread through an entire local community with one copycat suicide inspiring the next. Such a 'suicide contagion' is most likely to occur in impressionable and vulnerable population groups such as disaffected teenagers.

Suicide: Risk factors

At the individual level, a person's risk of committing suicide can be increased by a number of demographic and social risk factors (Table 6.1). Demographic risk factors for suicide, at least in the West, include being male; being relatively young; and being single, widowed, separated, or divorced. Social risk factors include having recently suffered a life crisis such as losing a close friend or relative; being unemployed, insecurely employed, or retired; and having a poor level of social support as is often the case for the elderly, prisoners, immigrants, refugees, and the bereaved. Certain occupational groups such as veterinary surgeons, farmers, pharmacists, and doctors have been found to be at a higher risk of suicide. This probably owes to their training and skills, and to their privileged access to highly lethal means such as prescription-only drugs and firearms.

As well as demographic and social risk factors, a person's risk of committing suicide can be significantly increased by a number of clinical risk factors (Table 6.2). Indeed, the most important predictor of suicide is a previous episode of self-harm, and a person's risk of completing suicide in the year following an episode of self-harm is approximately 100 times greater than average. Conversely, up to half of all people who complete suicide have a history of self-harm.

Suicidal behaviour tends to cluster in families, so a family history of suicide or self-harm also increases suicide risk. This might be because suicide is a learnt behaviour, or, more likely, because family members share a genetic predisposition to mental disorders such as schizophrenia and bipolar disorder that are associated with a higher risk of suicide.

Also at a higher risk of suicide are people with a mental disorder who are not responding to, or engaging with, their treatment; and people experiencing certain psychotic symptoms such as delusions of persecution, delusions of control, delusions of jealousy, delusions of guilt, second person auditory hallucinations (for example, a voice saying, 'Take that knife and kill yourself'), and passivity.

Physical illnesses also increase suicide risk. This is particularly true of physical illnesses that are terminal, that involve chronic pain or disability, or that affect the brain. Physical illnesses that have been associated with a significantly increased suicide rate include cancer, coronary heart disease, chronic obstructive pulmonary disease, early-onset diabetes, stroke, epilepsy, multiple sclerosis, AIDS, and endocrine and metabolic disorders.

Table 6.1: Sociodemographic risk factors for suicide

Sex	Completed suicide is four times more common in men.
Age	Recorded suicide is most common in middle-aged men and women.
Marital status	Single, widowed, or separated/divorced.
Employment status	Unemployed, insecurely employed, or retired.
Occupation	Veterinary surgeons, farmers, pharmacists, doctors.
Socioeconomic status	Lower socioeconomic status.
Poor social support	The elderly, prisoners, immigrants, refugees, the bereaved.
Other	Recent life crisis, victim of physical or sexual abuse, access to means.

Table 6.2: Clinical risk factors for suicide

Factor	Comments
History of DSH	A person's risk of completing suicide in the year following an episode of self-harm is approximately 100 times greater than average. Conversely, up to half of all people who complete suicide have a history of self-harm.
Family history of DSH	Suicidal behaviour clusters in families, although this may simply reflect a shared predisposition to mental disorder.
Mental disorder	Especially depressive disorders, substance misuse, schizophrenia, and personality disorders. Some of these disorders may, and often do, coexist. Treatment resistance or non-engagement/non-compliance raise risk further still. Specific factors in the mental state that raise risk are suicidal ideation and expressed intent, anger, hostility, revenge-seeking, suspiciousness, delusions of persecution, delusions of control, delusions of jealousy, delusions of guilt, second person command hallucinations, and passivity.
Physical illness	Notably cancer, coronary heart disease, chronic obstructive pulmonary disease, early-onset diabetes, stroke, epilepsy, multiple sclerosis, AIDS, and endocrine and metabolic disorders.

Talking about suicide

It is estimated that about two-thirds of people who commit suicide had told someone about their intentions, and that about half had visited a GP in the month prior to killing themselves. Talking about suicide can be uncomfortable, but health professionals must have the confidence to broach the subject.

Clinical skills: Assessing suicidal risk

To begin, explain to the patient that you are going to ask him some difficult questions about his thoughts and feelings. There is nothing to suggest that asking about suicide increases its risk, so do not hesitate to ask about suicide for fear of planting the idea.

Ask about the history of the current episode of self-harm (if any) to determine degree of suicidal intent (higher intent/lower intent—guidelines only):

- What was the precipitant for the attempt? (serious precipitant/trivial precipitant)
- Was it planned? (planned/unplanned)
- What was the method of self-harm, and did the patient expect it to be lethal? (violent method/non-violent method)
- Did he make a will or leave a suicide note? (suicide note/no suicide note)
- Was he alone? (alone/not alone)
- Did he take precautions against discovery? (precautions/no precautions)
- Was he intoxicated? (premeditated intoxication/incidental intoxication)
- Did he seek help after the attempt? (sought help/did not seek help)
- How did he feel when help arrived? (angry or disappointed/relieved)

Assess risk factors for suicide (Tables 6.1, 6.2):
- Previous suicide attempt(s).
- Recent life crisis.
- Male sex.
- Divorced, widowed, or single.
- Unemployed or in certain occupations such as medicine or farming.
- Poor level of social support.
- Physical illness.
- Psychiatric illness.
- Substance misuse.
- Family history of suicide, mental disorder, or substance misuse.

Carry out a mental state assessment. In particular, assess current mood and exclude psychosis.

Will the patient be returning to the same situation? What has changed? Are there any important protective factors?

Ask about current suicidal ideation. Has he made any plans?

Before taking any decisions, always discuss your assessment with a senior colleague.

Suicide: Management

The management plan should depend on the risk assessment, and should in all cases be discussed with a senior colleague or, ideally, a psychiatrist. In most cases, the patient can be discharged back into the community, particularly if he has a strong support network. In some cases, discharge can be facilitated by the crisis team or equivalent, which can step in to provide additional support and supervision. The patient should also be referred to his GP for follow-up, and, in some cases, also to the community mental health team or equivalent. If the patient is already under the care of mental health services, he should be referred to his care co-ordinator as soon as practicable, preferably by telephone or answerphone.

Clinical skills: Counselling for people with suicidal thoughts

If you are assailed by suicidal thoughts, the first thing to remember is that many people who have attempted suicide and survived ultimately feel relieved that they did not end their lives.

Some of the thoughts that you may be having include:
- I want to escape my suffering.
- I have no other options.
- I am a horrible person and do not deserve to live.
- I have betrayed those I love.
- Those I love would be better off without me.
- I want those I love to know how bad I am feeling.
- I want those I love to know how bad they have made me feel.

Whatever thoughts you are having, and however bad you are feeling, remember that you have not always felt this way, and that you will not always feel this way.

The risk of a person committing suicide is highest in the combined presence of (1) suicidal thoughts, (2) the means to commit suicide, and (3) the opportunity to commit suicide. If you are prone to suicidal thoughts, ensure that any means of committing suicide have been removed. For example, give tablets and sharp objects to a trusted person for safekeeping, or put them in a locked or otherwise inaccessible place. Also ensure that the opportunity to commit suicide is lacking by remaining in close contact with one or more people, for instance, by inviting them to stay with you. Share your thoughts and feelings with these people, and don't be reluctant to let them help you. If there's no one or no one seems suitable, there are a number of phone lines you can ring at any time. You can even take yourself to A&E or ring for an ambulance.

Do not use alcohol or drugs as these can make your behaviour more impulsive and significantly increase your likelihood of attempting suicide. In particular, do not drink or take drugs when alone, or when you're going to end up alone.

Make a list of all the positive things about yourself and all the positive things about your life, including the things that have so far kept you from suicide (you may need help with this). Keep the lists on you, and read them to yourself whenever you are assailed by suicidal thoughts. On a separate sheet of paper, write a safety plan for the times when you feel like acting on your suicidal thoughts. Your safety plan could involve delaying any suicidal attempt by at least 48 hours, and talking to someone about your thoughts and feelings as soon as possible. Discuss your safety plan with a health professional and commit yourself to it.

Sometimes even a single good night's sleep can completely change your outlook, so don't underestimate the importance of sleep. If you are finding it difficult to sleep, speak to your GP.

Once things are a bit more settled, try to address the cause or causes of your suicidal thoughts in as far as possible. Discuss this with your GP, care worker, or another heath professional.

My safety plan
- Read through the list of positive things about myself.
- Read through the list of positive things about my life and remind myself of the things that have so far prevented me from committing suicide.
- Distract myself from suicidal thoughts by reading a book, listening to jazz, or watching my favourite film or comedy.
- Get a good night's sleep. Take a sleeping tablet if necessary.
- Delay any suicidal attempt by at least 48 hours.
- Call Stan on (phone number). If he is unreachable, call Julia on (phone number). Or call my care worker on (phone number), or the crisis line on (phone number).
- Go to a place where I feel safe such as the sports or community centre.
- Go to A&E.
- Call for an ambulance.

Deliberate self-harm

> I slashed my wrist again and again, as deeply as I could. I knew perfectly well that it would not kill me, not like the times before. They have been something quite different. As my writing to you comes to a close, the pain is so unbearable inside me that a force of such strength has driven me to inflict a physical pain on myself in the hope of appeasing the other.
>
> —Sarah Ferguson, *A Guard Within*

Acts of self-harm such as self-cutting or overdosing that are neither suicide, attempted suicide, nor parasuicide may be carried out for a variety of reasons, most commonly to express and relieve bottled-up anger or tension, feel more in control of a seemingly desperate life situation, or punish oneself for being a 'bad' person.

For some people, the pain inflicted by self-harm is preferable to the numbness and emptiness that it replaces: it is something rather than nothing, and a salutatory reminder that one is still able to feel, that one is still alive. For others, the pain of self-harm merely replaces a different kind of pain that they can neither understand nor control.

Acts of self-harm reflect deep distress, and are most often used as a desperate and reluctant last resort—a means of surviving rather than dying, and sometimes also a means of attracting much-needed attention.

In general, it appears that teenagers, particularly teenage girls, are at the highest risk of self-harm. Perhaps this is because older people are more adept at dealing with their emotions; or because they are better at hiding their self-harming activity; or else because they self-harm only indirectly, for instance, by misusing alcohol or drugs.

Self-harm is reaching epidemic proportions in the UK. In a speech delivered to the Mental Health Conference in January 2015, the then Deputy Prime Minister Nick Clegg claimed that emergency departments see 300,000 cases of self-harm each year. This in itself is a gross underestimate of the true incidence of self-harm, as the vast majority of cases never present to hospital.

Is deliberate self-harm a culture-bound syndrome?

Deliberate self-harm is generally believed to be rare in many non-Western countries, suggesting that it is in fact a culture-bound syndrome (Chapter 7). Foreign doctors often claim never to have seen a case of self-harm prior to working in the UK.

The testimonial of Dr Eric Avevor in *The Psychiatrist* is fairly representative:

According to the British Psychological Association and the Guardian, the most recent Health Behaviour in School-Aged Children (HBSC) report is due to reveal that, of 6,000 young people aged 11, 13, and 15 surveyed across England, about 20% of the 15-year-olds reported self-harming within the last 12 months.

The last similar study of self-harm in England, published in the British Medical Journal in 2002, surveyed 6020 pupils aged 15 and 16. At the time, 'only' 6.9% of the pupils reported self-harming within the past 12 months, compared to about 20% in the 2013-14 HBSC study.

The vast majority of cases of self-harm that present to hospital involve either a tablet overdose or self-cutting, although self-cutting is much more common in the community at large. Occasionally, other forms of self-harm are also seen, such as banging or hitting body parts, scratching, hair pulling, burning or scalding, and strangulation. The drugs most commonly involved in tablet overdoses are painkillers, antidepressants, and sedatives.

According to the most recent report of self-harm in Oxford, England, of those people who present to hospital, about 25% report high suicidal intent, and about 40% are assessed as suffering from a 'major psychiatric disorder' excluding personality disorder and substance misuse. This suggests that many people who self-harm, though highly distressed, are not in fact mentally ill.

The problems most frequently cited at the time of presentation are problems with relationships, alcohol, employment or studies, finances, housing, social isolation, physical health, bereavement, and childhood emotional and sexual abuse.

For many people, self-harm is a one-off response to a severe emotional crisis. For others, it is a more long-term problem. People may carry on self-harming because they carry on suffering from the same problems, or they may stop self-harming for a time, sometimes several years, only to return to self-harm at the next major emotional crisis.

The subject [of self-harm] was hardly mentioned, let alone taught, as a topic throughout my undergraduate medical training in Ghana. In my medical school clinical years and throughout my work as a house officer in the largest teaching hospital in Ghana, I never saw or heard of a single case of self-harm. I later worked as a medical officer (hospital-based general practice) in a busy district hospital for three years and here too

I never encountered such a case ... I had a cultural shock in my first psychiatric senior house officer post in the UK when I quickly realised that self-harm was the 'bread and butter' of emergency psychiatric practice.

As Dr Avevor concedes, this stark difference could owe to under-reporting of cases in Ghana. But even if widespread, under-reporting seems unlikely to account for the full difference.

Clinical skills: Counselling for people with thoughts of self-harm

If you are plagued by thoughts of self-harm, try to take your mind off them by using one of several coping strategies and distraction techniques. An effective coping strategy is to find someone you trust, such as a friend, relative, or teacher, and to share your feelings with him or her. If you can't find anyone, or there is no one you feel comfortable sharing your feelings with, there are a number of phone lines you can ring at any time.

Engaging in creative activities such as writing, drawing, or playing a musical instrument can provide distraction, and also enable you to express and understand your feelings. Other coping strategies include reading a good book, listening to classical or jazz music, watching a comedy or nature programme, or even just cooking a simple meal or going out to the shops. Relaxation techniques like deep breathing can also help, as can yoga and meditation. However, avoid alcohol and drugs as these can make your behaviour more impulsive and uncontrollable.

In some cases, the urge to self-harm may be so great that all you can do is minimize the risks involved. Things to try: hold ice cubes in your palm and attempt to crush them, fit an elastic band around your wrist and flick it, or pluck off the hairs on your arms and legs.

If you have harmed yourself and are in pain or unable to control the bleeding, or if you have taken an overdose of whatever type or size, get someone to take you to A&E as soon as possible or call emergency services.

Once things are more settled, consider asking for a talking treatment such as counselling or cognitive behavioural therapy. Joining a local support group enables you to meet other people with similar problems, that is, people who are likely to accept and understand you, and with whom you may feel more comfortable sharing yourself. However, beware of joining unmonitored online forums and chat groups, which are open to all and sundry, and which can sometimes leave you feeling even worse than before.

6

Self-assessment

Answer by true or false.

1. The provision to a person of the means to end his life, by which he does end his life, is called assisted suicide.
2. The deliberate ending of the life of another person who has requested it and is physically unable to commit suicide is called voluntary euthanasia.
3. 'Parasuicide' is a synonym for 'attempted suicide'.
4. The majority of suicides are so-called 'rational suicides'.
5. The suicide rate is ten times higher in males than in females.
6. Suicide statistics are reliable.
7. In females, in the UK, poisoning is the most common method of suicide.
8. Leaving a suicide note suggests high suicidal intent.
9. The suicide rate peaks at Christmas time.
10. The onset of war might be expected to lead to an increase in the suicide rate.
11. Suicide rates among immigrants to the UK closely reflect those of their country of origin, highlighting the importance of cultural factors in the aetiology of suicide.
12. Two-thirds of people who complete suicide had visited a GP in the month prior to killing themselves.
13. Drug overdose is the most common form of deliberate self-harm.
14. The most important risk factor for deliberate self-harm is a history of deliberate self-harm.
15. In some cases, patients who self-harm should be taught to self-harm in less dangerous ways.

Answers

1. True.
2. True.
3. False. Strictly speaking, 'attempted suicide' is a subset of 'parasuicide'.
4. False. Only a small minority.
5. False. About four times higher.
6. False. Many suicides are unsuspected or difficult to determine, and suicide is taboo.
7. False. It is now 'hanging, strangulation and suffocation'.
8. True. As do phone messages, etc.
9. False. In the spring time.
10. False. A decrease.
11. True.
12. False. Half had visited a GP. Two-thirds had told someone of their intentions.
13. False. Cutting.
14. True.
15. True.

Anxiety, stress-related, and somatoform disorders

7

Anxiety can be defined as 'a state consisting of psychological and physical symptoms brought about by a sense of apprehension at a perceived threat'. Fear is similar to anxiety, except that with fear the threat is, or is perceived to be, more concrete, present, or imminent.

The psychological and physical symptoms of anxiety (Table 7.1) vary according to the nature and magnitude of the perceived threat, and from one person to another. Psychological symptoms may include feelings of fear and dread, an exaggerated startle reflex, poor concentration, irritability, and insomnia.

In mild to moderate anxiety, a surge in adrenaline gives rise to physical symptoms such as tremor, perspiration, muscle tension, tachycardia, and tachypnoea. Some people can also develop a dry mouth together with the irritating feeling of having a lump in the throat. This feeling, referred to in the jargon as *globus hystericus*, is associated with forced swallowing and a characteristic gulping sound that is often exploited in children's cartoons to signal fear.

In severe anxiety, hyperventilation can lead to a fall in the concentration of carbon dioxide in the blood. This gives rise to an additional set of physical symptoms, among which chest discomfort, numbness or tingling in the hands and feet, dizziness, and faintness.

Fear and anxiety can be a normal response to life experiences, a protective mechanism that has evolved both to prevent us from entering into potentially dangerous situations and to assist us in escaping from them should they befall us regardless. For instance, anxiety can prevent us from coming into close contact with disease-carrying or poisonous animals such as rats, snakes, and spiders; from engaging with a much stronger or angrier enemy; and even from declaring our undying love to someone who is unlikely to spare our feelings. If we do find ourselves in a potentially dangerous situation, the fight-or-flight response triggered by fear can help us to mount an appropriate response by priming our body for action and increasing our performance and stamina.

In short, the purpose of fear and anxiety is to preserve us from harm, and, above all, from death—whether it be literal or metaphorical, biological or psychosocial.

Table 7.1: Symptoms of anxiety

Psychological symptoms	Feelings of fear and impending doom, feelings of dizziness and faintness, restlessness, exaggerated startle response, poor concentration, irritability, insomnia and night terrors, depersonalization and derealization, *globus hystericus*.
Physical symptoms	Physical symptoms arise from autonomic arousal and hyperventilation.
Cardiovascular	Palpitations, tachycardia, chest discomfort
Gastrointestinal	Dry mouth, nausea, abdominal discomfort, frequent or loose motions
Respiratory	Tachypnoea, difficulty in catching breath, chest tightness
Genitourinary	Urinary frequency, impotence, amenorrhoea
Other/general	Hot flushes or cold chills, tremor, perspiration, headache and muscle pains, numbness and tingling sensations around the mouth and in the extremities, dizziness, faintness

Although some degree of anxiety can improve our performance on a range of tasks, severe or inappropriate anxiety can have the opposite effect and hinder our performance. Thus, whereas a confident actor may perform optimally in front of a live audience, a novice may suffer from stage fright and freeze. The relationship between anxiety and performance can be expressed graphically by a parabola or inverted 'U' (Figure 7.1).

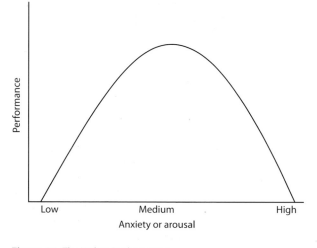

Figure 7.1. The Yerkes-Dodson curve.

According to the Yerkes-Dodson curve, our performance increases with arousal, but only up to a certain point, beyond which it begins to decline. The Yerkes-Dodson curve best applies to complex or difficult tasks, rather than simple tasks for which the relationship between arousal and performance is more linear.

Also important is the nature of the task. Generally speaking, intellectual challenges require a lower level of arousal for optimal performance than tasks that call for physical strength and stamina. This makes good sense, since those situations that trigger the greatest anxiety are generally those that call for the greatest strength and stamina, for instance, to face a foe or scamper up the nearest tree.

The Yerkes-Dodson curve indicates that very high levels of anxiety can result in handicap, even paralysis. From a medical standpoint, anxiety becomes problematic when it becomes so severe, frequent, or longstanding as to prevent us from fulfilling our occupational or social obligations. This often owes to a primary anxiety disorder, although in some instances the anxiety is secondary to another mental disorder such as depression or schizophrenia, or to a medical disorder such as hyperthyroidism or alcohol withdrawal.

Primary anxiety disorders are very common, affecting almost one in every five people in the US in any given year. As broadly conceived, they present in a great variety of forms, including phobic anxiety disorders, panic disorder, generalized anxiety disorder, post-traumatic stress disorder, conversion disorders, and culture-bound syndromes.

Epidemiology

Anxiety disorders generally take hold in early adulthood or, less commonly, in middle age. Although very common, many cases never present to medical attention, and so it is difficult to be precise about prevalence. Moreover, some of those cases that do present to medical attention might be misdiagnosed as depression or a medical disorder. According to the US National Institute of Mental Health (NIMH), anxiety disorders affect 18.1% of adults in the United States (Table 7.2). With the exceptions of social phobia and obsessive-compulsive disorder, females are more affected than males. Comorbidity is common, and anxiety disorders often co-present with depression or depressive symptoms, other anxiety disorders, personality disorder, or substance misuse.

Table 7.2: Prevalence of anxiety disorders and OCD in the US adult population (best estimate)

Phobic anxiety disorders	
Agoraphobia	0.8%
Social phobias	6.8%
Specific (simple) phobias	8.7%
Panic disorder	2.7%
Generalized anxiety disorder	3.1%
Post-traumatic stress disorder	3.5%
Obsessive-compulsive disorder	1.0%

Source: NIMH (2015)

Aetiology

Mental and medical disorders

Anxiety may overlie an anxiety disorder or a broad range of mental and medical disorders.

Mental disorders associated with anxiety include mood disorders, psychotic disorders, somatoform disorders, and eating disorders.

Medical disorders associated with anxiety include endocrine disorders such as hyperthyroidism, Cushing's disease, phaeochromocytoma, and hypoglycaemia, and drug and alcohol intoxication or withdrawal.

Genetic factors

Genetic factors play a predisposing role in the aetiology of anxiety disorder, and may manifest as 'neurotic' personality traits or neurotic cluster (cluster C) personality disorders.

Environmental factors

Anxiety disorders may be triggered and perpetuated by stress and stressful events, especially those involving a threat.

They may also result from traumatic events in childhood such as parental neglect or physical abuse.

Psychological theories

According to cognitive behavioural theories, anxiety disorders result from inappropriate thought processes.

According to psychoanalytic theory, anxiety disorders have their origins in childhood events such as separation or loss, and in unresolved childhood conflicts of psychosexual development. Phobias in particular may stem from the displacement of repressed fear onto an unrelated object or situation. The phobia is then perpetuated by avoidance behaviour that is negatively reinforced through fear reduction.

Neurochemical abnormalities

Noradrenergic neurones originating in the locus cœruleus and serotonergic neurones originating in the raphe nuclei act on the limbic system to increase anxiety, and an imbalance in these neurotransmitters, and in gamma aminobutyric acid (GABA), may contribute to symptoms. This imbalance may result from biological factors, environmental factors, or psychological factors, or, more likely, a combination of the three.

Neurosis

Neurosis is an old-fashioned but still useful term that derives from the Ancient Greek *neuron* (nerve) and loosely means 'disease of the nerves'. The core feature of neurosis is anxiety, but neurosis can manifest as a range of other problems such as irritability, depression, perfectionism, obsessive-compulsive tendencies, and even personality disorders such as anankastic personality disorder.

Although neurosis in some form or other is very common, it can prevent us from enjoying the moment, adapting usefully to our environment, and developing a richer, more complex, and more fulfilling outlook on life.

Jung believed that neurotic people fundamentally had issues with the meaning and purpose of their life. But, interestingly, he also believed that neurosis could be beneficial to some people in spite of its debilitating effects:

The reader will doubtless ask: What in the world is the value and meaning of a neurosis, this most useless and pestilent curse of humanity? To be neurotic—what good can that do? … I myself have known more than one person who owed his whole usefulness and reason for existence to a neurosis, which prevented all the worst follies in his life and forced him to a mode of living that developed his valuable potentialities. These might have been stifled had not the neurosis, with iron grip, held him to the place where he belonged.

—CG Jung, *Two Essays in Analytical Psychology*

Phobic anxiety disorders

Phobic anxiety disorders are the most common type of anxiety disorder, and involve the persistent and irrational fear of an object, activity, or situation. ICD-10 and DSM-5 recognize three types of phobic anxiety disorder: agoraphobia, social phobia, and specific phobia.

Agoraphobia

'Agoraphobia' derives from the Greek *phobos* ('fear') and *agora* ('market', 'marketplace'), and so literally means 'fear of the marketplace'. Contrary to popular belief, agoraphobia does not describe a fear of open spaces, but of places that are difficult or embarrassing to escape from, typically because they are confined, crowded, or far from home. In time, people with agoraphobia may become increasingly homebound and reliant on one or more trusted companions to accompany them on their outings.

Interestingly, there seems to be an association between agoraphobia and poor spatial orientation, suggesting that spatial disorientation, particularly in places where visual cues are sparse, may contribute to the development of the disorder. Spatial orientation is critical from an evolutionary standpoint, since it enables us not only to locate ourselves, but also our friends and foes, sources of food and water, and places of shelter and safety.

Agoraphobia may respond to cognitive behavioural techniques such as graded exposure and anxiety management. Relapse is common.

Social phobia

Social phobia is the fear of being judged by others and of being embarrassed or humiliated in one or more social or performance situations such as holding a conversation or delivering a speech.

Social phobia is not new, and Hippocrates himself once described someone who:

...through bashfulness, suspicion, and timorousness, will not be seen abroad; loves darkness as life and cannot endure the light or to sit in lightsome places; his hat still in his eyes, he will neither see, nor be seen by his good will. He dare not come in company for fear he should be misused, disgraced, overshoot himself in gesture or speeches, or be sick; he thinks every man observes him.

—Hippocrates, *The History of Epidemics, in Seven Books*

Social phobia (DSM-5: 'social anxiety disorder') has many features in common with shyness, and distinguishing between the two can be a cause of debate and controversy. Some critics claim that the label is no more than an attempt to pass off a problematic personality trait as a mental disorder and thereby legitimize its medical 'treatment'. Proponents retort that social phobia differs from simple shyness in that it usually starts at a later age and is more severe and debilitating, with much more prominent anxiety. In addition, whereas social phobia is invariably maladaptive, a certain degree of shyness can be adaptive in so far as it can protect our self-esteem and social standing, and preserve us from interacting too closely with potentially hostile or abusive strangers—which is no doubt why shyness is most pronounced in children and other vulnerable groups.

Social phobia may respond to cognitive behavioural techniques such as graded exposure and anxiety management. Alcohol and benzodiazepine misuse are more common than in other phobic anxiety disorders.

Specific phobia

Specific phobia is by far the most common of the three phobic anxiety disorders. As its name implies, it is the fear of a specific object, activity, or situation. Common specific phobias include arachnophobia (spiders), acrophobia (heights), claustrophobia (enclosed spaces), achluophobia (darkness), brontophobia (storms), and haematophobia (blood).

Unlike other anxiety disorders, which tend to begin in adulthood, specific phobias often trace their beginnings to early childhood. Moreover, we seem to have a strong innate predisposition for phobias of the natural dangers commonly faced by our ancestors such as spiders and heights, even if manmade hazards such as motor vehicles, electric cables, and text messaging now pose much greater threats to our chances of surviving and reproducing.

Specific phobias may respond to cognitive behavioural techniques such as graded exposure and anxiety management, flooding, and modelling.

Panic disorder

In a phobic anxiety disorder (whether agoraphobia, social phobia, or a specific phobia), exposure to the dreaded object, activity, or situation can trigger an attack of severe anxiety, or panic attack.

During a panic attack, symptoms of anxiety are so severe that the person fears that he is suffocating, having a heart attack, losing control, or even 'going crazy'. In time, he comes to develop a fear of the panic attacks themselves, which in turn sets off further panic attacks. A vicious circle takes hold, with the panic attacks becoming ever more frequent and ever more severe, and even occurring 'out of the blue'.

This pattern of recurrent panic attacks is referred to as 'panic disorder', and can superimpose itself onto any anxiety disorder as well as depression, substance misuse, and certain physical states and conditions such as hypoglycaemia and hyperthyroidism.

Panic disorder often leads to so-called secondary agoraphobia, in which the person becomes increasingly homebound so as to minimize the risk and consequences of suffering further panic attacks.

Panic disorder may respond to cognitive behavioural therapy (Figure 7.2).

7

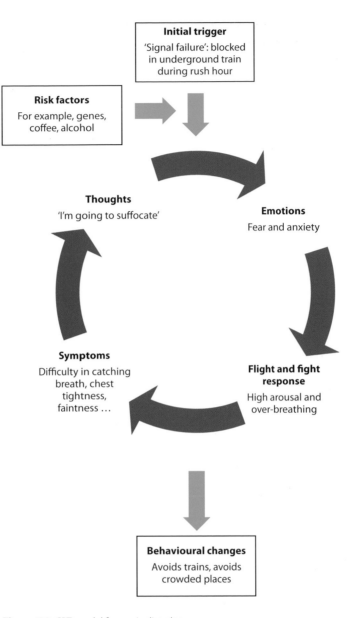

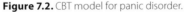

Figure 7.2. CBT model for panic disorder.

Generalized anxiety disorder (GAD)

GAD is characterized by long-standing free-floating anxiety that may fluctuate, but that is neither situational as in phobic anxiety disorders nor episodic as in panic disorder (Table 7.3). There is apprehension about a number of hypothetical events that is completely out of proportion to their actual likelihood or potential impact. People with GAD fear the future to such an extent that they behave in a manner that is overly cautious and risk-averse. They are, quite literally, 'paralyzed with fear'. Other common symptoms include symptoms of autonomic arousal, irritability, poor concentration, muscle tension, tiredness, and sleep disturbance.

The presence of prominent depressive symptoms may warrant a diagnosis of 'mixed anxiety and depressive disorder' (ICD-10).

GAD may respond to counselling and cognitive and behavioural techniques. Drugs, if they cannot be avoided, are best used on a short-term basis as an adjunct to psychological treatment.

Table 7.3: The three types of anxiety disorder compared

	Phobic anxiety	Panic disorder	GAD
Type of anxiety	Situational	Episodic	Free-floating
Associated cognitions	Fear of object or situation	Fear of symptoms	Fear of future
Associated behaviour	Avoidance	Escape	Inhibition

Clinical skills: Benzodiazepines

The Austrian scientist Leo Sternbach serendipitously discovered the first benzodiazepine in 1954, and benzodiazepines soon replaced barbiturates as the drug of choice for the treatment of anxiety and insomnia.

Benzodiazepines act at the $GABA_A$-BDZ receptor complex to enhance the inhibitory action of GABA, and they have anxiolytic, hypnotic, anticonvulsant, muscle relaxant, and amnesic properties.

They have found a clinical use in:
- Disabling anxiety disorders.
- Severe acute anxiety.
- Agitation.
- Insomnia.
- Detoxification from alcohol.
- Convulsive disorders.
- Spastic disorders.
- Involuntary movement disorders.
- Surgical pre-medication.

Potency and half-life vary considerably from one benzodiazepine to another, and choice of benzodiazepine is principally determined by the indication.

High potency, short half-life: alprazolam, lorazepam.
High potency, long half-life: clonazepam.
Low potency, short half-life: oxazepam, temazepam.
Low potency, long half-life: chlordiazepoxide.

Commoner adverse effects of benzodiazepines include psychomotor retardation, anterograde amnesia, and paradoxical reactions such as agitation or disinhibition.

Tolerance and dependence, including cross-tolerance to other benzodiazepines and to alcohol, may develop, so it is advisable to prescribe short courses and avoid repeat prescriptions. If the patient has become tolerant to benzodiazepines, their abrupt discontinuation may lead to anxiety-symptoms and rebound insomnia, and, rarely, to depression, psychosis, seizures, and *delirium tremens* (Chapter 11).

Benzodiazepines are relatively safe in overdose but toxic effects are enhanced by a number of drugs, including alcohol. The antidote to benzodiazepines is the benzodiazepine antagonist flumazenil.

Adjustment disorders and reactions to severe stress

Adjustment disorder

Adjustment disorder is a protracted response to a significant life change or life event such as a change of job, migration, or divorce. It is characterized by depressive symptoms and/or anxiety symptoms that are not severe enough to warrant a diagnosis of depressive disorder or anxiety disorder, but that nonetheless impact on social functioning.

The patient feels unable to cope and continue in the present situation, and may be prone to angry outbursts.

Supportive psychotherapy is often helpful, but adjustment disorders have a good prognosis and normally resolve within six months.

Abnormal bereavement reaction

Bereavement refers to the grief that often occurs after the loss of a loved one, and which can also occur after the loss of a pet or icon/celebrity, or the loss of an asset such as health or social status. Bereavement in such cases is normal, and varies greatly in duration and intensity from one individual to another, and from one culture to another. Various stages or phases of bereavement have been suggested, but they are neither consistent nor universal.

Sudden and unexpected loss tends to be associated with a longer and more severe bereavement reaction, as does the loss of someone who was particularly close, or with whom one had a dependent or ambivalent relationship.

A bereavement reaction is considered abnormal if it is either unusually intense or unusually prolonged, that is, if it meets the criteria for a depressive disorder or it lasts for more than six months. It is also considered abnormal if it is delayed, inhibited, or distorted. In such cases, it can be considered as a form of adjustment disorder (ICD-10).

Acute stress reaction

Acute stress reaction is an acute response to a highly threatening or catastrophic experience such as a road traffic accident, criminal assault, or natural catastrophe, which subsides in a matter of hours or days. Symptoms are variable but typically include an initial state of shock together with symptoms of anxiety and depression. Management is by removal of the stressor, reassurance, and support. Physical exhaustion and organic factors can increase vulnerability to acute stress reaction, as well as the severity of the reaction.

Post-traumatic stress disorder (PTSD)

Anxiety related to a traumatic event can also manifest in the form of post-traumatic stress disorder. PTSD is a protracted and sometimes delayed response to a highly threatening or catastrophic experience, most commonly combat exposure in men and sexual assault in women. Common symptoms include anxiety, of course, but also numbing, detachment, flashbacks, nightmares, partial or complete amnesia for the traumatic event, and avoidance of reminders of the traumatic event—although not all of these symptoms need be present for a diagnosis to be made. The symptoms can last for several years, and predispose to secondary mental disorders such as depression, other anxiety disorders, and alcohol and drug misuse.

There is little evidence to suggest that PTSD can be prevented through 'debriefing' in the aftermath of the trauma; indeed, this may even be harmful. The condition may respond to supportive therapy, cognitive behavioural therapy in the form of cognitive therapy and exposure therapy and relaxation, and group therapy. Antidepressants are sometimes prescribed, but benzodiazepines should be avoided because of the high risk of dependence. Prognosis is generally good but in some cases PTSD may persist for several years.

PTSD was first recognized in the aftermath of the First World War, and its historical epithets include 'shell shock', 'combat neurosis', and 'survivor syndrome'.

Culture-bound syndromes

Generally speaking, culture-specific, or culture-bound, syndromes are mental disturbances that only find expression in certain cultures or ethnic groups, and that are not comfortably accommodated by Western psychiatric classifications. DSM-IV defined them as 'recurrent, locality-specific patterns of aberrant behavior and troubling experience...'

There are perhaps hundreds of culture-bound syndromes. One example is dhat, which is seen in men from South Asia, and involves sudden anxiety about loss of semen in the urine, whitish discoloration of the urine, and sexual dysfunction, combined with feelings of weakness and exhaustion. The syndrome may originate in the Hindu belief that it takes forty drops of blood to create a drop of bone marrow, and forty drops of bone marrow to create a drop of semen, and thus that semen is a concentrated essence of life.

DSM-5 replaces the notion of culture-bound syndromes with three 'cultural concepts of distress': cultural syndromes, cultural idioms of distress, and cultural explanations for distress. Rather than merely listing specific cultural syndromes, DSM-5 adopts a broader approach to cultural issues, and acknowledges that all mental disorders, including DSM disorders, can be culturally shaped.

Psychiatric imperialism

Some mental disorders are, it seems, much more culturally shaped than others. For instance, PTSD, anorexia nervosa, bulimia nervosa, depression, and deliberate self-harm can all be understood as cultural syndromes. Yet, for being listed in influential classifications such as ICD-10 and DSM-5, they are usually seen, and largely legitimized, as biological and therefore universal expressions of human distress.

Thus, one criticism of classifications of mental disorders such as DSM and ICD is that, arm in arm with pharmaceutical companies, they encourage the wholesale exportation of Western mental disorders, and, more than that, the wholesale exportation of Western accounts of mental disorder, Western approaches to mental disorder, and, ultimately, Western values such as biologism, individualism, and the medicalization of distress and deviance.

In her recent book, *Depression in Japan*, anthropologist Junko Kitanaka writes that, until relatively recently, depression (*utsubyō*) had remained largely unknown to the lay population of Japan. Between 1999 and 2008, the number of people diagnosed with depression more than doubled as psychiatrists and pharmaceutical companies urged people to re-interpret their distress in terms of depression. Depression, says Kitanaka, is now one of the most frequently cited reasons for taking sick leave, and has been 'transformed from a rare disease to one of the most talked about illnesses in recent Japanese history'.

7

In *Crazy Like Us: The Globalization of the American Psyche*, journalist Ethan Watters shows how psychiatric imperialism is leading to a pandemic of Western disease categories and treatments. Watters argues that changing a culture's ideas about mental disorder actually changes that culture's disorders, and depletes the store of local beliefs and customs which, in many cases, provided better answers to people's problems than antidepressants and anti-psychotics. For Watters, the most devastating consequence of our impact on other cultures is not our golden arches, but the bulldozing of the human psyche itself.

He writes:

Looking at ourselves through the eyes of those living in places where human tragedy is still embedded in complex religious and cultural narratives, we get a glimpse of our modern selves as a deeply insecure and fearful people. We are investing our great wealth in researching and treating this disorder because we have rather suddenly lost other belief systems that once gave meaning and context to our suffering.

Distressed people are subconsciously driven to externalize their suffering, partly to make it more manageable, and partly so that it can be recognized and legitimized. According to medical historian Edward Shorter, our culture's beliefs and narratives about illness provide us with a limited number of templates or models of illness by which to externalize our distress. If authorities such as psychiatrists and celebrities appear to endorse or condone a new template such as ADHD or deliberate self-harm, the template enters into our culture's 'symptom pool' and the condition starts to spread. At the same time, tired templates seep out of the symptom pool, which may explain why conditions such as 'hysteria' and catatonic schizophrenia (schizophrenia dominated by extreme agitation or immobility and odd mannerisms and posturing) have become so rare.

The incidence of bulimia nervosa rose in 1992, the year in which journalist Andrew Morton exposed Princess Diana's 'secret disease', and peaked in 1995, when she revealed her eating disorder to the public. It began to decline in 1997, the year of her tragic death. This synchronology suggests that Princess Diana's status and glamour combined with intense press coverage of her bulimia and bulimia in general led to an increase in the incidence of the disorder.

An alternative explanation is that Princess Diana's example encouraged people to come forward and admit to their eating disorder. By the same token, it could have been that the Japanese had always suffered from depression, but had been hiding it, or had not had a template by which to recognize or externalize it. The danger for health professionals when treating people with mental disorder is to treat the template without addressing or even acknowledging the very real distress that lies beneath.

Obsessive-compulsive disorder (OCD)

According to ICD-10, OCD can be classified as predominantly obsessional thoughts, predominantly compulsive acts, or mixed obsessional thoughts and acts.

An obsessional thought is a recurrent idea, image, or impulse that is perceived as being senseless, that is unsuccessfully resisted, and that results in marked anxiety and distress. Unlike passivity phenomena such as thought insertion, an obsessional thought is recognized as being one's own, even though it might be violent or obscene. Common obsessional themes include doubt, contamination, orderliness or symmetry, safety, physical symptoms, aggression, and sex. According to the thought avoidance paradox, the more you try to avoid thinking about something, the more you actually think about it. For example, try not to think about a pink elephant. Paradoxically, the only way not to think about a pink elephant is to think about it!

A compulsive act is a recurrent stereotyped behaviour that is not useful or enjoyable but that reduces anxiety and distress. It is usually perceived as being senseless but is unsuccessfully resisted. A compulsive act may be a response to an obsessional thought or according to rules that must be applied rigidly. Common compulsive acts include washing and cleaning, arranging and ordering, checking, and other ritualistic behaviours; and mental rituals such as counting or repeating a particular phrase.

> ### Key features of obsessions and compulsions
>
> An obsession:
> - Is a recurrent idea, image, or impulse.
> - Is recognized as being a product of one's own mind.
> - Is usually perceived as being senseless.
> - Is unsuccessfully resisted.
> - Results in marked anxiety and distress, as well as functional impairment.
>
> A compulsion:
> - Is a recurrent stereotyped behaviour.
> - Reduces anxiety but is neither useful nor enjoyable.
> - Is usually perceived as being senseless.
> - Is unsuccessfully resisted.
> - Results in marked anxiety and distress, as well as functional impairment.

7

Case study: Mr MD

Mr MD is a 30-year-old father of two presenting with a nine-year history of obsessions and compulsions. He is terrified of being inadvertently responsible for harm befalling his loved ones and so checks 'dangerous' electrical appliances repeatedly to make sure that they have been switched off.

Over the years, the doubt about having switched off all the appliances has gradually increased. Simply looking at the stove no longer provides enough reassurance: instead, he must stare at each knob to make sure that it is aligned in the *off* position, and say to himself, 'It's off' over and over again. He must then place his hand on each hotplate and count to ten to make sure that the hotplate is cold. If this ritual is interrupted, or if he loses concentration, he has to start all over again, and it can take him up to fifteen minutes just to check the stove.

After that, he also has to check the kettle, toaster, and iron to make sure that they have been turned off and unplugged, and the doors and windows to make sure that they have been secured. Leaving home can take up to an hour, and the rituals leave him feeling anxious, upset, and exhausted. As he is constantly running late, he has been given several warnings at work and may well end up losing his job. Although he recognizes that his rituals are senseless, he becomes extremely distressed whenever he tries to resist them.

According to biological models of OCD, OCD results from pathology of the caudate nucleus, which fails to suppress signals from the orbitofrontal cortex. As a result, the thalamus becomes overexcited and sends strong signals back to the orbitofrontal cortex, and so on. Such a neuronal loop model of OCD is supported by MRI and PET studies, and by the documented associations between OCD and Tourette's syndrome and Sydenham's chorea, which both involve pathology of the basal ganglia.

The differential diagnosis of OCD is from depressive disorders, anxiety disorders, anankastic personality disorder, Tourette syndrome, psychotic disorders, and organic mental disorders. Comorbid mental disorders, especially depression, are common.

OCD may respond to cognitive behavioural techniques such as exposure and response prevention (ERP) or to medication in the form of high doses of an SSRI or clomipramine (a tricyclic antidepressant that also behaves as a serotonin reuptake inhibitor), with or without augmentation. Obsessive-compulsive symptoms are common

in depressive disorders, and treatment of the underlying depressive disorder may lead to improvement in the obsessive-compulsive symptoms. OCD may run a relapsing and remitting course, but untreated prognosis is poor. Neurosurgery, usually in the form of anterior cingulotomy or capsulotomy, might be indicated for very severe or refractory cases.

Clinical skills: CBT techniques for anxiety disorders and OCD

CBT is commonly used in the treatment of anxiety disorders. In CBT for phobias, the patient makes a list of problems to overcome, and then breaks each problem down into a series of tasks that can be attempted in ascending order of difficulty. For instance, a patient with arachnophobia may first think about spiders, then look at pictures of spiders, then look at real spiders from a safe distance, and so on. Relaxation techniques may also be taught to help the patient manage his or her anxiety at each stage.

One common and effective relaxation technique, called deep breathing, involves regulating one's breathing by:
- Breathing in through the nose and holding one's breath for several seconds.
- Pursing the lips and gradually releasing as much air as possible.
- Repeating this cycle *ad lib*.

CBT for panic disorder also involves graded exposure and relaxation, with an added emphasis on cognitive therapy. For instance, the patient may learn to interpret a fast heart rate as a symptom of anxiety rather than a heart attack. He may also be taught how to control his breathing and avoid hyperventilating.

CBT for OCD typically involves exposure and response prevention: the patient is taught to delay responding to his compulsive urges for increasingly long periods, while distracting himself from the tension and anxiety provoked by the delay.

Other psychological treatments for anxiety disorders include supportive therapy, counselling, psychodynamic therapy, and family therapy.

Dissociative (conversion) disorders

In a dissociative disorder, a traumatic event leads to a disruption of the usually integrated functions of consciousness, memory, identity, or perception. The patient may deny the impact of the traumatic event and/or lack concern for his disability. This lack of concern is sometimes referred to as *la belle indifférence* ('beautiful indifference').

Compared to anxiety disorders and OCD, dissociative disorders are relatively rare. They are sometimes called conversion disorders, reflecting the theory that they result from the conversion of anxiety into more tolerable symptoms (primary gain) that attract the benefits of the sick role (secondary gain). Although dissociative symptoms lack an organic basis, they are no less real than organic symptoms, and are not simply 'put on' by the patient. Another name for dissociative disorders is hysteria, but this term has largely been abandoned owing to its sexist and pejorative connotations.

According to ICD-10, dissociative disorders may involve amnesia, fugue, stupor, trance and possession, motor loss, sensory loss, convulsions, Ganser's syndrome, and multiple personalities (Table 7.4).

The differential diagnosis of dissociative disorders is from physical causes for the disturbance, other mental disorders including somatoform disorder and factitious disorder (see later), substance misuse, and malingering. It is important to exclude physical causes, but this can prove difficult and involve extensive and exhaustive investigations.

Management involves acceptance and support, physical rehabilitation if indicated, and treatment of comorbid mental disorders. Prognosis is good.

Table 7.4: ICD-10 dissociative disorders

Dissociative amnesia	Loss of memory, most commonly for a traumatic or stressful event.
Dissociative fugue	Sudden, unexpected journey that may last several months. There is memory loss and confusion about personal identity or assumption of another identity. Once the fugue ends, the memory of it is lost.
Dissociative stupor	Although conscious, the patient is motionless and mute and does not respond to stimulation. Important differential diagnoses include affective disorders, schizophrenia, and organic brain diseases.
Trance and possession disorders	Temporary replacement of a patient's identity by a spirit, ghost, deity, other person, animal, or inanimate object that is not accepted by the patient's culture as a normal part of a collective cultural or religious experience.
Dissociative motor disorders	Dissociative motor disorders may include the full range of organic motor disorders and more, but most commonly involve paralysis of muscle groups, for instance, paralysis of a limb or hemiparesis. *Atasia abasia* is a type of dissociative motor disorder involving an inability to stand or walk.
Dissociative anaesthesia	Dissociative sensory loss may accompany dissociative motor disorders and is most commonly of the 'glove and stocking' distribution. Less common are hemianaesthesia and loss of the special senses.
Dissociative convulsions	Seizures that have no organic basis. They are sometimes called 'pseudo-seizures' or 'psychogenic non-epileptic seizures'.
Ganser syndrome	A very rare syndrome characterized by *vorbeireden* or 'approximate answers' (for instance, 2 + 2 = 5), absurd statements, confusion, hallucinations, and psychogenic physical symptoms. First described in three prisoners by psychiatrist Sigbert Ganser (1853-1931) in 1898, it has been suggested that Ganser syndrome is in fact a factitious disorder.
Multiple personality disorder (MPD)	Two or more distinct identities that successively take control of the same shared body, and memory loss of each identity for the other. MPD, if it does in fact exist, is very rare.

Case study: Agatha Christie

The mystery writer Agatha Christie, who is outsold only by Shakespeare and the Bible, disappeared from her home in Berkshire, England, on the evening of December 3, 1926. Her mother, to whom she had been close, had died some months earlier, and her husband Colonel Archibald Christie (Archie) was having an affair with one Nancy Neele. Archie made little effort to disguise this affair, and on the day that Agatha disappeared he had gone to the home of some friends in Surrey to be reunited with Nancy.

Before vanishing, Agatha had written several confused notes to Archie and others: in one, she wrote that she was simply going on holiday to Yorkshire, but in another that she feared for her life. The following morning, her abandoned car was discovered in Surrey, not far from a lake called Silent Pool in which she had drowned one of her fictional characters. Inside the green Morris Cowley, she had left her fur coat, a suitcase with her belongings, and an expired driver's license. Fearing suicide, the police dredged the lake, organized as many as 15,000 volunteers to beat the surrounding countryside, and even, for the first time in England, sent up aeroplanes to scour the landscape.

In fact, Agatha had checked into a health spa in Harrogate, Yorkshire, not under her own name but—significantly—under that of 'Teresa Neele'. Her disappearance soon made the national headlines: several people at the spa thought to have recognized her, but she stuck to her story of being a bereaved mother from Cape Town. She was only reliably identified on December 14, when the police brought Archie up to her in Harrogate. As Archie entered the spa, Agatha simply said, 'Fancy, my brother has just arrived.'

Agatha never discussed this perplexing episode and excluded it from her biography. Perhaps she contrived it as an act of revenge, maybe even as a publicity stunt, but a dissociative fugue is an equally likely explanation and also the one upheld by her then doctors.

In any case, just like dissociative fugue, revenge and fame can also be construed as ego defences. In Agatha's own words, 'Most successes are unhappy. That's why they are successes—they have to reassure themselves about themselves by achieving something that the world will notice.'

Somatoform disorders

Somatoform disorders (DSM-5: somatic symptom and related disorders) and dissociative disorders are often confused. In essence, somatoform disorders are characterized by physical symptoms that cannot be accounted for (or, by DSM-5, sufficiently account for) by a physical disorder or other mental disorder. As with dissociative disorders, the symptoms are nonetheless real, and, moreover, are frequently accompanied by symptoms of anxiety or depression.

Somatoform disorders include somatization disorder, hypochrondriacal disorder, and persistent somatoform pain disorder (Table 7.5).

Table 7.5: ICD-10 somatoform disorders

Somatization disorder (Briquet's syndrome, St. Louis hysteria)	A long history of multiple, severe physical symptoms that cannot be accounted for by a physical disorder or other mental disorder. Somatization is more common in females.
Hypochondriacal disorder (Hypochrondriasis)	A fear or belief of having a serious physical disorder despite medical reassurance to the contrary. In ICD-10, body dysmorphic disorder (dysmorphophobia) is included under hypochondriacal disorder. Risk factors for hypochrondriacal disorder include being a medical student, especially a male one.
Persistent somatoform pain disorder	Chronic pain that cannot be accounted for by a physical disorder or other mental disorder.

Management of somatoform disorders involves acceptance, although it is also important not to reinforce any false beliefs. All healthcare professionals involved in the patient's care need to provide him or her with a clear and consistent explanation for the symptoms. Investigations should be kept to a minimum and guided only by clinical necessity. Cognitive behavioural techniques and treatment of comorbid mental disorders may be helpful, even if patients with a somatoform disorder are often reluctant to accept psychiatric treatment.

7

Distinguishing somatoform disorders from factitious disorders and malingering

Somatoform disorders are characterized by physical symptoms that cannot be accounted for by a physical disorder or other mental disorder, but that are nonetheless real.

Factitious disorders are characterized by psychological or physical symptoms that are manufactured or exaggerated for the purpose of assuming the sick role. DSM-5 distinguishes 'factitious disorder imposed on self' (Munchausen syndrome) from 'factitious disorder imposed upon another' (Munchausen syndrome by proxy), in which the perpetrator and the patient or victim are separate individuals. Munchausen syndrome is named after an 18th century Prussian cavalry officer, Baron von Munchausen (1720-1797), who was one of the greatest liars in recorded history. One of his many 'hair-raising' claims was to have pulled himself up from a swamp by his hair, or, in an alternative version, by the strap of his boots.

Malingering is characterized by psychological and physical symptoms that are manufactured or exaggerated for a purpose other than assuming the sick role, such as evading the police, claiming compensation, or obtaining shelter for the night. Malingering is not a mental disorder.

A philosophical cure for anxiety

In his paper of 1943, *A Theory of Human Motivation*, psychologist Abraham Maslow (1908-1970) proposed that healthy human beings had a certain number of needs, and that these needs are arranged in a hierarchy, with some needs (such as physiological and safety needs) being more primitive or basic than others (such as social and ego needs). Maslow's so-called 'hierarchy of needs' is often presented as a five-level pyramid (Figure 7.3), with higher needs coming into focus only once lower, more basic needs have been met.

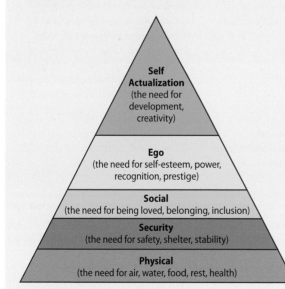

Figure 7.3. Maslow's hierarchy of needs.

Maslow called the bottom four levels of the pyramid 'deficiency needs' because we do not feel anything if they are met, but become anxious or distressed if they are not. Thus, physiological needs such as eating, drinking, and sleeping are deficiency needs, as are safety needs, social needs such as friendship and sexual intimacy, and ego needs such as self-esteem and recognition. On the other hand, he called the fifth, top level of the pyramid a 'growth need' because our need to self-actualize enables us to fulfil our true and highest potential as human beings.

Once we have met our deficiency needs, the focus of our anxiety shifts to self-actualization, and we begin, even if only at a sub- or semi-conscious level, to contemplate our bigger picture. However, only a small minority of people is able to self-actualize because self-actualization requires uncommon qualities such as honesty, independence, awareness, objectivity, creativity, and originality.

Maslow's hierarchy of needs has been criticized for being overly schematic and lacking in scientific grounding, but it presents an intuitive and potentially useful theory of human motivation. After all, there is surely some truth in the popular saying that one cannot philosophize on an empty stomach, or in Aristotle's observation that, 'all paid work absorbs and degrades the mind'.

Many people who have met all their deficiency needs do not self-actualize, instead inventing more deficiency needs for themselves, because to contemplate the meaning of their life and of life in general would lead them to entertain the possibility of their meaninglessness and the prospect of their own death and annihilation.

A person who begins to contemplate his bigger picture may come to fear that life is meaningless and death inevitable, but at the same time cling on to the cherished belief that his life is eternal or important or at least significant. This gives rise to an inner conflict that is sometimes referred to as 'existential anxiety' or, more colourfully, 'the trauma of non-being'.

While fear and anxiety and their pathological forms (such as agoraphobia, panic disorder, or PTSD) are grounded in threats to life, existential anxiety is rooted in the brevity and apparent meaninglessness or absurdity of life. Existential anxiety is so disturbing and unsettling that most people avoid it at all costs, constructing a false reality out of goals, ambitions, habits, customs, values, culture, and religion so as to deceive themselves that their lives are special and meaningful and that death is distant or delusory.

However, such self-deception comes at a heavy price. According to philosopher Jean-Paul Sartre (1905-1980), people who refuse to face up to 'non-being' are acting in 'bad faith', and living out a life that is inauthentic and unfulfilling. Facing up to non-being can bring insecurity, loneliness, responsibility, and consequently anxiety, but it can also bring a sense of calm, freedom, and even nobility. Far from being pathological, existential anxiety is a sign of health, strength, and courage, and a harbinger of bigger and better things to come.

For theologian Paul Tillich (1886-1965), refusing to face up to non-being leads not only to a life that is inauthentic but also to pathological (or neurotic) anxiety.

In *The Courage to Be*, Tillich asserts:

He who does not succeed in taking his anxiety courageously upon himself can succeed in avoiding the extreme situation of despair by escaping into neurosis. He still affirms himself but on a limited scale. Neurosis is the way of avoiding nonbeing by avoiding being.

According to this outlook, pathological anxiety, though seemingly grounded in threats to life, in fact arises from repressed existential anxiety, which itself arises from our uniquely human capacity for self-consciousness.

Facing up to non-being enables us to put our life into perspective, see it in its entirety, and thereby lend it a sense of direction and unity. If the ultimate source of anxiety is fear of the future, the future ends in death; and if the ultimate source of anxiety is uncertainty, death is the only certainty. It is only by facing up to death, accepting its inevitability, and integrating it into life that we can escape from the pettiness and paralysis of anxiety, and, in so doing, free ourselves to make the most out of our lives and out of ourselves.

Some philosophers have gone even further by asserting that the very purpose of life is none other than to prepare for death. In Plato's *Phaedo*, Socrates, who is not long to die, tells the philosophers Simmias and Cebes that absolute justice, absolute beauty, or absolute good cannot be apprehended with the eyes or any other bodily organ, but only by the mind or soul. Therefore, the philosopher seeks in as far as possible to separate body from soul and become pure soul. As death is the complete separation of body and soul, the philosopher aims at death, and indeed can be said to be almost dead.

Self-assessment

Answer by true or false.

1. Anxiety disorders are discrete, well-defined disorders that rarely blur.
2. Depersonalization and derealization are delusions.
3. Globus hystericus is the fear that the world is mad or going mad.
4. Females are twice as likely to suffer from obsessive-compulsive disorder as males.
5. According to cognitive behavioural theories, anxiety disorders have their origins in childhood events such as separation and loss, and in unresolved childhood conflicts of psychosexual development.
6. According to psychoanalytic theory, phobias arise from intrapsychic conflicts that are repressed and then displaced onto the feared object, activity, or situation.
7. Some people are far more prone to acute stress reaction than others.
8. A phobia is usually recognized as being irrational.
9. Specific phobias most often have their onset in adolescence or early adulthood.
10. Agoraphobia is the most common type of phobic anxiety disorder.
11. Most agoraphobia is secondary to panic disorder.
12. In social phobia, there is persistent irrational fear of places that are difficult or embarrassing to escape from.
13. Panic attacks are characterized by gradual onset of severe anxiety lasting for about 20-30 minutes.
14. Generalized anxiety disorder is characterized by long-standing anxiety that does not fluctuate in intensity, and that is neither situational nor episodic.
15. Evidence suggests that debriefing in the aftermath of a trauma can help to prevent the development of PTSD.
16. PTSD can be understood in terms of a culture-bound syndrome.
17. Adjustment disorder is a protracted response to a highly threatening or catastrophic experience.
18. With dissociative disorders, the patient may deny the impact of the traumatic event and/or lack concern for his disability. This lack of concern is sometimes referred to as Briquet's syndrome.
19. In a somatoform disorder, the patient's symptoms are real.
20. Somatization disorder is more common in males.
21. One of the principal factors distinguishing hypochondriasis from persistent delusional disorder is the fixity with which the belief is held.
22. One of the principal factors distinguishing an obsession from thought insertion is that an obsession is recognized as a product of one's own mind.
23. Whereas obsessive-compulsive disorder is said to be egodystonic (opposed to one's own self-image), anankastic personality disorder is said to be egosyntonic (consistent with one's own self-image).

24. Egosyntonic disorders such as anorexia nervosa, paranoid personality disorder, narcissistic personality disorder, and persistent delusional disorder are particularly difficult to manage.
25. Factitious disorder is the American term for malingering.
26. Choice of benzodiazepine is principally determined by half-life and adverse effects.

27. Commoner adverse effects of benzodiazepines include psychomotor retardation, memory impairment, and disinhibitory reactions.
28. Tolerance and dependence to benzodiazepines are common.
29. The toxic effects of benzodiazepines are enhanced by alcohol.
30. The antidote to benzodiazepines is the benzodiazepine antagonist naltrexone.

Answers

1. False.
2. False.
3. False. It is the irritating feeling of having a lump in the throat.
4. False. In social phobia and OCD, the male:female ratio is closer to 1:1.
5. False. This is according to psychoanalytic theory.
6. True.
7. True.
8. True.
9. False. Unlike other anxiety disorders, specific phobias usually trace their beginnings to early childhood.
10. False. Specific phobias.
11. True.
12. False. This describes agoraphobia.
13. False. Sudden onset.
14. False. It does fluctuate in intensity.
15. False.
16. True.
17. False. This describes PTSD.
18. False. It is sometimes referred to as *la belle indifférence*.
19. True.
20. False.
21. True
22. True.
23. True.
24. True.
25. False. These are not synonyms.
26. False. Half-life and potency.
27. True.
28. True.
29. True.
30. False. Flumazenil.

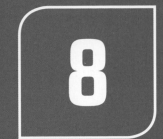

Personality disorders

History of personality disorders

The study of human personality or 'character' (from the Greek *charaktêr*, the mark impressed upon a coin) dates back at least to antiquity. In his *Characters*, Tyrtamus (371-287 BC)—nicknamed Theophrastus or 'divinely speaking' by his friend Aristotle—divided the people of ancient Athens into thirty different personality types. The *Characters* exerted a strong influence on subsequent studies of human personality such as those of Thomas Overbury (1581-1613) in England and Jean de la Bruyère (1645-1696) in France.

Table 8.1: Theophrastus' 30 personality types

The ironical man	The superstitious man
The flatterer	The grumbler
The garrulous man	The distrustful man
The boor	The offensive man
The complaisant man	The unpleasant man
The reckless man	The man of petty ambition
The chatty man	The mean man
The gossip	The boastful man
The shameless man	The arrogant man
The penurious man	The coward
The gross man	The oligarch
The unseasonable man	The late-learner
The officious man	The evil-speaker
The stupid man	The patron of rascals
The surly man	The avaricious man
	The aristocratic temper

The concept of personality disorder itself is much more recent and tentatively dates back to Philippe Pinel's 1801 description of *manie sans délire*, a condition which he characterized as outbursts of rage and violence (*manie*) in the absence of any symptoms of psychosis such as delusions and hallucinations (*délires*).

Across the English Channel, physician JC Prichard (1786-1848) coined the term 'moral insanity' in 1835 to refer to a larger group of people characterized by 'morbid perversion of the natural feelings, affections, inclinations, temper, habits, moral dispositions and natural impulses', but the term, probably considered too broad and non-specific, soon fell into disuse.

Some 60 years later, in 1896, Emil Kraepelin described seven forms of antisocial behaviour under the umbrella of 'psychopathic personality', a term later broadened by Kraepelin's younger colleague Kurt Schneider to include those who 'suffer from their abnormality'. Schneider's seminal volume of 1923, *Die psychopathischen Persönlichkeiten* (*Psychopathic Personalities*), still forms the basis of current classifications of personality disorders.

Classification of personality disorders

ICD-10 defines personality disorder as 'a severe disturbance in the personality and behavioural tendencies of the individual; not directly resulting from disease, damage, or other insult to the brain, or from another psychiatric disorder; usually involving several areas of the personality; nearly always associated with considerable personal distress and social disruption; and usually manifest since childhood or adolescence and continuing throughout adulthood.'

According to DSM-5, a personality disorder can be diagnosed if there are significant impairments in self and interpersonal functioning together with one or more pathological personality traits. In addition, these must be:

- Relatively stable across time and consistent across situations.
- Not better understood as normative for the individual's developmental stage or social and cultural environment.
- Not solely due to the direct effects of a substance or general medical condition.

DSM-5 lists ten personality disorders, and allocates each to one of three groups or 'clusters': A, B, or C (Table 8.2).

Table 8.2: DSM-5 classification of personality disorders

Cluster	Description	Personality disorders in the cluster
A	Odd, bizarre, eccentric	Paranoid Schizoid Schizotypal*
B	Dramatic, erratic	Antisocial (Dissocial) Borderline (Emotionally unstable) Histrionic Narcissistic
C	Anxious, fearful	Avoidant Dependent Anankastic

* In ICD-10, schizotypal personality disorder is classified alongside schizophrenia as 'schizotypal disorder'.

Before going on to characterize these ten personality disorders, it should be emphasized that they are more the product of historical observation than scientific study, and thus that they are rather vague and imprecise constructs. As a result, they rarely present in their classic 'textbook' form, but rather tend to blur into one another. Their division into three clusters in DSM-5 is intended to

reflect this tendency, with any given personality disorder most likely to blur with other personality disorders within its cluster.

Characterizing the ten personality disorders is hard enough, but diagnosing them reliably is even more so. For instance, how far from the norm must personality traits deviate before they can be counted as disordered? How significant is 'significant impairment'? And how is 'impairment' to be defined? Whatever the answers to these questions, they are bound to include a large part of subjectivity. Personal dislike, prejudice, or a clash of values can all play a part in arriving at a diagnosis of personality disorder, and it has been argued that the diagnosis amounts to little more than a convenient label for undesirables and social deviants.

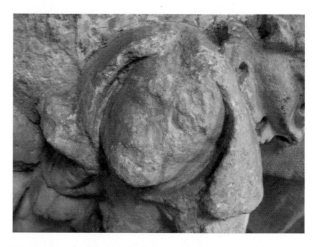

Figure 8.1. Stone face at Dorchester Abbey. 'Personality' derives from the Ancient Greek 'persona', meaning 'mask'.

Epidemiology

It is estimated that the prevalence of personality disorders is about 10% in the normal population, and considerably higher in psychiatric out- and in-patients—although the exact figures ultimately depend on where clinicians draw the line between 'normal' and 'abnormal' personality.

The high prevalence of personality disorders or deviations underscores the importance of assessing personality as part of the psychiatric history.

Several epidemiological studies have uncovered an excess of personality disorder in males, younger adults, and urban dwellers.

Aetiology

Personality disorders are generally thought to arise from a combination of genetic factors and adverse early life experiences such as parental loss or emotional, physical, or sexual abuse.

Although personality is usually acquired or 'fixed' in childhood and adolescence, profound and enduring personality change can occasionally occur in adulthood after exposure to a highly threatening or catastrophic experience, or after recovery from a mental disorder. Organic causes of significant personality change include brain disease and head injury.

Otherwise, personality can only evolve incrementally as we acquire greater experience and understanding, including self-understanding.

Clinical features

The majority of people who meet the diagnostic criteria for a personality disorder never come into contact with mental health services, and those who do usually do so in the context of another mental disorder or at a time of crisis, commonly after self-harming or falling foul of the law.

Nonetheless, personality disorders are important to health professionals because they predispose to mental disorder and affect the presentation and management of existing mental disorder. They also result in considerable distress and impairment, and so may need treatment 'in their own right'.

Whether this ought to be the remit of the health professions is a matter of debate and controversy, especially with regard to those personality disorders which predispose to criminal activity and which are treated with the primary purpose of preventing crime.

Paranoid personality disorder

Paranoid personality disorder (PD) is characterized by a pervasive distrust of others, including even friends, family, and partner. As a result, the person is guarded and suspicious, and constantly on the lookout for clues or suggestions to validate his fears. He also has a strong sense of personal rights: he is overly sensitive to setbacks and rebuffs, easily feels shame and humiliation, and persistently bears grudges. Unsurprisingly, he tends to withdraw from others and to struggle with building close relationships. The principal ego defence in paranoid PD is projection, which involves attributing one's unacceptable thoughts and feelings to other people. A large long-term twin study found that paranoid PD is modestly heritable, and that it shares a portion of its genetic and environmental risk factors with schizoid PD and schizotypal PD.

Schizoid personality disorder

The term 'schizoid' designates a natural tendency to direct attention toward one's inner life and away from the external world. A person with schizoid PD is detached and aloof and prone to introspection and fantasy. He has no desire for social or sexual relationships, is indifferent to others and to social norms and conventions, and lacks emotional response. A competing theory about people with schizoid PD is that they are in fact highly sensitive with a rich inner life: they experience a deep longing for intimacy but find initiating and maintaining close relationships too difficult or distressing, and so retreat into their inner world. People with schizoid PD rarely present to medical attention because, despite their reluctance to form close relationships, they are generally well functioning and untroubled by their apparent oddness.

Schizotypal personality disorder

Schizotypal PD is characterized by oddities of appearance, behaviour, and speech, unusual perceptual experiences, and anomalies of thinking similar to those seen in schizophrenia. These latter can include odd beliefs, magical thinking (for instance, thinking that speaking of the devil can make him appear), suspiciousness, and obsessive ruminations. People with schizotypal PD often fear social interaction and think of others as harmful. This may lead them to develop so-called ideas of reference, that is, beliefs or intuitions that events and happenings are somehow related to them. So whereas people with schizotypal PD and people with schizoid PD both avoid social interaction, with the former it is because they fear others, whereas with the latter it is because they have no desire to interact with others or find interacting with others too difficult or disappointing. People with schizotypal PD have a higher than average probability of developing schizophrenia, and, indeed, the condition used to be called 'latent schizophrenia'.

Antisocial personality disorder

Until Schneider broadened the concept of personality disorder to include those who 'suffer from their abnormality', personality disorder was more or less synonymous with antisocial personality disorder. Antisocial PD is much more common in men than in women, and is characterized by a callous unconcern for the feelings of others. The person disregards social rules and obligations, is irritable and aggressive, acts impulsively, lacks guilt, and fails to learn from experience. In many cases, he has no difficulty finding relationships—and can even appear extremely charming (the so-called 'charming psychopath')—but these relationships are usually fiery, turbulent, and short-lived. As antisocial PD is the mental disorder most closely correlated with crime, he is likely to have a criminal record or a history of being in and out of prison.

Although a personality disorder should not be firmly diagnosed before adulthood, the presence of three types of behaviour in children—sometimes referred to as Macdonald's triad—is thought to predict the later development of antisocial PD: bedwetting, cruelty to animals, and pyromania (impulsive fire-setting for gratification or relief).

Clinical skills: Antisocial personality disorder

Possible findings in the history of a person with antisocial personality disorder include:
- History of bedwetting, cruelty to animals, and pyromania (Macdonald's triad).
- History of truanting, bullying, being expelled or suspended from school, or leaving school early.
- Poor employment history with several job changes and long periods of unemployment.
- Convictions for assault and damage to property.
- Brief relationships, often with violence to partners.
- Substance misuse, especially sedatives such as alcohol and benzodiazepines.

Psychopathy

About 20% of people with antisocial personality disorder also meet the more restrictive criteria for psychopathy, as defined by Hare's Psychopathy Checklist-Revised (PCL-R). PCL-R is a clinical rating scale of 20 items, each scored on a three-point gradation. In addition to lifestyle and criminal behaviour, it measures aspects such as grandiosity, callousness, impulsivity, lack of remorse, pathological lying, and glib and superficial charm.

Borderline personality disorder

In borderline PD (or emotionally unstable PD), the person essentially lacks a sense of self, and, as a result, experiences feelings of emptiness and fears of abandonment. There is a pattern of intense but unstable relationships, emotional instability, outbursts of anger and violence (especially in response to criticism), and impulsive behaviour. Suicidal threats and acts of self-harm are common, for which reason many people with borderline PD frequently come to medical attention.

Borderline PD was so-called because it was thought to lie on the 'borderline' between neurotic (anxiety) disorders and psychotic disorders such as schizophrenia and bipolar disorder.

Case study: Miss GL

Twenty-eight-year old Miss GL was brought to A&E after taking an impulsive overdose. The overdose was prompted by an argument with her boyfriend, Jack, during which he threatened to end their relationship. Jack reported that Miss GL took an overdose of 16 paracetamol tablets just as he had his foot in the front door. As she swallowed the tablets, she screamed out, 'I hate you! Look at me, I'm going to die and it's all your fault!'

Medical records reveal that Miss GL last took an overdose only three months ago, in the heat of an argument with her mother. They also reveal that she has used all kinds of drugs, and that she had a road traffic accident only nine months ago. Upon further questioning, it transpires that she has dropped out of two college courses, and has never held down a job for more than six months.

By the time she left A&E, Miss GL was no longer angry but excited at the prospect of going out for a meal with Jack.

Is borderline personality disorder sexist?

It has been suggested that borderline personality disorder often results from childhood sexual abuse, and that it is more common in women in part because women are more likely to suffer sexual abuse. However, feminists have argued that borderline PD is more common in women because women presenting with angry and promiscuous behaviour tend to be labelled with it, whereas men presenting with similar behaviour tend instead to be labelled with antisocial PD.

Histrionic personality disorder

People with histrionic personality disorder lack a sense of self-worth, and depend for their wellbeing on attracting the attention and approval of others. They often seem to be dramatizing or 'playing a part' in a bid to be heard and seen. Indeed, 'histrionic' derives from the Latin *histrionicus*, 'pertaining to the actor'. People with histrionic PD may take great care of their appearance and behave in a manner that is overly charming or inappropriately seductive. As they crave excitement and act on impulse or suggestion, they can place themselves at risk of accident or exploitation. Their dealings with others often seem insincere or superficial, which, in the longer term, can adversely impact on their social and romantic relationships. This is especially distressing to them, as they are sensitive to criticism and rejection, and react badly to loss or failure. A vicious circle may take hold in which the more rejected they feel, the more histrionic they become; and the more histrionic they become, the more rejected they feel. It can be argued that a vicious circle of some kind is at the heart of every personality disorder, and, indeed, every mental disorder.

Narcissistic personality disorder

In narcissistic personality disorder, the person has an excessively high regard for his own importance, a sense of entitlement, and a need to be admired. He is envious of others and expects them to be the same of him. He lacks empathy and readily exploits others to achieve his aims. To others, he may seem self-absorbed, controlling, intolerant, selfish, or insensitive. If he feels obstructed or ridiculed, he can fly into a fit of destructive anger and revenge. Such a reaction is sometimes called 'narcissistic rage', and can have disastrous consequences for all those involved.

The alchemist picked up a book that someone in the caravan had brought. Leafing through the pages, he found a story about Narcissus.

The Alchemist knew the legend of Narcissus, a youth who daily knelt beside a lake to contemplate his own beauty. He was so fascinated by himself that, one morning, he fell into the lake and drowned. At the spot where he fell, a flower was born, which was called the narcissus.

But this was not how the author of the book ended the story. He said that when Narcissus died, the Goddesses of the Forest appeared and found the lake, which had been fresh water, transformed into a lake of salty tears.

'Why do you weep?' the Goddesses asked.

'I weep for Narcissus,' the lake replied.

'Ah, it is no surprise that you weep for Narcissus,' they said, 'for though we always pursued him in the forest, you alone could contemplate his beauty close at hand.'

'But… was Narcissus beautiful?' the lake asked.

'Who better than you to know that?' the Goddesses said in wonder, 'After all, it was by your banks that he knelt each day to contemplate himself!'

The lake was silent for some time. Finally it said: 'I weep for Narcissus, but I never noticed that Narcissus was beautiful. I weep because, each time he knelt beside my banks, I could see, in the depths of his eyes, my own beauty reflected.'

'What a lovely story,' the Alchemist thought.

—Paulo Coehlo, Prologue to *The Alchemist*.

Translated from the Portuguese by Clifford Landers and reproduced with the permission of Paulo Coehlo.

Avoidant personality disorder

People with avoidant personality disorder believe that they are socially inept, unappealing, or inferior, and constantly fear being embarrassed, criticized, or rejected. They avoid meeting others unless they are certain of being liked, and are restrained even in their intimate relationships. Avoidant PD is strongly associated with anxiety disorders, and may also be associated with actual or felt rejection by parents or childhood peers. Research suggests that people with avoidant PD excessively monitor internal reactions, both their own and those of others, which prevents them from engaging naturally or fluently in social situations. A vicious circle takes hold in which the more they monitor their internal reactions, the more inept they feel; and the more inept they feel, the more they monitor their internal reactions. Self-oblivion is often all that is required to carry the day.

Dependent personality disorder

Dependent personality disorder is characterized by a lack of self-confidence and an excessive need to be looked after. The person needs a lot of help in making everyday decisions and surrenders important life decisions to the care of others. He greatly fears abandonment and may go to considerable lengths to secure and maintain relationships.

A person with dependent PD sees himself as inadequate and helpless, and so surrenders personal responsibility and submits himself to one or more protective others, whom he idealizes as competent and powerful, and towards whom he behaves in a manner that is subservient and ingratiating.

People with dependent PD often end up with people with a cluster B personality disorder, who feed on the unconditional high regard in which they are held.

Overall, people with dependent PD maintain a naïve and childlike perspective, and have limited insight into themselves and others. This entrenches their dependency, and leaves them vulnerable to abuse and exploitation.

Anankastic personality disorder

Anankastic personality disorder is characterized by excessive preoccupation with details, rules, lists, order,

organization, or schedules; perfectionism so extreme that it prevents a task from being completed; and devotion to work and productivity at the expense of leisure and relationships. A person with anankastic PD is typically doubting and cautious, rigid and controlling, humourless, and miserly. His underlying anxiety arises from a perceived lack of control over a world that eludes his understanding; and the more he tries to exert control, the more out of control he feels. In consequence, he has little tolerance for complexity or nuance, and tends to simplify the world by seeing things as either all good or all bad—an ego defence called 'splitting'. His relationships with colleagues, friends, and family are often strained by the rigid and unreasonable demands that he makes upon them.

Can personality disorder be good for you?

While personality disorders may lead to 'severe impairment', they may also lead to extraordinary achievement. A 2005 study by Board and Fritzon found that histrionic, narcissistic, and anankastic personality disorders are *more* common in high-level executives than in mentally disordered criminal offenders at the high security Broadmoor Hospital.

This suggests that people often benefit from non-normative and potentially maladaptive personality traits. For instance, people with histrionic personality disorder may be more adept at charming and cajoling others, and therefore at building and exercising professional relationships. People with narcissistic personality disorder may be highly ambitious, confident, and self-motivated, and able to employ people and situations to maximum advantage. And people with anankastic personality

disorder may get quite far up their career ladder simply by being so devoted to work and productivity. Even people with borderline personality disorder may at times be bright, witty, and the life and soul of the party.

In their study, Board and Fritzon described the executives with a personality disorder as 'successful psychopaths' and the criminal offenders as 'unsuccessful psychopaths', and it may be that highly successful people and disturbed psychopaths have more in common than first meets the eye. As psychologist and philosopher William James (1842-1910) put it, 'When a superior intellect and a psychopathic temperament coalesce… in the same individual, we have the best possible condition for the kind of effective genius that gets into the biographical dictionaries.'

Differential diagnosis

The principal differential diagnosis of personality disorder is from affective disorders, substance misuse, psychotic disorders, anxiety disorders (especially phobia and panic disorder), obsessive-compulsive disorder, intellectual disability, dementia, and autism.

Management

Psychotropic drugs and in-patient admissions should be minimized. A long-term management plan that spells out realistic and mutually agreed goals should be communicated to everyone involved, or potentially involved, in the patient's care. The plan may include emo-

tional and practical support, psychological treatments, monitoring, and crisis contingencies. Psychological treatments may take the form of individual therapy, group therapy, or milieu therapy. Milieu therapy emphasizes the patient's treatment environment and everyday occurrences and interactions, and is epitomized by the therapeutic communities pioneered by the Cassel and Henderson Hospitals (see below). Dialectical behavioural therapy (DBT) is an effective psychological treatment for borderline personality disorder and recurrent self-harm based on Buddhist teachings, cognitive and behavioural therapy, and dialectics.

The Complex Needs Service (CNS) caters for people with long-standing and intractable emotional problems or interpersonal difficulties—often although not invariably people with a diagnosis of personality disorder. A person may be referred to the CNS, but in most cases is encouraged to self-refer by proactively calling or emailing. He then meets with a CNS staff member to discuss the CNS and his problems and dispositions. After this initial meeting, he may decide to join a weekly 'options' group, which aims to prepare him to join a therapeutic community (TC). He may attend the options group for up to one year, during which time he can decide whether or not to join the TC.

Joining the TC involves committing to attend a daily programme every weekday for 18 months. The idea behind a TC is that the best way of improving is by interacting positively with others, that is, by forming relationships that enable all parties to feel mutually accepted, valued, and supported. A TC is governed by a set of values and beliefs about how people should treat one another based on the principles of self-awareness, interdependence, respect, and responsibility. Apart from offering a trusting environment, the TC also offers a daily programme of therapeutic activities including individual therapy, group therapy, creative therapies, social and cultural events, and education and work placements. Members participate in the running of the TC, and may even get involved in chores such as cooking, cleaning, and gardening. Members and staff meet regularly to receive feedback from one another and discuss and decide upon the running of the community.

Prognosis

Personality disorders are lifelong disorders, but tend to mitigate in middle and old age as people grow in wisdom. For instance, at 15-year follow-up, most people with borderline personality disorder no longer meet the criteria for the disorder. Important complications of personality disorder include depression, substance misuse, accidents, and deliberate self-harm and suicide; and social complications such as isolation, unemployment, and crime.

Forensic psychiatry

It has been estimated that the prevalence of personality disorders in the prison population is as high as 75%. Often described as the interface between mental health and the law, forensic psychiatry is the sub-specialism of psychiatry dedicated to the assessment, treatment, and rehabilitation of mentally disordered people who have come into contact with the criminal justice system. Forensic psychiatrists care for their in-patients in locked wards, including the four national high security hospitals: Ashworth, Broadmoor, and Rampton in England, and Carstairs in Scotland. They also deliver out-patient care in prisons and communities, and advise local general psychiatrists on such matters as risk and the management of antisocial behaviour. An important aspect of their job is to provide evidence in court and prepare legal reports on medico-legal issues such as fitness to plead and diminished responsibility.

8

The psychology of self-deception

In psychoanalytic theory, ego defences are unconscious processes that we deploy to diffuse the fear and anxiety that arise when who we think we are or who we think we should be (our conscious 'superego') comes into conflict with who we really are (our unconscious 'id').

For instance, at an unconscious level a man may find himself attracted to another man, but at a conscious level he may find this attraction flatly unacceptable. To diffuse the anxiety that arises from this conflict, he may deploy one or several ego defences. For example, (1) he might refuse to admit to himself that he is attracted to this man. Or (2) he might superficially adopt ideas and behaviours that are diametrically opposed to those of a stereotypical homosexual, such as going out for several pints with the lads, banging his fists on the counter, and peppering his speech with loud profanities. Or (3) he might transfer his attraction onto someone else and then berate him for being gay (young children can teach us much through playground retorts such as 'mirror, mirror' and 'what you say is what you are'). In each case, the man has used a common ego defence, respectively, repression, reaction formation, and projection.

Repression can be thought of as 'motivated forgetting': the active, albeit unconscious, 'forgetting' of unacceptable drives, emotions, ideas, or memories. Repression is often confused with denial, which is the refusal to admit to certain unacceptable or unmanageable aspects of reality. Whereas repression relates to mental or internal stimuli, denial relates to external stimuli. That said, repression and denial often work together, and can be difficult to disentangle.

Repression can also be confused with distortion, which is the reshaping of reality to suit one's inner needs. For instance, a person who has been beaten black and blue by his father no longer recalls these traumatic events (repression), and instead sees his father as a gentle and loving man (distortion). In this example, there is a clear sense of the distortion not only building upon but also reinforcing the repression.

Reaction formation is the superficial adoption—and, often, exaggeration—of emotions and impulses that are diametrically opposed to one's own. A possible high-profile case of reaction formation is that of a particular US congressman, who, as chairman of the Missing and Exploited Children's Caucus, introduced legislation to protect children from exploitation by adults over the Internet. The congressman resigned when it later emerged that he had been exchanging sexually explicit electronic messages with a teenage boy. Other, classic, examples of reaction formation include the alcoholic who extolls the virtues of abstinence and the rich student who attends and even organizes anti-capitalist rallies.

Projection is the attribution of one's unacceptable thoughts and feelings to others. Like distortion, projection necessarily involves repression as a first step, since unacceptable thoughts and feelings need to be repudiated before they can be attributed to others. Classic examples of projection include the envious person who believes that everyone envies him, the covetous person who lives in constant fear of being dispossessed, and the person with fantasies of infidelity who suspects that his partner is cheating on him.

Just as common is splitting, which can be defined as the division or polarization of beliefs, actions, objects, or people into good and bad by selectively focusing on either their positive or negative attributes. This is often seen in politics, for instance, when left-wingers caricature right-wingers as selfish and narrow-minded, and right-wingers caricature left-wingers as irresponsible and self-serving hypocrites. Other classic examples of splitting are the religious zealot who divides people into blessed and damned, and the child of divorcees who idolizes one parent while shunning the other. Splitting diffuses the anxiety that arises from our inability to grasp a complex and nuanced state of affairs by simplifying and schematizing it so that it can more readily be processed or accepted.

Splitting also arises in groups, with people inside the group being seen in a positive light, and people outside the group in a negative light. Another phenomenon that occurs in groups is groupthink, which is not strictly speaking an ego defence, but which is so important as to be worthy of mention. Groupthink arises when members of a group unconsciously seek to minimize conflict by failing to critically test, analyse, and evaluate ideas. As a result, decisions reached by the group tend to be more irrational than those that would have been reached by any one member of the group acting alone. Even married couples can fall into groupthink, for instance, when they decide to take their holidays in places that neither wanted, but thought that the other wanted. Groupthink arises because members of a group are afraid both of criticizing and of being criticized, and also because of the hubristic sense of confidence and invulnerability that arises from being in a group.

An ego defence similar to splitting is idealization. Like the positive end of splitting, idealization involves overestimating the positive attributes of a person, object, or idea while underestimating its negative attributes. More fundamentally, it involves the projection of our needs and desires onto that person, object, or idea. A paradigm of idealization is infatuation, when love is confused with the need to love, and the idealized person's negative attributes are glossed over or even imagined as positive. Although this can make for a rude awakening, there are few better ways of relieving our existential anxiety than by manufacturing something that is 'perfect' for us, be it a piece of equipment, a place, country, person, or god.

If in love with someone inaccessible, it might be more convenient to intellectualize our love, perhaps by thinking of it in terms of idealization! In intellectualization, uncomfortable feelings associated with a problem are repressed by thinking about the problem in cold and abstract terms. I once received a phone call from a junior doctor in psychiatry in which he described a recent in-patient admission as 'a 47-year-old mother of two who attempted to cessate her life as a result of being diagnosed with a metastatic mitotic lesion'. A formulation such as '…who tried to kill herself after being told that she is dying of cancer' would have been better English, but all too effective at evoking the full horror of this poor lady's predicament.

Intellectualization should not be confused with rationalization, which is the use of feeble but seemingly plausible arguments either to justify something that is painful to accept ('sour grapes') or to make it seem 'not so bad after all' ('sweet lemons'). For instance, a person who has been rejected by a love interest convinces himself that she rejected him because she did not share in his ideal of happiness (sour grapes), and also that her rejection is a blessing in disguise in that it has freed him to find a more suitable partner (sweet lemons).

While no one can altogether avoid deploying ego defences, some ego defences are thought to be more 'mature' than others, not only because they involve some degree of insight, but also because they can be adaptive or useful. If a person is angry at his boss, he may go home and kick the dog, or he may instead go out and play a good game of tennis. The first instance (kicking the dog) is an example of displacement, the redirection of uncomfortable feelings towards someone or something less important, which is an immature ego defence. The second instance (playing a good game of tennis) is an example of sublimation, the channelling of uncomfortable feelings into socially condoned and often productive activities, which is a much more mature ego defence.

There are a number of mature ego defences like sublimation that can be substituted for the more primitive ones. Altruism, for instance, can in some cases represent a form of sublimation in which a person copes with his anxiety by stepping outside himself and helping others. By concentrating on the needs of others, people in altruistic vocations such as medicine or teaching may be able to permanently push their own needs into the background. Conversely, people who care for a disabled or elderly person may experience profound anxiety and distress when this role is suddenly removed from them.

Another mature ego defence is humour. By seeing the absurd or ridiculous aspect of an emotion, event, or situation, a person is able to put it into a less threatening context and thereby diffuse the anxiety that it gives rise to. In addition, he is able to share, and test, his insight with others in the benign and gratifying form of a joke. If man laughs so much, it is no doubt because he has the most developed unconscious in the animal kingdom. The things that people laugh about most are their errors and inadequacies; the difficult challenges that they face around personal identity, social standing, sexual relationships, and death; and incongruity, absurdity, and meaninglessness. These are all deeply human concerns: just as no one has ever seen a laughing dog, so no one has ever heard of a laughing god.

Further up the maturity scale is asceticism, which is the denial of the importance of that which most people fear or strive for, and so of the very grounds for anxiety and disappointment. If fear is, ultimately, for oneself, then the denial of the self removes the very grounds for fear. People in modern societies are more anxious than people in traditional or historical societies, no doubt because of the strong emphasis that modern societies place on the self as an independent and autonomous agent.

In the Hindu *Bhagavad Gita*, the god Krishna appears to Arjuna in the midst of the Battle of Kurukshetra, and advises him not to succumb to his scruples but to do his duty and fight on. In either case, all the men on the battlefield are one day condemned to die, as are all men. Their deaths are trivial, because the spirit in them, their human essence, does not depend on their particular incarnations for its continued existence. Krishna says, 'When one sees eternity in things that pass away and infinity in finite things, then one has pure knowledge.'

There has never been a time when you and I have not existed, nor will there be a time when we will cease to exist … the wise are not deluded by these changes.

There are a great number of ego defences, and the combinations and circumstances in which we use them reflect on our personality. Indeed, one could go so far as to argue that the self is nothing but the sum of its ego defences, which are constantly shaping, upholding, protecting, and repairing it.

The self is like a cracked mask that is in constant need of being pieced together. But behind the mask there is nobody at home.

While we cannot entirely escape from ego defences, we can gain some insight into how we use them. This self-knowledge, if we have the courage for it, can awaken us to ourselves, to others, and to the world around us, and free us to express our full potential as human beings.

The greatest oracle of the ancient world was the oracle at Delphi, and inscribed on the forecourt of the temple of Apollo at Delphi was a simple two-word command:

Know thyself.

Self-assessment

Answer by true or false.

1. Personality disorders are clear-cut, discrete disorders that do not blur.
2. The prevalence of personality disorders in psychiatric in- and out-patients is about 10-15%.
3. Antisocial personality disorder is significantly more common in males.
4. Borderline personality disorder is more common in females.
5. Personality disorders usually trace their beginnings to childhood or adolescence.
6. DSM-5 cluster B personality disorders can be described as 'odd, bizarre, eccentric'.
7. Anankastic personality disorder is a DSM-5 cluster C personality disorder.
8. In ICD-10, schizotypal personality disorder is not listed as a personality disorder, but alongside schizophrenia as 'schizotypal disorder'.
9. Schizoid personality disorder is characterized by eccentric behaviour and anomalies of thinking and affect similar to those seen in schizophrenia.
10. People with antisocial personality disorder find it hard to find relationships.
11. Antisocial personality disorder is synonymous with psychopathy.
12. People with paranoid personality disorder are suggestible, especially to people in a position of authority.
13. The main ego defence in paranoid personality disorder is splitting.
14. Avoidant personality disorder is characterized by a lack of self-confidence and an excessive need to be taken care of.
15. Anankastic personality disorder is related to obsessive-compulsive disorder.
16. Personality disorder should never be diagnosed on the basis of a single interview.
17. Important complications of personality disorders include depressive disorder, substance misuse, and deliberate self-harm.
18. Drugs play an important role in the treatment of some personality disorders.
19. People who stand to benefit from the complex needs service are best advised to self-refer.
20. Personality disorders are lifelong disorders, but tend to mellow with increasing age.

Answers

1. False.
2. False. It is probably much higher.
3. True.
4. True.
5. True.
6. False. Cluster A.
7. True.
8. True.
9. False. This describes schizotypal disorder.
10. False. They find it hard to keep them.
11. False. Psychopathy is a similar but narrower construct.
12. False. This describes histrionic personality disorder.
13. False. It is projection.
14. False. This describes dependent personality disorder.
15. False.
16. True. The diagnosis ought to be confirmed over time.
17. True.
18. False.
19. True.
20. True.

Organic disorders (delirium and dementias)

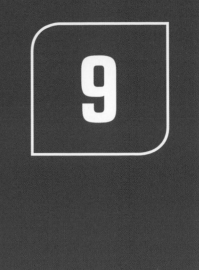

9

Pray, do not mock me:
I am a very foolish fond old man,
Four score and upward, not an hour more nor less;
And, to deal plainly,
I fear I am not in my perfect mind.
Methinks I should know you, and know this man;
Yet I am doubtful: for I am mainly ignorant
What place this is: and all the skill I have
Remembers not these garments; nor I know not
Where I did lodge last night. Do not laugh at me;
For, as I am a man, I think this lady
To be my child Cordelia.

—Shakespeare, *King Lear*

Introduction

Organic mental disorders are so-called because they obviously result from biological organic causes such as pathological lesions, medical disorders, and drugs.

Organic mental disorders are contrasted with so-called 'functional' mental disorders such as schizophrenia and bipolar disorder, which, historically, have been thought to result from altered 'functioning' in the brain.

The brain is unusual among bodily organs in that it is the concern of not one but two medical specialisms, neurology and psychiatry. What exactly is the difference between neurology and psychiatry? If mental disorders can be both 'functional' and organic, then, clearly, that is not the difference. Disorders falling under the remit of neurology tend principally to affect motor and sensory function, whereas those falling under the remit of psychiatry tend principally to affect the higher functions such as

belief, emotion, and desire. As may be expected, there are a number of overlaps and grey areas.

Organic disorders can sometimes present as a 'functional' mental disorder. For instance, hypothyroidism can present as a depressive disorder, or a brain tumour as a psychotic disorder. These 'functional' presentations of organic disorders are not classified under mood disorders or psychotic disorders, but under organic psychiatric disorders as 'organic mood disorder due to hypothyroidism' or 'organic delusional disorder due to a brain tumour'. 'Functional' presentations of organic disorders are not uncommon, and it is important to consider them, and either uncover them or rule them out. In this book, they are covered in the chapters on 'functional' mental disorders, leaving this chapter to focus on the principal organic mental disorders: delirium and the dementias.

Delirium

Deadly delirium

Delirium is a condition that falls between the stools of general medicine, geriatrics, psychiatry, and neurology, and so risks being ignored. However, it is both common and deadly, and all medical students and junior doctors must have a thorough grasp in particular of its prevention and early detection.

Definition

Delirium (Latin, *off the track*), or acute confusional state, is common in in-patients, particularly the elderly and young children. It affects up to 40% of in-patients over the age of 65.

ICD-10 defines it as 'an aetiologically non-specific syndrome characterized by concurrent disturbances of consciousness and attention, perception, thinking, memory, psychomotor behaviour, emotion, and the sleep-wake cycle (that is) transient and of fluctuating intensity...'

Clinical features

Delirium usually has a rapid onset of hours to days, and typically lasts for days to weeks—although it can last for several months, especially with conditions such as chronic liver disease, carcinoma, or subacute bacterial endocarditis. In many cases, the course is diurnally fluctuating, with the patient relatively settled during the daytime and most agitated in the evening ('sundowning'). In some cases, the patient may not be agitated ('hypoactive delirium'), which makes diagnosis much more difficult.

Delirium is characterized by:

- Impairment of consciousness and difficulty focusing, maintaining, and shifting attention.
- Impairment of abstract thinking and comprehension, and, in some cases, transient delusions.
- Impairment of immediate recall and recent memory, with remote memory relatively spared.
- Disorientation in time and, in severe cases, also in place and person.
- Perceptual abnormalities including distortions, illusions, and hallucinations, most commonly in the visual modality.
- Hyperactivity or hypoactivity, and sudden shifts from one to the other.

- Disturbance and, in severe cases, reversal of the sleep-wake cycle.
- Emotional disturbances and lability.

> ### Case study: Mrs DS
>
> 73-year-old Mrs DS is admitted in an acute confusional state after taking an overdose of eight tablets of temazepam 10mg. She has no significant medical or psychiatric history, but her son reports that her beloved dog died three months ago, leaving her bereft. Urine dipstick reveals a urinary tract infection and she is started on antibiotics.
>
> The medical team ask for a psychiatric opinion as to Mrs DS's suicidal risk. The psychiatrist, who is having a busy day, arrives at 6pm to find her very agitated. She says she is seeing spiders on the curtains and implores the psychiatrist to 'call the fire brigade before the petrol station shuts'. As the psychiatrist cannot make an accurate assessment of her suicidal risk, he asks the medical team to call him back once she is more settled. Unfortunately, three days later, she dies of septicaemic shock.
>
> Diagnosis: delirium (probably) owing to multiple aetiologies, including old age, bereavement, temazepam overdose, change in environment, distress and agitation, and urinary tract infection.

Differential diagnosis

- Dementia (Table 9.1).
- Delirium superimposed upon dementia (dementia being an important risk factor for delirium, although not a cause as such).
- Substance misuse.
- Affective disorder.
- Psychotic disorder.

Table 9.1: Delirium versus dementia

	Delirium	Dementia
Onset	Rapid	Insidious
Course	Fluctuating	Progressive
Duration	Days to weeks (reversible)	Months to years (irreversible)
Consciousness	Altered	Clear
Attention	Impaired	Usually normal
Memory	Immediate recall impaired	Immediate recall usually normal
Pyschomotor changes	Hyperactivity or hypoactivity	Usually none
Sleep-wake cycle	Disturbed	Often normal

Aetiology

Table 9.2 lists the commoner causes of delirium. Any form of stress can cause delirium, which ultimately results from excessive neurotransmitter release (especially acetylcholine and dopamine) and abnormal signal conduction.

Table 9.2: Commoner causes of delirium

Drugs (commonest)	Alcohol, opiates, sedatives, anticholinergics, diuretics, steroids, digoxin, anticonvulsants, lithium, tricyclic antidepressants, L-dopa, 'polypharmacy'
Metabolic	Renal failure, hepatic failure, respiratory failure, cardiac failure, disorders of electrolyte balance (especially hyponatraemia and hypercalcaemia), dehydration, porphyria
Infective	Urinary tract infection (remove unnecessary urinary catheters), pneumonia, septicaemia, endocarditis, encephalitis, meningitis, cerebral abscess, HIV, malaria
Endocrine	Hypoglycaemia, diabetic ketoacidosis, hypothyroidism, hyperthyroidism, Cushing's syndrome
Neurological	Stroke, sub-arachnoid haemorrhage, head injury, space-occupying lesions, epilepsy
Other	Other hypoperfusion states (e.g. anaemia, cardiac arrhythmias), post-operative states, stress and sleep deprivation, change in environment, faecal impaction, urinary retention, vitamin deficiencies (B1, B3, B12)

Investigations

It is important to maintain a high degree of suspicion for delirium in susceptible patients, and to carry out daily assessments of their cognitive status and mental state. If delirium is suspected, a psychiatric assessment, full physical examination (including vital signs), and delirium screen (Table 9.3) should be undertaken to confirm the diagnosis and identify one or more physical causes. In a minority of cases, no cause will be found.

Table 9.3: Investigations in delirium (minimum investigations in bold)

Blood tests	**FBC, U&Es**, LFTs, TFTs, glucose, thiamine level, drug screen
Infection screens	**Urinary dipstick**, **MSU**, sputum samples, blood cultures, lumbar puncture
Imaging	**CXR**, AXR, CT head, MRI head
Other	**ECG**, EEG*, urinary drug screen

* Characteristic changes in delirium include slowing of the posterior dominant rhythm and generalized slow-wave activity.

Management and prognosis

In susceptible patients, delirium should be actively prevented. Simple measures that are all too often overlooked include:

- Carrying out regular cognitive assessments.
- Rationalizing the drug chart.
- Ensuring that sensory aids such as spectacles and hearing aids are available.
- Encouraging fluids and nutrition, and correcting any electrolyte imbalances and nutritional deficiencies.
- Encouraging gentle mobilization.
- Encouraging relatives and carers to spend time at the bedside.

If delirium supervenes despite these preventive measures, the cause of the delirium must be sought and treated.

The patient should be nursed in a consistent, comfortable, and familiar environment on a medical (rather than psychiatric) ward. Relatives, who may well be alarmed, should be educated about their loved one's condition, and encouraged to remain at his or her bedside to provide reorientation and reassurance. Clocks, calendars, and familiar objects from home can be brought in to act as memory cues.

Tranquillizers should be avoided, but can find a role if the patient is agitated or psychotic. Haloperidol is the drug of choice (except if the cause of the delirium is alcohol or benzodiazepines, in which case it is a benzodiazepine) because of its minimal anticholinergic adverse effects. Doses should be kept to a minimum (e.g. haloperidol 0.5mg QDS, but *not* PRN to avoid precipitating alternating episodes of agitation and sedation), and stopped as soon as it is no longer indicated.

Complications of delirium can sometimes be prevented; if not, they should be actively identified and addressed. They include:

- Prolonged hospital stay and increased risk of nosocomial infections.
- Accelerated cognitive decline.
- Aspiration pneumonia.
- Fluid and electrolyte imbalance.
- Malnutrition.
- Falls.
- Injuries.
- Decreased mobility.
- Pressure sores.

Mortality is high, both in hospital and following discharge. One-year mortality has been estimated to be as high as 50%.

Dementia

What do they think has happened, the old fools,
To make them like this? Do they somehow suppose
It's more grown-up when your mouth hangs open and drools,
And you keep pissing yourself, and can't remember
Who called this morning? Or that, if they only chose,
They could alter things back to when they danced all night,
Or went to their wedding, or sloped arms some September?
Or do they fancy there's really been no change,
And they've always behaved as if they were crippled or tight,
Or sat through days of thin continuous dreaming
Watching the light move? If they don't (and they can't), it's strange;
Why aren't they screaming?

—Philip Larkin (1922-1985), from *The Old Fools*

Definition

According to ICD-10, dementia is 'a syndrome due to disease of the brain, usually of a chronic or progressive nature, in which there is disturbance of multiple higher cortical functions, including memory, thinking, orientation, comprehension, calculation, learning capacity, language, and judgement. Consciousness is not clouded… Dementia produces an appreciable decline in intellectual functioning, and usually some interference with personal activities of daily living, such as washing, dressing, eating, personal hygiene, excretory and toilet activities.'

Diagnosis

Again according to ICD-10, 'the primary requirement for diagnosis is evidence of a decline in both memory and thinking sufficient to impair personal activities of daily living, as described above. The impairment of memory typically affects the registration, storage, and retrieval of new information, but previously learnt and familiar material may also be lost, particularly in later stages. Dementia is more than dysmnesia: there is also impairment of thinking and reasoning capacity, and a reduction in the flow of ideas.'

The type of dementia in question is determined on clinical grounds, and the diagnosis can only be verified by brain biopsy or at post-mortem (in other words, it cannot be verified).

Clinical features

The principal clinical features of dementia are outlined in Table 9.4. Clinical features vary according to the type and severity of the dementia, as different types of dementia affect different parts of the brain (Table 9.5).

Table 9.4: Principal clinical features of dementia
(In approximate order of progression in Alzheimer's disease, from 1 to 7)

1. Memory loss	Short-term memory is more affected than long-term memory, with impaired learning and disorientation (first in time and then in place and person)
2. Impaired thinking	Poor judgement, decreased fluency, dyscalculia, concrete thinking and impaired abstraction, lack of ability to plan or sequence behaviour, delusions
3. Language impairments	Expressive and receptive dysphasia/aphasia
4. Deterioration in personal functioning	Deterioration in occupational and social functioning and self-care. Severe senile self-neglect is referred to as Diogenes syndrome (named after Diogenes the Cynic), which may be accompanied by syllogomania, a tendency to hoard rubbish
5. Disturbed personality and behaviour	Euphoria and emotional lability or apathy and irritability, disinhibition leading to aggressive or inappropriate behaviour, inattention and distractability, obsessive and stereotyped behaviours

9

Table 9.4: Principal clinical features of dementia – *contd*
(In approximate order of progression in Alzheimer's disease, from 1 to 7)

6. Perceptual abnormalities	Visual and auditory agnosia, visuospatial difficulties, body hemi-neglect, inability to recognize faces (prosopagnosia), illusions, hallucinations (often visual), cortical blindness
7. Motor impairments	Apraxia, spastic paresis, urinary incontinence

Table 9.5: Focal lobe deficits

Frontal lobe	**Orbitofrontal syndrome**: disinhibition, aggressive and inappropriate behaviour, obsessive or repetitive stereotyped behaviours, euphoria, emotional lability, poor insight **Dorsolateral prefrontal syndrome**: apathy, irritability, lack of ability to plan or sequence behaviour, decreased fluency, impaired abstraction
Temporal lobe	**Dominant (left) temporal lobe:** verbal agnosia, visual agnosia, receptive aphasia, hallucinations **Non-dominant (right) temporal lobe:** visuospatial deficiencies, inability to recognize faces (prosopagnosia), hallucinations **Bilateral disease:** blunted emotional reactivity, apathy, Korsakov syndrome, Klüver-Buçy syndrome (a rare syndrome consisting of hyperorality and hypersexuality)
Parietal lobe	**Dominant (left) parietal lobe**: receptive aphasia, agnosia, apraxia, Gerstmann syndrome (finger agnosia, dyscalculia, dysgraphia, left-right disorientation) **Non-dominant (right) parietal lobe**: body hemineglect, visuospatial difficulties, anosognosia or denial of deficits, constructional apraxia **Bilateral disease**: visuospatial imperception, spatial disorientation, Balint syndrome (a rare disorder of visuo-spatial processing)
Occipital lobe	Visual perception defects such as visual agnosia, alexia, and prosopagnosia, progressing to cortical blindness, illusions, and visual hallucinations, and Anton syndrome (a form of anosognosia involving the denial of cortical blindness)

Case study: Phineas Gage

On September 13, 1848, one Phineas Gage was working on the construction of the Rutland and Burlington Railroad when he accidentally ignited some gunpowder with a large tamping iron. The iron was blown through his head (Figure 9.1) with such force that it landed several yards behind him.

Although Gage survived and was even talking and walking moments after the accident, his friends described him as 'no longer Gage'. The local doctor, JM Harlow, later reported in the *Boston Medical and Surgical Journal* that:

Gage was fitful, irreverent, indulging at times in the grossest profanity (which was not previously his custom), manifesting but little deference for his fellows, impatient of restraint or advice when it conflicts with his desires, at times pertinaciously obstinate, yet capricious and vacillating, devising many plans of future operations, which are no sooner arranged than they are abandoned in turn for others appearing more feasible. A child in his intellectual capacity and manifestations, he has the animal passions of a strong man. Previous to his injury, although untrained in the schools, he possessed a well-balanced mind, and was looked upon by those who knew him as a shrewd, smart businessman, very energetic and persistent in executing all his plans of operation. In this regard his mind was radically changed, so decidedly that his friends and acquaintances said he was 'no longer Gage'.

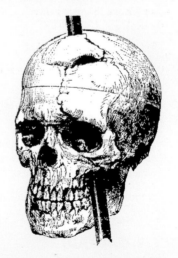

Figure 9.1. The tamping iron passed through the ventromedial areas of the prefrontal cortex.

Harlow JM (1848): Passage of an iron rod through the head, *Boston Med. Surg. J.* 39:389-393.
Harlow JM (1868): Recovery from the passage of an iron bar through the head, *Publ. Mass. Med. Soc.* 2:327-347.

Types

Dementias can be classified as either primary (or degenerative) or secondary.

The principal primary dementias are:

- Alzheimer's disease.
- Dementia with Lewy bodies and Parkinson's disease.
- Pick's disease and other frontotemporal dementias.
- Huntington's disease.

Secondary dementias are listed in Table 9.6.

Overall, the commonest dementias are Alzheimer's disease, dementia with Lewy bodies, vascular dementia, and frontotemporal dementias.

Table 9.6: Secondary dementias

Vascular (common)	Vascular infarction, vascular disease
Infective	AIDS, Lyme disease, neurosyphilis, prion diseases, encephalitis
Inflammatory	Systemic lupus erythematosus, cranial arteritis, encephalopathy, multiple sclerosis
Neoplastic	Primary or secondary tumour, paraneoplastic syndrome
Metabolic	Cardiac, hepatic, and renal failure, anaemia, chronic hypoglycaemia, vitamin B12 deficiency, thiamine deficiency, Wilson's disease
Endocrine	Hyper- and hypo-thyroidism, hyper- and hypo-parathyroidism, Addison's disease, Cushing's syndrome
Toxic	Alcohol, heavy metals, organic solvents, organophosphates
Traumatic	Severe single head injury, repeated head injury (punch-drunk syndrome, *dementia pugilistica*), subdural haematoma
Other	Normal pressure hydrocephalus, radiation, anoxia

Alzheimer's disease (AD)

Epidemiology

Alzheimer' disease is the commonest cause of dementia, accounting for more than 50% of all cases and affecting over 500,000 people in the UK. Prevalence approximately doubles for every five years of age from the ages of 65 (prevalence 1%) to 90 (prevalence 30-40%). AD is more common in females, even after accounting for their longer life expectancy.

Aetiology

Risk factors for AD include:

- Age (up to about age 90).
- Female sex (the female to male ratio is about 2:1).
- Family history (overall relative risk of 4).
- Down's syndrome.
- Head injury.

In terms of genetics:

- Inheritance of the ε4 allele of apolipoprotein E on chromosome 19 is a risk factor for the common sporadic, late-onset form of the disease. The ε2 allele on the other hand is protective.
- Mutations in the beta-amyloid precursor protein (APP) gene on chromosome 21, in the presenilin-1 gene on chromosome 14, and in the presenilin-2 gene on chromosome 1 are involved in the rare, early-onset familial forms of the disease. The inheritance pattern in this case is autosomal dominant.

Factors that may protect against late-onset AD include a healthy and engaged lifestyle, high educational attainment, (although this may simply delay detection), non-steroidal anti-inflammatory drugs (NSAIDs), hormone replacement therapy (HRT), and vitamins C and E.

Neuropathology

Selective neuronal and synaptic loss leads to neuro-chemical abnormalities (notably a cholinergic deficit) and symmetrical cortical atrophy that is initially more pronounced in the temporal and parietal lobes.

Extracellular senile plaques and intracellular neurofibrillary tangles are seen in normal ageing, but are more numerous in AD and closely related to the degree of cognitive impairment. Senile plaques consist of a core of beta-amyloid surrounded by filamentous material. Neurofibrillary tangles consist of coiled filaments of abnormally phosphorylated microtubule-associated protein tau (note that tau is also found in Pick bodies—see later).

Other histopathological findings include glial proliferation, granulovascular degeneration, and Hirano inclusion bodies.

Clinical features

AD is characterized by insidious onset and progression of memory loss and personality changes. Other spheres of cognitive and non-cognitive impairment are added over the course of several years (Table 9.4). Life expectancy from the time of diagnosis is about eight years. The felt experience and consequences of suffering with Alzheimer's disease are accurately depicted in the film *Iris*, about the life of the writer and philosopher Iris Murdoch (Dame Judi Dench).

Dementia with Lewy bodies (DLB)

Epidemiology
DLB overlaps with AD and parkinsonian dementia. It is the second most common cause of dementia, accounting for about 20% of all cases.

Aetiology
Aetiology is uncertain. DLB may form part of a spectrum of Lewy body disorders that includes Parkinson's disease. In DLB, Lewy bodies are more numerous in cortical areas (especially in cortical layers V and VI of the temporal lobe), the cingulate gyrus, and the insular cortex, whereas in Parkinson's disease they are more numerous in the basal ganglia.

Neuropathology
Both cortical and subcortical structures are involved. Lewy bodies are intracellular eosinophilic inclusions consisting of abnormally phosphorylated neurofilament proteins aggregated with ubiquitin and alpha-synuclein. There is associated neuronal loss leading to cholinergic deficit and other chemical abnormalities. However, there is only minimal cortical atrophy. Compared to Alzheimer's disease, senile plaques may be present but neurofibrillary tangles are not a marked feature.

Clinical features
DLB is mostly characterized by:
* Marked fluctuations in alertness and cognitive impairment.
* Vivid visual hallucinations and other psychotic symptoms.
* Early parkinsonism and neuroleptic sensitivity.
* Frequent faints and falls.

Memory loss itself may not be a marked feature in the early stages of DLB.

Life expectancy from the time of diagnosis is about six years.

Frontotemporal dementias (using Pick's disease as the archetypal form)

Epidemiology
Pick's disease is a type of frontotemporal dementia accounting for about 5% of all cases of dementia. It is more common in females, with peak age of onset at 45-60 years.

Aetiology
Aetiology is unclear. Familial forms are more common in people of Scandinavian descent.

Neuropathology
Pick's disease leads to selective, often asymmetrical 'knife-blade' atrophy, neuronal loss, and gliosis affecting the frontal and temporal lobes. There are characteristic 'ballooned' neurones called Pick cells and tau-positive neuronal inclusions called Pick bodies, but no senile plaques or neurofibrillary tangles as in AD.

Clinical features
Pick's disease is characterized by insidious and progressive dementia with early and prominent personality changes and behavioural disturbances, eating disturbances, mood changes, cognitive impairment, language abnormalities, and motor signs.

Huntington's disease

Epidemiology
The prevalence of Huntington's disease, or Huntington's chorea, in Caucasians is 5-10 per 100,000. Onset is usually although not invariably in the fourth or fifth decade.

Aetiology
Huntington's disease is an autosomal dominant neuro-degenerative disorder that manifests in the presence of 36 or more glutamine-encoding CAG trinucleotide repeats in the huntingtin gene on chromosome 4. The age of onset decreases as the number of CAG trinucleotide repeats increases: this occurs from one generation to the next in the paternal line, a phenomenon referred to as anticipation.

Neuropathology
Abnormal huntingtin protein leads to degeneration of neurones, notably in the caudate nucleus and putamen and in the cerebral cortex. Degeneration in the caudate nucleus and putamen is associated with movement disorders, and degeneration in the cerebral cortex with dementia.

Clinical features

Clinical features of Huntington's disease include choreiform ('dance-like') movements, progressive dementia, and other psychiatric disturbances. In the later stages, there is increasing dementia with cognitive impairment, behavioural changes, and depressive symptoms. Insight is often retained until late, and, as a result, the suicide rate is very high—in the order of 10%.

Vascular dementia

Epidemiology

Vascular dementia, which is a secondary dementia, is the third commonest cause of dementia after AD and DLB, accounting for about 20% of all dementias. In Japan, it is the commonest form of dementia, accounting for about half of all dementias. In so-called 'mixed dementia', there is evidence of both AD and vascular dementia. Vascular dementia is more common in males.

Aetiology

Risk factors for vascular dementia include:

- Older age.
- Male sex.
- Cardiovascular disease.
- Cerebrovascular disease.
- Valvular heart disease.
- Hypercoagulation disorders.
- Hypertension.
- Hypercholesterolaemia.
- Diabetes.
- Smoking.
- Alcohol misuse.

Neuropathology

Focal and diffuse disease often co-exist. Focal disease may result from single or, more commonly, multiple thrombotic or embolic infarcts. Diffuse disease (Binswanger disease and lacunar state), on the other hand, results from small vessel disease.

Clinical features

Owing to its aetiology, vascular dementia classically has an abrupt onset and step-wise progression. Clinical features vary according to the location of the infarcts. However, mood and behavioural changes are common. Insight is usually retained until late. Significant comorbidity leads to a shorter mean life expectancy than in AD.

Other dementias and amnestic syndrome

Normal pressure hydrocephalus

Normal pressure hydrocephalus is a potentially reversible or partially reversible form of dementia that accounts for about 5% of all dementias. It is understood as a form of communicating hydrocephalus with impaired cerebrospinal fluid (CSF) reabsorption at the arachnoid villi. CSF formation eventually equilibrates with reabsorption, and so intracranial pressure (ICP) is only slightly raised. Signs of raised ICP such as headache, vomiting, and altered consciousness are absent. The classic triad consists of, in order of progression, abnormal gait and ataxia, dementia, and urinary incontinence. Lumbar puncture and lumbar tapping and brain imaging are useful in securing the diagnosis. A ventriculoperitoneal shunt can be surgically implanted to drain excess CSF into the abdomen from where it can be absorbed.

HIV-related dementia

HIV-related dementia or AIDS dementia complex is usually observed in the late stages of AIDS in up to one third of AIDS patients. It is in fact a metabolic encephalopathy resulting from a direct effect of the HIV virus. The virus enters the central nervous system by infecting macrophages and monocytes that cross the blood brain barrier. These cells invite an inflammatory response that ultimately leads to neuronal loss. Clinical features include cognitive impairment progressing to dementia, behavioural changes, and motor involvement.

Neurological complications of HIV other than HIV-related dementia include opportunistic infections, cerebral lymphoma and metastasis of AIDS-related cancers, toxic effects of drug treatments, and malnutrition.

Creutzfeldt-Jakob disease and other prion-related diseases

Prions are protein particles that can be infectious despite containing no RNA or DNA. Prion diseases are a group of related neurodegenerative diseases that affect both humans and animals, and that result from the deposition of the prion protein (PrP) to form amyloid sheets. In humans, they include Creutzfeldt-Jakob disease (CJD), Gerstmann-Sträussler syndrome (GSS), and kuru.

Prion diseases can occur sporadically, as in most cases of CJD which result from spontaneous PrP^C to PrP^{Sc} conversion or somatic mutation. Or they can be inherited, as in GSS which results from the autosomal dominant inheritance of a mutation in the PrP gene on chromosome 20. Or they can be contracted by infection, as in new variant CJD (nvCJD), which results from the ingestion of bovine spongiform encephalopathy (BSE)-infected beef products; or kuru, which results from the cannibalism of neural tissue, as described in the Fore people of Papua New Guinea.

All these human prion diseases are very rare. The most common by far is CJD, which has an incidence of about one in a million. Prion diseases tend to affect grey matter, producing neuronal loss, gliosis, and characteristic spongiform change. In CJD there is rapidly progressive dementia associated with myoclonic jerks and a variable constellation of pyramidal, extrapyramidal, and cerebellar signs. Mean age of onset is 62 years and death occurs in the space of about eight months. In contrast, the mean age of onset for nvCJD is just 28 years. The first cases of nvCJD were reported in 1995, and so far most cases have been circumscribed to the United Kingdom. In contrast to sporadic CJD, psychiatric symptoms are common at the time of first presentation, and there are no characteristic EEG changes. Death occurs in about 12 months.

Amnestic syndrome

Amnestic syndrome is rare, and results from damage to the mammillary bodies, hippocampus, or thalamus. The most common cause is thiamine deficiency secondary to chronic alcoholism (see Wernicke-Korsakov syndrome, Chapter 11), and other causes include thiamine deficiency owing to other causes, head injury, hypoxia, carbon monoxide poisoning, herpes simplex encephalitis, and brain tumours. There is selective loss of recent memory with disorientation and confabulation, and relative sparing of immediate and long-term memory and other intellectual faculties. Amnestic syndrome is usually irreversible.

Differential diagnosis

Dementia is a clinical diagnosis, and its differential includes:

- Mild cognitive impairment (see below).
- Amnestic syndrome.
- Delirium.
- Delirium superimposed upon dementia.
- Depressive disorder ('pseudodementia')—although depressive and anxiety disorders are found in about half of people with dementia.

- Late-onset schizophrenia (paraphrenia).
- Intellectual disability/mental retardation.
- Substance misuse.
- Iatrogenic causes, particularly drugs.
- Dissociative disorder.
- Factitious disorder.
- Malingering.

Mild cognitive impairment (MCI) refers to subtle but measurable memory difficulties that are more severe than in normal ageing but less so than in AD. There is no deterioration in overall thinking and judgement or in level of functioning. However, the risk of conversion to Alzheimer's disease is about 15% per year.

Investigations

Physical examination aims at identifying any underlying causes of a possible secondary dementia (Table 9.6), and any complications such as malnutrition, burns, falls, and so on.

Investigations should include full blood count (FBC), urea and electrolytes (U&Es), calcium, serum cholesterol, liver function tests (LFTs), thyroid function tests (TFTs), serum B12 and folate, serum glucose, and chest X-ray (CXR). Neuroimaging such as computed tomography (CT) and magnetic resonance imaging (MRI) can be helpful, particularly to exclude potentially treatable causes such as tumour, subdural haematoma, and hydrocephalus. Further investigations should be ordered on a case-by-case basis, and might include HIV testing, syphilis serology, copper studies, cerebrospinal fluid (CSF) examination, and genetic testing, as well as vasculitic, autoimmune, neoplastic, and toxicological screens. Brain biopsy itself is rarely indicated.

Detailed neurocognitive testing by a clinical psychologist is helpful in identifying and delineating cognitive impairments and confirming a diagnosis. The Montreal Cognitive Assessment (MoCA) or Mini Mental State Examination (MMSE) are often used as a screening and monitoring tool.

Management

Secondary dementias may be partially reversed if the underlying cause can be identified and treated. Otherwise, the aim of management is to improve or maintain the quality of life of patient and carers by treating symptoms and complications (e.g. depression, chest infection, urinary tract infection...) of the dementia, addressing functional and social problems, and providing carers with education and support.

With regards to functional problems, the first step is careful assessment of the patient's functional abilities and risk exposure. Care should be taken to ensure personal hygiene and adequate nutrition. Functional abilities can be maintained and even improved by a regular daily routine, environmental modifications, and graded assistance. The patient should be reoriented and reassured, and encouraged to partake in physical and mental activity, including attending a group cognitive stimulation programme. Memory aids such as clocks, calendars, notebooks, and photographs and reality orientation and reminiscence therapies may also be helpful, particularly in the early stages of the disease. Behavioural problems can be addressed, and quality of life improved, by simple measures such as aromatherapy, music, animal-assisted therapy, and massage.

With regards to social problems, areas to consider include accommodation, social isolation, and financial and legal matters such as power of attorney, curatorship, and wills.

Carers should be educated about the condition and advised about its broader management. Caring for someone with dementia is physically and emotionally exhausting and carers should be encouraged to seek support from a carer support group. Ultimately, carers may have little choice but to fall back on day care, respite care, or long-term care in a residential or nursing home.

There may also be a small role for drug treatment, principally in the form of a cholinesterase inhibitor. In AD and DLB, usually, a cholinesterase inhibitor should be tried first. Other drugs should be used as infrequently and sparingly as possible. A benzodiazepine such as diazepam or lorazepam might be indicated for anxiety or agitation, and an antipsychotic such as quetiapine for psychosis.

> **Antipsychotics in dementia** (!)
>
> Antipsychotics should never be used to manage behavioural problems as they may accelerate cognitive decline and increase the risk of stroke.
>
> In DLB and some frontotemporal dementias, antipsychotics are associated with severe extrapyramidal symptoms, and special care should be taken in their use.

Cholinesterase inhibitors include donepezil, rivastigmine, and galantamine. These drugs act by increasing neurotransmission and can modestly and temporarily ameliorate cognitive performance and behavioural problems in a minority of patients with mild to moderate AD and DLB. Dose-related gastrointestinal adverse effects are common; other adverse effects are relatively rare.

An anticholinesterase inhibitor should initially be prescribed after thorough assessment in a specialist clinic if the MMSE is 10 or greater. The prescription should be reassessed after two-to-four months and continued only if there is demonstrable improvement or lack of decline. Thereafter, the prescription should be reassessed at six monthly intervals.

Memantine is a N-methyl-d-aspartate (NMDA) receptor antagonist that protects neurones from glutamate-mediated neurotoxicity. It may be of modest benefit in moderate to severe AD.

Other drugs that are sometimes used to offset cognitive or functional decline include antioxidants such as vitamin E.

Self-assessment

Answer by true or false.

1. Infection is the commonest cause of delirium.
2. Delirium can be caused by urinary retention or faecal impaction.
3. In delirium, consciousness is not clouded.
4. In delirium, recent memory is relatively spared.
5. Typically, in delirium, the patient is most agitated during the day and least agitated at night.
6. Simple measures that can prevent delirium, such as rationalizing the drug chart and correcting electrolyte disturbances, are often overlooked.
7. Haloperidol is the drug of choice in delirium. Doses should be kept to a minimum and the drug stopped as soon as it is no longer required.
8. Delirium superimposed upon dementia can accelerate cognitive decline.
9. In delirium, long-term prognosis is good.
10. A diagnosis of dementia requires evidence of a decline in either memory or thinking that is sufficiently severe to impair activities of daily living.
11. Lesions in the non-dominant temporal lobe can lead to verbal agnosia, visual agnosia, receptive aphasia, and hallucinations.
12. Lesions in the non-dominant parietal lobe can lead to body hemineglect and visuospatial disorders.
13. Risk factors for Alzheimer's disease include age, male sex, family history, and head injury.
14. Inheritance of the ε2 allele of apolipoprotein E on chromosome 19 is a risk factor for the common sporadic, late-onset form of Alzheimer's disease.
15. Neurofibrillary tangles seen in Alzheimer's disease consist in a core of beta-amyloid surrounded by filamentous material.
16. In mild cognitive impairment, the risk of conversion to Alzheimer's disease is about 15% per year.
17. Dementia with Lewy bodies is a recently recognized entity that overlaps with Alzheimer's disease and parkinsonian dementias, and may form part of a spectrum of Lewy body disorders that includes Parkinson's disease.
18. Dementia with Lewy bodies classically features an abrupt onset and step-wide progression.
19. A person has mental capacity so long as he has the ability to understand and retain relevant information for long enough to reach a reasoned decision, regardless of the actual decision reached.
20. If capacity is lacking, the next-of-kin has the responsibility to act in the best interests of the patient, although it is good practice for him to involve the doctor in charge and other relatives and carers in the decision-making.

Answers

1. False. Drugs are the commonest cause of delirium.
2. True. Delirium has a multitude of causes.
3. False. Consciousness is not clouded in dementia.
4. False. Remote memory is relatively spared.
5. False. The opposite is true.
6. True.
7. True.
8. True.
9. False. Mortality is high.
10. False. There should be evidence of a decline in *both* memory and thinking sufficient to impair activities of daily living.
11. False. Lesions in the non-dominant temporal lobe can lead to visuospatial difficulties, prosopagnosia, and hallucinations. Lesions in the dominant temporal lobe can lead to verbal agnosia, visual agnosia, receptive aphasia, and hallucinations.
12. True. Lesions in the dominant parietal lobe lead to receptive aphasia, agnosia, apraxia, and Gerstmann syndrome.
13. False. Female sex.
14. False. Inheritance of the ε4 allele of apolipoprotein E on chromosome 19 is a risk factor for the common sporadic, late-onset form of Alzheimer's disease. The ε2 allele is protective.
15. False, this describes senile plaques. Neurofibrillary tangles consist of coiled filaments of abnormally phosphorylated microtube-associated protein tau.
16. True.
17. True.
18. False. This best describes vascular dementia.
19. True.
20. False. If capacity is lacking, the doctor in charge has the responsibility to act in the best interests of the patient, although it is good practice for him to involve relatives and carers in the decision-making.

9

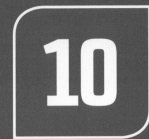

Intellectual disability

The problem with IQ scores

An important problem with grading the severity of ID by IQ score is that people from deprived socioeconomic backgrounds or minority cultural or linguistic backgrounds, as well as people with sensory, motor, or communication handicaps, often obtain spuriously depressed IQ scores.

Definition

ICD-10 defines 'mental retardation' as 'a condition of arrested or incomplete development of the mind, which is especially characterized by impairment of skills manifested during the developmental period, skills which contribute to the overall level of intelligence, i.e. cognitive, language, motor, and social abilities.'

ICD-10 further specifies that 'retardation can occur with or without any other mental or physical condition'.

In DSM-IV, 'mental retardation' was defined as:

- IQ of 70 or less.
- Significant limitations in adaptive functioning in at least two areas.
- Onset before the age of 18.

DSM-5 drops the term 'mental retardation' in favour of 'intellectual disability' (ID) or 'intellectual developmental disorder' (IDD). More importantly, it grades the severity of ID no longer by IQ score but according to adaptive functioning.

In both DSM-5 and ICD-10, severity of ID is classified as mild, moderate, severe, or profound (Table 10.1).

Table 10.1: Subtypes of intellectual disability

Mild	Needs only limited assistance and support, for instance, with finding appropriate accommodation and paying the bills. Can otherwise become self-sufficient and live independently.
Moderate	Needs variable degrees of assistance or support. Typically, can live in a supervised environment such as a group home, and work in a sheltered workshop.
Severe	Can master basic self-care and communication skills, but nonetheless needs continuous care.
Profound	Not capable of self-care, needs continuous care.

Epidemiology

The prevalence of ID is about 2-3%. Declines in incidence have been matched by increases in life expectancy, leading to large changes in the age structure of the patient population, but only small changes in the overall prevalence rate. Mild ID accounts for about 85% of cases of ID, moderate ID for about 10%, and severe and profound ID for about 5%. The male to female ratio for severe ID is about 6:5, but is higher for mild ID owing in part to a larger variance in IQ in males.

Aetiology

Many cases of mild ID represent the tail end of the normal distribution curve, and result from an interaction of genetic factors and environmental factors such as nutritional deficiency and psychosocial deprivation. With severe ID, it is much more common to find a specific cause. Specific causes can be classified as genetic, pre-natal, peri-natal, and post-natal (Tables 10.2, 10.3).

Table 10.2: Common specific causes of intellectual disability

Genetic	Table 10.3
Pre-natal	Pre-eclampsia
	Placental insufficiency
	Hydrocephalus
	Myelomeningocoele
	Congenital hypothyroidism
	Infections such as rubella, toxoplasmosis, cytomegalovirus, syphilis, HIV
	Foetal alcohol syndrome
Peri-natal	Brain trauma and hypoxia
	Intraventricular haemorrhage
	Hyperbilirubinaemia
	Infections
Post-natal	Head injury
	Brain infections
	Brain tumours
	Hypoxia
	Chronic lead poisoning
	Neglect and abuse
	Malnutrition and general poverty

Table 10.3: Genetic causes of intellectual disability

Chromosomal abnormalities

Trisomy 21 (Down's syndrome)	Down's syndrome is the most common cause of ID. Incidence is about 1 in 700 births overall but rises to about 1 in 30 births in mothers aged 45. 95% of cases result from non-disjunction of chromosome 21, and the remaining 5% from Robertsonian translocations (4%) or mosaicism (1%). ID is accompanied by characteristic physical abnormalities including oblique or almond-shaped palpebral fissures, Brushfield spots on the irises, flat nasal bridge, protruding tongue, short neck, shortened limbs, and single transverse palmar creases ('Simian creases'). There is increased risk of deafness, cataracts, respiratory infections, cardiovascular malformations, gastrointestinal abnormalities, haematological abnormalities, hypothyroidism, epilepsy, and early-onset Alzheimer's disease.
Fragile X syndrome (Martin-Bell syndrome)	Fragile X syndrome is the second most common cause of ID, with an incidence of about 1 in 1500 births. It results from CGG trinucleotide repeats in the FMR1 gene on the long arm of chromosome X, and so is commoner in males. ID is accompanied by characteristic physical abnormalities including elongated face, large or protruding ears, prognathism, macro-orchidism, and hypotonia. As with all trinucleotide repeat disorders (Huntington's disease, Lesch Nyhan syndrome…) disease severity increases in successive generations ('anticipation').
Other chromosomal abnormalities	Other chromosomal abnormalities include other trisomies and deletions such as *Cri du chat* syndrome (deletion of the short arm of chromosome 5).
	NB. Numerical sex chromosome abnormalities such as Klinefelter's syndrome, triple X syndrome, and Turner's syndrome are not typically associated with ID.

Single gene disorders

Phenylketonuria	Phenylketonuria is the commonest metabolic disorder, with an incidence of about 1 in 10,000 births. The autosomal recessive inheritance of a defect in the phenylalanine hydroxylase enzyme results in a high serum phenylalanine. ID is accompanied by short stature, hyperactivity, irritability, epilepsy, lack of pigment, and eczema. Treatment is by diet control.

Table 10.3: Genetic causes of intellectual disability – *contd*

Other metabolic disorders	Other metabolic disorders include other disorders of amino acid metabolism such as homocysteinuria, disorders of carbohydrate metabolism such as galactosaemia, disorders of lipid metabolism such as Tay Sachs disease, and mucopolysaccharidoses such as Hunter syndrome.
Neurofibromatosis	The incidence of neurofibromatosis is about 1 in 3000 births. A mutation in the *NF1* gene on chromosome 17 (type I neurofibromatosis or Von Recklinghausen syndrome) leads to mild ID accompanied by *café au lait* spots, multiple neurofibromas, and other abnormalities of the skin, soft tissues, nervous system, and bone. Joseph Merrick, the 'Elephant Man', probably suffered from type I neurofibromatosis and Proteus syndrome, not Elephantiasis.
Tuberous sclerosis	The incidence of tuberous sclerosis is about 1 in 6000 births. A mutation in the tumour suppressor gene TSC1 on chromosome 9 or TSC2 on chromosome 16 can lead to ID accompanied by autism, epilepsy, characteristic skin changes, and tumours of the brain and other organs. Both mutations can be inherited in an autosomal dominant pattern.

Clinical features

Case study: Lennie Small

…His hands went quickly into his side coat pockets. He said gently, "George… I ain't got mine. I musta lost it." He looked down at the ground in despair.

"You never had none, you crazy bastard. I got both of 'em here. Think I'd let you carry your own work card?"

Lennie grinned with relief. "I… I thought I put it in my side pocket." His hand went into the pocket again.

George looked sharply at him. "What'd you take outa that pocket?"

…

Lennie held his closed hand away from George's direction. "It's on'y a mouse, George."

"A mouse? A live mouse?"

"Uh-uh. Jus' a dead mouse, George. I didn't kill it. Honest! I found it. I found it dead.

"Give it here!" said George.

"Aw, leave me have it, George."

…

"What do you want of a dead mouse, anyways?"

"I could pet it with my thumb while we walked along," said Lennie.

"Well, you ain't petting no mice while you walk with me. You remember where we're goin' now?"

Lennie looked startled and then in embarrassment hid his face against his knees. "I forgot again."

"Jesus Christ," George said resignedly. "Well—look, we're gonna work on a ranch like the one we come from up north."

"Up north?"

"In Weed."

"Oh, sure. I remember. In Weed."

"That ranch we're goin' to is right down there about a quarter mile. We're gonna go in an' see the boss. Now, look—I'll give him the work tickets, but you ain't gonna say a word. You jus' stand there and don't say nothing. If he finds out what a crazy bastard you are, we won't get no job, but if he sees ya work before he hears ya talk, we're set. Ya got that?"

—John Steinbeck (1902-1968), *Of Mice and Men*

ID is characterized by uniformly impaired cognitive, language, motor, and social skills, and failure to meet expected developmental milestones—even if, in some cases, ID is not evident until the preschool years. Alternatively, the clinical picture may be dominated by behavioural disturbances such as hyperactivity, aggression, inattention, and abnormal movements, including repeated self-harming behaviours. People with ID are often suggestible and impulsive, and, as a result, are more likely to engage in criminal behaviours such as arson and exhibitionism.

Physical disorders including motor and sensory disabilities, epilepsy, and incontinence are common, but the full range of physical disorders depends on the underlying cause of ID (Tables 10.2, 10.3).

Mental disorders such as schizophrenia, mood disorders, anxiety disorders, adjustment disorders, dissociative disorders, delirium, dementia, and autism are all more common than in the normal population. However, they are more difficult to diagnose because symptoms may be modified by ID or poorly articulated by the patient. For instance, in psychosis, hallucinations and delusions may be less elaborate and manifest as behavioural changes such as fearfulness and head- or ear-banging (Table 10.4).

Table 10.4: Possible presentations of mental disorders in ID

Schizophrenia	• Deterioration from previous level of functioning • Behaviour that seems out of character • Indirect evidence of hallucinations and delusions
Hypomania	• Giggling • Overactivity • Disinhibition
Depression	• Loss of appetite • Sleep disturbance • Speech and motor retardation • Anhedonia

Clinical skills: Impairment, disability, or handicap?

Impairment: Any loss or abnormality of psychological, physiological, or anatomical structure or function.

Disability: Any restriction or lack, owing to an impairment, in ability to perform an activity in a way that is more or less normal for a human being.

Handicap: Any disadvantage suffered from being unable, owing to an impairment or disability, to adequately fulfil a normal role or function.

Assessment

The aim of assessment is not only to diagnose ID, but also to identify its cause (assistance from a paediatric neurologist may be required), uncover any associated physical and mental disorders, and map out functional deficits.

A patient with an established diagnosis of ID may be referred to a psychiatrist to investigate a suspected mental disorder or decline in functioning, or to carry out a forensic or risk assessment relating to criminal behaviour.

Assessment of ID calls for patience and tolerance of uncertainty. The approach to the patient should be flexible and adapted to his cognitive abilities and communications skills, with greater emphasis on direct observation and informant histories from parents and carers. In the history and mental state examination, particular attention should be paid to obstetric complications, neurodevelopmental delays, and behavioural disturbances. Other important areas include past medical history, family history, and social history. Physical examination should encompass sensory assessment, developmental assessment, and functional-behavioural assessment. Selected investigations may include standardized assessment instruments, metabolic studies, cytogenetic studies, and neuroimaging.

Management

The management of moderate to severe ID usually involves an individualized habilitation plan co-ordinated by a community intellectual disability team or equivalent. The elements of this habilitation plan depend upon the patient's specific problems and needs. Health professionals that may be co-opted into the patient's care include psychiatrists and other medical professionals, educational psychologists, specialist teachers, speech and language therapists, occupational therapists, behavioural therapists, and family therapists, among others. Social services may also be involved, particularly if the family is of modest means.

Medical management is seldom transformative, except perhaps in certain patients such as those with phenylketonuria. Psychotropic drugs are used in the management of mental disorders and behavioural problems, as in other patient groups. Although care in the community should be privileged, day care may be required to provide respite for the family, and a small minority of patients may need to be considered for residential care.

Prevention of ID involves improved obstetric and perinatal care, earlier detection of genetic disorders by amniocentesis and chorionic villus sampling, and, if appropriate, genetic counselling.

Self-assessment

Answer by true or false.

1. Historically, intellectual disability (ID) has been understood as a form of mental illness.
2. In DSM-5, severity of ID is graded by a combination of IQ score and adaptive functioning.
3. A person with profound ID can master basic self-care and communication skills, but nonetheless needs continuous care.
4. The prevalence of ID is about 1%.
5. Declines in the incidence of ID have been followed by declines in its overall prevalence.
6. Mild ID accounts for 85% of ID.
7. The male to female ratio in severe ID is about 2:1.
8. With severe ID, it is much more uncommon to find a specific cause.
9. Fragile X syndrome, which results from CGG trinucleotide repeats in the FMR1 gene on the long arm of chromosome X, is the most common cause of ID.
10. In 5% of cases, Down's syndrome results from non-disjunction of chromosome 21.
11. *Cri du chat* syndrome is a disorder of amino acid metabolism.
12. Turner syndrome is a common cause of mild ID in females.
13. A handicap is any restriction or lack, owing to an impairment, in ability to perform an activity in a way that is more or less normal for a human being.
14. In some cases of ID, behavioural disturbances may dominate the clinical picture.
15. A patient with ID and depression may not display or articulate any of the psychological symptoms of depression.

Answers

1. False.
2. False. Adaptive functioning only.
3. False. A person with profound ID is not capable of self-care.
4. False. The prevalence of ID is about 2-3%.
5. False. Declines in incidence have been matched by increases in life expectancy.
6. True.
7. False. The male to female ratio for severe ID is about 6:5, but is higher for mild ID.
8. False. It is much more common to find a specific cause.
9. False. Down's syndrome is the most common cause of ID.
10. False. 95% of cases of Down's syndrome result from non-disjunction of chromosome 21, and the remaining 5% from Robertsonian translocations (4%) or mosaicism (1%).
11. False. *Cri du chat* syndrome results from deletion of the short arm of chromosome 5.
12. False. Most girls with Turner syndrome are of normal intelligence.
13. False. This describes a disability.
14. True.
15. True.

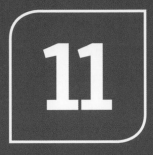

Substance misuse (alcohol and drugs)

Classification and diagnosis

In both ICD-10 and DSM-5, the first step in diagnosis is to specify the substance or class of substance involved (Table 11.1).

Table 11.1: First specify the substance or class of substance involved

ICD-10

F10	Alcohol
F11	Opioids
F12	Cannabinoids
F13	Sedatives or hypnotics
F14	Cocaine
F15	Other stimulants, including caffeine
F16	Hallucinogens
F17	Tobacco
F18	Volatile solvents
F19	Multiple drug use and other

The second step is to specify the type of disorder involved (Table 11.2).

Table 11.2: Then specify the type of disorder involved

ICD-10

.0	Acute intoxication
.1	Harmful use
.2	Dependence syndrome
.3	Withdrawal state
.4	Withdrawal state with delirium
.5	Psychotic disorder
.6	Amnestic syndrome
.7	Residual and late-onset psychotic disorder
.8	Other mental and behavioural disorders

For instance, for heroin dependence the ICD-10 coding is F11.2 (opioids, dependence syndrome), for Othello syndrome it is F10.5 (alcohol, psychotic disorder), and for Korsakov syndrome it is F10.6 (alcohol, amnestic syndrome).

Alcohol

Drinking guidelines

Since 2016, the UK government recommends that both men and women drink no more than 14 units of alcohol a week, spread over three or more days with some alcohol-free days. Beyond this, there is a significant risk of alcohol-related health and social problems. A unit is about 8g of alcohol, equivalent to half a pint of ordinary beer, one glass of table wine, one conventional glass of sherry or port, or one single bar measure of spirits (Figure 11.1). As a rough measure, one bottle of wine is equivalent to about 12 units, and one bottle of spirits to 40 units.

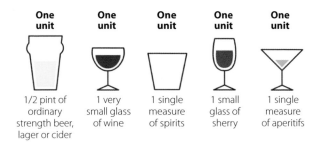

Figure 11.1. Equivalences for one unit of alcohol.

Epidemiology

It is estimated that 7% of US adults suffer from an alcohol use disorder. In the UK, the prevalence of alcohol dependence is about 6% in men and 2% in women. However, these figures mask much higher rates of harmful drinking and hazardous drinking, with about one third of men and one sixth of women in England drinking in a way that could be harmful. UK deaths from alcohol liver disease have more than doubled since 1980, while in England and Wales alcohol-related injury and illness has come to account for about 14% of attendances at Accident & Emergency departments.

Although alcohol misuse is most prevalent among young men, in recent years there has been a disproportionate increase in the numbers of women misusing alcohol. Compared to men, women are more likely to suffer with the physical complications of alcohol.

There are important international variations in the prevalence of alcohol misuse and dependence. Broadly speaking, compared to the UK, alcohol-related disorders are more prevalent in Russia and Latin America, and less so in the Middle East, Africa, and South and South-East Asia.

Aetiology

Choose life. Choose a job. Choose a career. Choose a family. Choose a f***ing big television, choose washing machines, cars, compact disc players, and electrical tin can openers. Choose good health, low cholesterol and dental insurance. Choose fixed interest mortgage repayments. Choose a starter home. Choose your friends. Choose leisure wear and matching luggage. Choose a three-piece suite on hire purchase in a range of f***ing fabrics. Choose DIY and wondering who the f*** you are on a Sunday morning. Choose sitting on that couch watching mind-numbing spirit-crushing game shows, stuffing f***ing junk food into your mouth. Choose rotting away at the end of it all, p***ing your last in a miserable home, nothing more than an embarrassment to the selfish, f***ed up brats you have spawned to replace yourselves. Choose your future. Choose life … But why would I want to do a thing like that? I chose not to choose life: I chose something else. And the reasons? There are no reasons. Who needs reasons when you've got heroin?

—Renton, quoted in the film *Trainspotting* (1996)

Social factors

Life events and circumstances: Life events and circumstances such as separation, bereavement, loss of employment, discrimination, loneliness, and homelessness can lead to alcohol misuse and dependence.

Occupation: Certain occupational groups are at a significantly higher risk of alcohol misuse, including publicans and bar staff, seafarers, butchers, builders, musicians, cooks, barbers, sales people, and entertainers.

Availability and attitudes: Average alcohol consumption in a given population is closely related to prevalence of alcohol-related disorders, for example, number of deaths by cirrhosis. Average alcohol consumption in a population can be controlled by three levers: price, availability, and social attitudes to alcohol.

Cormorbidity

Mental disorders such as depression and anxiety and stress-related disorders, and medical disorders and their complications such as terminal illness and chronic pain, commonly lead to alcohol misuse and dependence. Conversely, alcohol misuse and dependence commonly lead to other mental and medical disorders (Table 11.3).

'Dual diagnosis' refers to the co-occurrence of mental disorder and alcohol or drug misuse—although, strictly speaking, the term does not encompass those mental states that are fully contingent upon substance misuse, for instance, cocaine-induced psychosis. The failure to uncover co-morbid substance misuse can lead to an incorrect diagnosis and inappropriate management plan.

Psychological theories

There is no such thing as an 'alcoholic personality', although depression, anxiety and stress-related disorders, borderline personality disorder, antisocial personality disorder, and a history of childhood conduct disorder are associated with alcohol misuse and dependence.

According to cognitive behavioural theories, alcohol misuse can result from positive reinforcement (seeking out the pleasant effects of alcohol) and negative reinforcement (drowning negative thoughts and feelings, or avoiding the negative effects of alcohol withdrawal), from a conditioned response to one or more cues or circumstances (such as being in a pub or hotel, or having a row), or from modelling the drinking behaviour of relatives, peers, and media icons.

According to psychodynamic theories, alcohol misuse can result from such factors as maternal deprivation, childhood abuse, and unconscious gains from intoxication, the license that it provides, and the damage that it causes.

11

Genetics

The concordance rate for alcohol dependence in monozygotic twins is 70% in males and 43% in females, versus 43% in males and 32% in females in dizygotic twins. First-degree relatives of alcohol dependent persons have a seven-fold increased risk of developing alcohol dependence. Adoption studies of sons of alcohol dependent parents suggest that this increased risk is largely maintained after adoption by non-alcohol dependent parents.

The genetic influence in alcohol dependence may exert itself through heritable personality factors, or else through single genes that modulate the body's response to alcohol. In particular, East Asian populations are much less likely to develop alcohol dependence because many individuals have a particular isoenzyme of aldehyde dehydrogenase which, upon alcohol ingestion, leads to an accumulation of acetaldehyde and an unpleasant 'flushing reaction' consisting of flushing, nausea, palpitations, headache, and other symptoms.

Neurochemical abnormalities

Alcohol has a variety of effects on a number of neurotransmitters, including gamma aminobutyric acid (GABA), dopamine, serotonin, and glutamate. The reinforcing effects of alcohol are mediated by GABA, dopamine, and serotonin. In alcohol dependence, there is compensatory up-regulation of glutamate to counterbalance the GABAergic central nervous system (CNS) depressant effects of alcohol: suddenly withdrawing the alcohol therefore leads to symptoms of CNS hyperexcitation.

Clinical features and complications

Alcohol dependence

The following are seven key features of alcohol dependence:

1. Compulsion to drink or craving.
2. Primacy of drinking over other activities.
3. Stereotyped pattern of drinking, e.g. narrowing of drinking repertoire.
4. Increased tolerance to alcohol, i.e. needing more and more to produce the same effect.
5. Repeated withdrawal symptoms.
6. Relief drinking to avoid withdrawal symptoms, e.g. 'eye opener' first thing in the morning.
7. Reinstatement after abstinence.

For a diagnosis of alcohol dependence to be made, ICD-10 requires at least three from a similar list of features occurring at any time during a 12-month period.

Withdrawal syndrome

Withdrawal symptoms usually occur after several years of heavy drinking, and range from mild anxiety and sleep disturbance to life-threatening delirium tremens (see later). They are most likely to occur first thing in the morning, which is why some people with alcohol dependence go so far as to sleep with a straw in their mouth. Common symptoms include agitation, tremor ('the shakes'), perspiration, nausea, and vomiting. Unless relieved by alcohol or medical treatment, these symptoms can last for several days and progress to transient perceptual distortions and hallucinations, seizures, and/or delirium tremens.

> ### Veisalgia (alcoholic hangover)
>
> 'Hangover' effects peak several hours following alcohol intoxication, and subside within 8-24 hours. They include thirst, headache, dizziness and vertigo, increased sensitivity to light and sound, irritability, anxiety, dysphoria, sympathetic hyperactivity, red eyes, muscle ache, lethargy, sleep disturbance, and hypothermia.
>
> Hangover effects are thought to result from dehydration, the toxic effects of alcohol metabolites acetaldehyde and acetate, the toxic effects of congeners (impurities produced during alcohol fermentation), irritation of the gastric lining, hypoglycaemia, and vitamin B12 deficiency.
>
> There is no compelling evidence for any of the interventions currently used for preventing or treating hangovers, and the best approach is probably one involving fluids, food, and sleep. Non-steroidal anti-inflammatory drugs (NSAIDs) and paracetamol ought to be avoided as their deleterious effects on (respectively) the stomach lining and liver are compounded by alcohol. Caffeine may increase the effect of analgesics used, but it is also a diuretic and promotes dehydration.
>
> "I never get a hangover with fine wine": because it contains fewer congeners; because it is more intense, complex, and long and takes longer to drink; because it is usually drunk with food; and because it is poured in smaller amounts.

Delirium tremens

Delirium tremens is a medical emergency that occurs in about 5% of alcohol dependent people after one-to-three days without alcohol. Untreated mortality rate is around 10%.

Delirium tremens is a delirious disorder characterized by:

- Clouding of consciousness.
- Disorientation in time and place.
- Impairment of recent memory.
- Fear, agitation, and restlessness.
- Vivid hallucinations (most commonly visual) and delusions (most commonly paranoid).
- Insomnia.
- Autonomic disturbances (tachycardia, hypertension, hyperthermia, perspiration, dilated pupils).
- Coarse tremor.
- Nausea and vomiting.
- Dehydration and electrolyte imbalances.
- Seizures.

Important differentials include hypoglycaemia, drug overdose, and other causes of delirium such as urinary tract infection; and the condition should also be distinguished from alcohol hallucinosis and Wernicke's encephalopathy (see below).

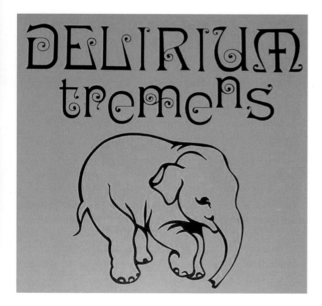

Figure 11.2. 'Delirium Tremens' is also the name of an award-winning beer. Reproduced with the permission of Brewery Huyghe NV, Melle, Belgium.

Prevention and treatment involve benzodiazepines, correction of fluid and electrolyte imbalances, treatment of concurrent infections, and parenteral multivitamin injections.

Delirium tremens is not uncommon in in-patients who cannot drink while in hospital, and often complicates other states and conditions. The diagnosis is easy to miss in people who conceal their drinking habits. Fever and shock are poor prognostic indicators.

Wernicke-Korsakov syndrome

Wernicke encephalopathy is a medical emergency. It is a disorder of acute onset characterized by impaired consciousness, confusion, episodic memory impairment, ataxia, nystagmus, abducens and conjugate gaze palsies, pupillary abnormalities, and peripheral neuropathy (the 'classic triad' that students are sometimes asked about is confusion, ataxia, and ocular palsy). Wernicke encephalopathy results from thiamine (vitamin B_1) deficiency, most commonly secondary to alcohol dependence. Other causes of thiamine deficiency include starvation, malabsorption, hyperemesis, and carbon monoxide poisoning. The differential diagnosis is principally from hypoglycaemia, hepatic encephalopathy, and subdural haemorrhage. Treatment involves parenteral thiamine, but only 20% of sufferers recover, and 10% die from haemorrhages in the brainstem and hypothalamus.

The remainder develop Korsakov syndrome, which results from neuronal loss, gliosis, haemorrhage in the mammillary bodies, and damage to the dorsomedial nucleus of the thalamus. Korsakov syndrome is an irreversible amnestic syndrome characterized by impairment of recent and, to a lesser extent, remote memory. Confabulation—the falsification of memory in clear consciousness—may be a marked feature, but immediate recall, perception, and other cognitive functions are usually intact. For a case study of Korsakov syndrome, see *The Lost Mariner* in *The Man Who Mistook His Wife for a Hat* by Oliver Sacks.

Other complications of alcohol misuse and dependence are outlined in Table 11.3.

Table 11.3: Other complications of alcohol misuse and dependence

Psychiatric	• Mood and anxiety disorders. • Suicide and deliberate self-harm. • Partially reversible cognitive impairment. • Alcoholic hallucinosis: Auditory hallucinations, first of fragmentary sounds then of derogatory voices, usually in the third person. Hallucinations can persist even after several months of abstinence, and can lead to secondary delusions. • Othello syndrome: Pathological jealousy is often compounded by sexual problems and the partner's lack of interest in an intoxicated partner. If may be necessary for the couple to separate to protect the spouse. • Pathological intoxication (*manie à potu*): An uncommon and idiosyncratic reaction to even small amounts of alcohol marked by maladaptive changes in behaviour.
Neurological	• Episodic anterograde amnesia. • Seizures. • Peripheral neuropathy. • Cerebellar degeneration. • Optic atrophy (rare). • Central pontine myelinolysis (rare). • Marchiafava-Bignami disease (rare): Demyelination of the corpus callosum, optic tracts, and cerebral peduncles manifesting as dysarthria, ataxia, seizures, and impaired consciousness, and, later, dementia and limb paralysis.
Gastrointestinal	• Oesophagitis. • Oesophageal varices. • Gastritis. • Peptic ulceration. • Acute and chronic pancreatitis. • Alcoholic hepatitis. • Cirrhosis: 10-20% of alcohol-dependent people develop cirrhosis. • Cancer of the oesophagus, stomach, and liver.
Cardiovascular	• Hypertension with increased risk of stroke and ischaemic heart disease. • Cardiac arrhythmias. • Cardiomyopathy.
Other medical	• Episodic hypoglycaemia. • Vitamin deficiencies and anaemia. • Accidents, especially head injury. • Hypothermia. • Respiratory depression. • Aspiration pneumonia. • Increased susceptibility to infections. • Sexual problems: decreased libido, impotence.
Social	• Family and marital difficulties. • Employment difficulties. • Financial problems. • Vagrancy and homelessness. • Crime and its repercussions.

11

Alcohol in pregnancy

The amount of alcohol that can be safely consumed in pregnancy is uncertain, so it is probably best to advise pregnant women to avoid it altogether. Drinking alcohol in pregnancy increases the rate of stillbirths and other obstetric complications. It also leads to foetal alcohol syndrome (FAS), which is characterized by growth retardation, dysmorphology (particularly midfacial anomalies), and CNS damage (cognitive impairment, learning difficulties, behavioural problems). FAS affects around 0.1-0.2% of live births, but milder forms of FAS, sometimes referred to as foetal alcohol effects (FAE) or alcohol-related neurodevelopmental disorder (ARND), with problems mostly circumscribed to CNS involvement, are probably much more common.

Clinical skills: Alcohol risk assessment

Before starting
- Introduce yourself to the patient and establish a rapport.
- Explain that you would like to ask him some questions about his drinking habits, and check if this is OK. Remember to be especially sensitive and tactful in your questioning.

Alcohol history
Ask about
- Alcohol intake in a typical day:
  - type (enquire separately into beer, wine, and spirits)
  - amount
  - place
  - time
- Onset and duration of alcohol problem, e.g. *When do you think it got out of hand? Have you ever tried going dry?*
- Features of alcohol dependence:
  - compulsion to drink
  - primacy of drinking over other activities
  - stereotyped pattern of drinking
  - increased tolerance to alcohol
  - withdrawal symptoms
  - relief drinking to avoid withdrawal symptoms
  - reinstatement after abstinence

Psychiatric and medical history
Ask about depression and anxiety and the common medical complications of alcohol misuse such as peptic ulceration, oesophageal varices, pancreatitis, liver disease, ischaemic heart disease, stroke, and peripheral neuropathy.

Drug history
Ask about prescription and recreational drug use. Co-morbid abuse of recreational drugs is common, as is abuse of certain prescription drugs such as benzodiazepines. Bear in mind that alcohol interacts with many prescription drugs including NSAIDs, anti-epileptics, antidepressants, antibiotics, and warfarin.

Family and social history
Ask about:
- Alcohol misuse in other family members.
- The effect of alcohol misuse on relationships, particularly with the partner and children, if any.
- The effects of alcohol misuse on employment, finances, and housing.
- Any problems with the authorities, e.g. for brawling or drink driving.

Informant history
An informant history can sometimes provide a more accurate account of the patient's drinking habits and problems.

After finishing
- Give the patient feedback on his drinking habits (e.g. number of units drunk versus guidelines), and, if appropriate, suggest ways for him to cut down his intake.
- Ask if he has any questions or concerns.
- Thank him for his co-operation.

Management

Alcohol misuse is common, and clinicians in all specialisms should routinely ask about alcohol intake and, if appropriate, alcohol-related problems. Rapid screening questionnaires such as the CAGE questionnaire may be useful in this context, even if they are not as sensitive as a comprehensive alcohol risk assessment (see above). If drinking habits are difficult to assess, take an informant history or ask the patient to keep an alcohol diary.

Clinical skills: CAGE questionnaire

C Have you ever felt you should **C**ut down on your drinking?
A Have people **A**nnoyed you by criticizing your drinking?
G Have you ever felt bad or **G**uilty about drinking?
E Have you ever had a drink first thing in the morning (**E**ye opener) to steady your nerves or nurse a hangover?

A positive response to one or more of the four questions ought to trigger further questioning.

Blood tests may be helpful both in uncovering alcohol misuse and in monitoring progress. Gamma-glutamyltransferase (GGT) is raised in about 80% of heavy drinkers, alkaline phosphatase (ALP) in about 60%, and mean corpuscular volume (MCV) in about 50%. Of the three, MCV has the highest specificity for alcohol misuse but, owing to the long half-life of red blood cells (120 days), may remain elevated for a long time after the patient has stopped drinking. Carbohydrate-deficient transferrin has an even higher specificity than MCV, but is not routinely available. The sensitivity and specificity of GGT, ALP, and MCV can be improved by studying them together.

Early management of alcohol misuse is often delivered in primary care, and involves simple advice and support together with an appraisal of social, psychological, and medical problems. It can be useful to agree a goal-oriented management plan with the patient.

If alcohol misuse has reached the stage of dependence, detoxification is required. Detoxification involves a reducing course of a benzodiazepine in lieu of alcohol, for instance, chlordiazepoxide 20mg QDS reducing daily over five to seven days and supplemented with thiamine 200mg OD (often in the form of a multivitamin preparation). Detoxification can usually be carried out in the community under the aegis of the GP practice or community drug and alcohol service, but hospital admission should be considered if the patient has a comorbid medical or mental disorder or a history of convulsions or delirium tremens, or lacks social support. A drug regimen similar to the one outlined above can also be used for the early stages of alcohol withdrawal.

Following detoxification, the patient should be advised to abstain from alcohol as abstention has a better prognosis than controlled drinking. Abstention can be encouraged by maintenance treatments such as naltrexone, acamprosate, or disulfiram. Naltrexone is a μ–opioid receptor antagonist which reduces the reinforcing euphoric effects of alcohol. Acamprosate is a structural analogue of GABA which mimics the CNS depressant effects of alcohol and reduces alcohol cravings. Disulfiram is an irreversible aldehyde dehydrogenase inhibitor which, upon drinking, leads to an accumulation of acetaldehyde and an unpleasant flushing reaction. It is, in effect, a chemical form of aversion therapy. Complications of disulfiram include seizures, coma, and death.

Maintenance treatments require close supervision, often by a nominated 'supervisor' such as the patient's spouse, and are not a substitute for psychosocial interventions. These latter include attendance at groups run by the community drug and alcohol service or Alcoholic Anonymous, supportive therapy, cognitive behavioural therapy, and marital and family therapy.

Social skills training is a type of behavioural therapy which aims to improve the patient's responses in social situations. It involves a variety of interventions such as focused instruction, modelling, role-playing (for example, declining the offer of an alcoholic drink, or going to a bar and ordering a non-alcoholic drink), and assertiveness training.

Alcohol dependence is a chronic relapsing condition, and only a minority of patients remain abstinent one year after detoxification. Predictors of relapse include poor motivation, lack of employment and social support, and co-morbid mental disorder.

Alcoholic Anonymous

Founded in 1935 in Ohio, Alcoholic Anonymous is a spiritually oriented community of alcoholics whose aim is to stay sober and, through shared experience and understanding, to help other alcoholics to do the same, 'one day at a time', by avoiding that first drink.

The essence of the programme involves a 'spiritual awakening' that is achieved by 'working the steps', usually with the guidance of a more experienced member or 'sponsor'. Members attend initially daily meetings in which they share their experiences of alcoholism and recovery and engage in prayer or meditation.

This is the short version of the Serenity prayer, which is usually recited at every meeting:

God grant me the serenity to accept the things I cannot change,
Courage to change the things I can,
And the wisdom to know the difference.

11

Clinical skills: Motivational interviewing

Scenario A

Doctor: According to your blood tests, you are drinking rather too much alcohol.

Patient: I suppose I do enjoy the odd drink.

Doctor: Are you sure it's just the odd drink? Alcohol is very bad for you, and I think that if you're drinking too much you really need to stop.

Patient: You sound like my wife!

Doctor: Well, she's right, you know. Alcohol can cause liver and heart problems and many other nasty things besides. So you really need to stop drinking, OK?

Patient: Yes, doctor, thank you.

(Patient never returns.)

Scenario B, with motivational interviewing

Doctor: We all enjoy a drink now and then, but sometimes alcohol can do us a lot of harm. What do you know about the harmful effects of alcohol?

Patient: Quite a bit, I'm afraid. My best friend, well he used to drink a lot. Last year he spent three months in hospital. I visited him often, but most of the time he wasn't with it. Then he died from internal bleeding.

Doctor: I'm sorry to hear that, alcohol can really do us a lot of damage.

Patient: It does a lot of damage to the liver, doesn't it?

Doctor: That's right, but it doesn't just do harm to our body, it also does harm to our lives: our work, our finances, our relationships…

Patient: Funny you should say that. My wife's been at my neck...

(...)

Doctor: So, you've told me that you're currently drinking about 16 units of alcohol a day. This has placed severe strain on your marriage and on your relationship with your daughter Emma, not to mention that you haven't been to work since last Tuesday and have started to fear for your job. But what you fear most is ending up lying on a hospital bed like your friend Tom. Is that a fair summary of things as they stand?

Patient: Things are completely out of hand, aren't they? If I don't stop drinking now, I might lose everything I've built over the past 20 years: my job, my marriage, even my daughter.

Doctor: I'm afraid you might be right.

Patient: I really need to quit drinking.

Doctor: You sound very motivated to stop drinking. Why don't we make another appointment to talk about the ways in which we can support you?

Recreational drugs

A brief history of recreational drugs

Opiates

The Sumerians cultivated the opium poppy as early as 3400 BC, and referred to it as *Hul Gil* or 'joy plant'. In the 18th century, the British East India Company secured a monopoly on the increasingly important opium trade, and in 1839 China's efforts to suppress it triggered a series of belligerent attacks from the British that culminated in a Chinese defeat. The British not only maintained their opium trade, but also gained a piece of China called Hong Kong. The first synthetic opiate, diamorphine, appeared at the end of that century. In 1896, Bayer Pharmaceuticals began marketing it under the name of 'heroin', 'the hero of medicines'.

Stimulants

In 1859, Paolo Mantegazzo (1831-1910) first isolated cocaine from the coca leaf, which was chewed upon by native South Americans to relieve fatigue. The drug became so popular as to be included in an American drink called Coca-Cola, or Coke, which only became a 'soft' drink in 1914, following a number of deaths by overdose. In 1887, Lazar Edeleanu (1861-1941) first synthesized 'phenylisopropylamine' or amphetamine. By the 1930s, amphetamine had found use as an over-the-counter nasal decongestant and in the treatment of narcolepsy and attention deficit hyperactivity disorder. It only became popular as a recreational drug in the 1940s, after having been given to soldiers to improve their performance. First synthesized in 1912, the psychedelic amphetamine MDMA or ecstasy only became available in the 1960s, but soon replaced cocaine as the drug of choice in bars and clubs.

Hallucinogens (Psychedelics)

In 1938, Albert Hofmann (1906-2008) discovered lysergic acid diethylamide (LSD), a derivative of ergot, a fungus that attacks rye. In 1943, he took it by accident and described the experience as 'an uninterrupted stream of fantastic pictures, extraordinary shapes with intense kaleidoscopelike play of colours'. LSD quickly established itself as a street drug, but Hofmann strongly disapproved of its use in this context, commenting:

11

'In old times psychedelic substances were considered sacred and they were used with the right attitude and in a ritual and spiritual context. And what a difference if we compare it with the careless and irresponsible use of LSD in the streets and in the discotheques of New York City and everywhere in the West. It is a tragic misunderstanding of the nature and the meaning of these kind of substances.'

Epidemiology

According to the 2014/15 Crime Survey for England and Wales, 34.7% of adults aged 16 to 59 said that they had taken an illicit drug in their lifetime, and 15.5% that they had taken a Class A drug.

In the last year, 8.6% (11.9% of men and 5.4% of women) had taken an illicit drug, versus 11.2% in 2004/5. 3.2% had taken a Class A drug (Table 11.4), and 2.2% could be classed as frequent drug users. 6.7% had used cannabis, 2.3% had used powder cocaine, and 1.7% had used ecstasy.

In the last year, the level of any drug use was 18.8% in 16 to 19 year olds and 19.8% in 20 to 24 year olds, compared to just 2.4% in 55 to 59 year olds. 2.8% of 16 to 24 year olds had taken a designer drug, but only 0.9% of 16 to 59 year olds.

Table 11.4: Controlled substances under the UK Misuse of Drugs Act 1971

Class A	Cocaine, crack, metamphetamine, any class B drug that is prepared for injection, ecstasy, LSD, phencyclidine, magic mushrooms, opium, heroin, morphine, pethidine, methadone…
Class B	Amphetamine, cannabis, codeine, ketamine, methoxetamine, methylphenidate…
Class C	Gamma hydroxybutyrate (GHB), diazepam, flunitrazepam and most other tranquillizers, sleeping tablets, and benzodiazepines, as well as anabolic steroids.

Aetiology

I don't do drugs, I am drugs.

—Salvador Dali

The aetiology of drug misuse is similar to that of alcohol misuse, and highly multi-factorial. Social factors such as the availability of the drug and attitudes to drug taking in the peer group are important in determining the likelihood of experimentation. About 10% of experimenters go on to develop problems, usually at a young age. These are more likely to come from a dysfunctional family and to have a history of delinquency or truancy. Other risk factors for drug misuse include having a mental disorder, having certain personality traits such as poor self-esteem, sensation seeking, and impulsivity, having a physical disability or illness, having a family history of drug misuse, being young, being male, being single, being or feeling socially isolated, being unemployed, living in a deprived or inner city area, and frequenting nightclubs.

Positive and negative reinforcement of drug misuse can be both physiological, such as euphoria or warding off a withdrawal reaction, and social, such as enhanced peer status or escaping from a noxious home, school, or marriage. Once a pattern of drug misuse is established, neuroadaptive changes in the brain lead to the phenomena of tolerance and withdrawal, and increased amounts of the drug are required to experience sought-after effects and ward off withdrawal symptoms.

Table 11.5: Some street names

Cannabis	Marijuana, Aunt Mary, Mary Jane, pot, dope, hash, skunk, grass, herb, weed, leaf, reefer, green, smoke, gunga
Cocaine	Charlie, coke, cola, candy, freeze, snow, blow, blast, white lady, white dust, ivory flakes, freebase, crack, rock, 'C'
Ecstasy	'E', Adam, blue kisses, hug drug, love drug, clarity, bickies, disco biscuits, dolphins, Mercedes, Rolexes, vitamins, XTC
Amphetamines	Speed, whizz, crank, crystal, ice, cartwheels, leapers, uppers, go, zip, dexies, bennies, black beauties
LSD	Acid, paper acid, microdots, dots, blotters, tabs, trips, trippers, cheer, smilies, Elvis, golden dragon, ying yang, hawk, blaze, flash, lightening, stars, rainbows
Heroin	'H', Big 'H', brown, brown sugar, hammer, scat, skag, smack, gear

11

Clinical features and management

Case study: Thomas de Quincey

It will occur to you often to ask, Why did I not release myself from the horrors of opium, by leaving it off, or diminishing it! To this I must answer briefly; it might be supposed that I yielded to the fascinations of opium too easily; it cannot be supposed that any man can be charmed by its terrors. The reader may be sure, therefore, that I made attempts innumerable to reduce the quantity. I add, that those who witnessed the agonies of those attempts, and not myself, were the first to beg me to desist.

—Thomas de Quincey (1785-1859), *Confessions of an English Opium-Eater*

Under the connecting feeling of tropical heat and vertical sunlights, I brought together all creatures, birds, beasts, reptiles, all trees and plants, usages and appearances, that are found in all tropical regions, and assembled them together in China or Indostan. From kindred feelings, I soon brought Egypt and all her gods under the same law. I was stared at, hooted at, grinned at, chattered at, by monkeys, by paroquets, by cockatoos. I ran into pagodas, and was fixed, for centuries, at the summit, or in secret rooms: I was the idol; I was the priest; I was worshipped; I was sacrificed. I fled from the wrath of Brama through all the forests of Asia: Vishnu hated me; Seva laid wait for me. I came suddenly upon Isis and Osiris: I had done a deed, they said, which the ibis and the crocodile trembled at. I was buried for a thousand years, in stone coffins, with mummies and sphinxes, in narrow chambers at the heart of eternal pyramids. I was kissed, with cancerous kisses, by crocodiles; and laid, confounded with all unutterable slimy things, amongst reeds and Nilotic mud.

—Thomas de Quincey, *Confessions of an English Opium-Eater*

This section describes the sought after and adverse effects of commonly misused drugs, including opioids such as heroin and morphine, cocaine, amphetamines, ecstasy, LSD, cannabis, benzodiazepines, and volatile substances.

In addition to drug-specific adverse effects, drug misuse in general is associated with a plethora of medical, psychiatric, and social complications. Intravenous drug use predisposes to septicaemia, bacterial endocarditis, hepatitis B and C, and HIV; and local complications such as infection of the injection site and venous thrombosis. Drug misuse in early pregnancy can lead to foetal abnormalities, and in late pregnancy to dependence in the foetus and withdrawal in the newborn. Associated psychiatric complications are common, especially depressive disorders, anxiety disorders, and personality disorders, and are often precipitated or perpetuated by the drug use and associated lifestyle. An inability to fulfil social obligations can result in unemployment, marital strife, and child neglect. Other social consequences include motoring offences, accidents, and criminal activity.

Use and abuse of the Mental Health Act

The Mental Health Act cannot be invoked for substance misuse and dependence, but associated or concurrent mental disorder may constitute grounds for compulsory admission and treatment of the disorder under the Act.

Cannabis

- Related compounds: Cannabis derives from the hemp plant *Cannabis sativa* and refers to marijuana ('grass', dried flower buds), hashish (resin), hashish oil (various extracts), and sinsemilla (highly potent form of marijuana obtained from unpollinated, seedless female plants). The main active ingredient is Δ-9-tetrahydrocannabinol.
- Route of administration: Usually smoked, but can also be eaten or drunk as an infusion.
- Mechanism of action: Acts on specific cannabinoid receptor in the CNS. The endogenous ligand for this receptor is the neurotransmitter anadamide.
- Effects: Variable according to dose and circumstances; the pre-existing mood tends to be exaggerated. The effects include heightened aesthetic experiences, altered perception of time and space, impaired short-term memory, attention, and motor skills, bloodshot eyes, irritation of the respiratory tract, dry mouth, tachycardia—and, less commonly, anxiety, paranoid ideation, gynaecomastia, reduced spermatogenesis, and carcinoma of the bronchus.
- Overdose: Higher doses may lead to confusion and psychosis.
- Withdrawal syndrome: Generally mild and short-lived symptoms including restlessness, irritability, nausea, anorexia, and insomnia. Tolerance and dependence can occur but are uncommon.
- Management: Management is aimed at reducing use and promoting abstinence. Advise users not to drive or operate machinery.

Cocaine

- Related compounds: Crack or freebase cocaine, speedball (a mixture of cocaine and heroin). Crack cocaine, so named for the sound it makes upon burning, produces a short-lived high that promotes dependence.
- Routes of administration: Oral ('chewing'), intranasal ('snorting'), intravenous ('mainlining'), and inhalation ('smoking', crack cocaine and freebase).
- Mechanism of action: Blocks reuptake of serotonin and catecholamines, especially dopamine.
- Effects: Euphoria, increased energy and confidence, disinhibition, decreased need for food and sleep, mydriasis (pupil dilatation), tachycardia, hypertension, hyperthermia. In higher doses, hallucinations, paranoid ideation, aggression. Formication ('cocaine bugs') describes the sensation of having insects crawling under one's skin. Violence is common.
- Overdose: Tremor, confusion, seizures, stroke, cardiac arrhythmias, myocardial infarction, myocarditis, cardiomyopathy, respiratory arrest.
- Withdrawal symptoms: Generalized malaise, intense craving, dysphoria, anxiety, irritability, agitation, fatigue, hypersomnolence, vivid and unpleasant dreams, suicidal ideation.
- Management: Cognitive behavioural therapy and treatment of comorbid mental disorder. In acute intoxication, consider benzodiazepines and antipsychotics to treat symptoms, and treat complications.

Amphetamines

- Related compounds: Methamphetamine, dextroamphetamine, methylphenidate, ecstasy.
- Routes of administration: Oral, intravenous, inhalation. The pure form of methamphetamine called 'ice' can be inhaled or injected.
- Mechanism of action: Blocks reuptake of noradrenaline and dopamine.
- Effects: Increased energy and confidence, insomnia, anorexia, dry lips, mouth and nose (frequent lip licking), mydriasis, tachycardia, hypertension, hyperthermia—and, less commonly, irritability, anxiety, dysphoria, confusion. Prolonged use in high doses can lead to stereotyped repetitive behaviour and paranoid psychosis.

- Overdose: Cardiac arrhythmias, severe hypertension, stroke, circulatory collapse, seizures, coma.
- Withdrawal syndrome: Dysphoria and decreased energy, and sometimes craving, anxiety, depression, fatigue, nightmares.
- Management: Cognitive behavioural therapy, treat comorbid mental disorder. In acute intoxication, consider benzodiazepines and antipsychotics to treat symptoms, and treat complications.

Ecstasy (3,4 methylenedioxymethamphetamine, MDMA)

- Related compounds: Amphetamines.
- Route of administration: Oral.
- Mechanism of action: Increased serotonergic, dopaminergic, and noradrenergic neurotransmission.
- Effects: Euphoria, sociability, intimacy, heightened perceptions, loss of appetite, nausea, tachycardia, hypertension, hyperthermia, perspiration, dehydration, bruxism (teeth grinding). High lasts 4-6 hours.
- Overdose: Still unclear, but similar to amphetamines.
- Withdrawal syndrome: Dysphoria and fatigue ('coming down'), which limits abuse potential.
- Management: Education to avoid hyperthermia by replacing lost fluids and taking breaks from dancing (ecstasy is typically used in nightclubs and at rave parties).

LSD (Lysergic acid diethylamide)

- Related compounds: Other synthetic hallucinogens include dimethyltryptamine and ecstasy. Naturally occurring hallucinogens include psilocybin (magic or psychedelic mushrooms) and mescaline (peyote cactus).
- Route of administration: Oral.
- Mechanism of action: Partial agonism at serotonin 5-HT$_{2A}$ receptors.
- Effects: Mydriasis, tachycardia, hypertension, mood changes (euphoria, distress, or anxiety), distortion or intensification of sensory experience, synaesthesia (cross-referencing of the senses, for instance, seeing sounds, hearing colours), and, in some cases, distortion of body image. Psychological effects last from 8 to 14 hours. 'Bad trips' occur if the user is not relaxed or if the setting is overly stimulating.

- Overdose: Overdose is rare but manifests as nausea and vomiting, autonomic overactivity, hyperthermia, coma, and respiratory arrest.
- Withdrawal syndrome: A withdrawal syndrome has not been described, although a minority of users experience distressing flashbacks. Tolerance can occur but dependence is rare.
- Management: Consider benzodiazepines for acute intoxication and distressing flashbacks.

Opioids

- An opioid is any agent that binds to opioid receptors, including endogenous opioid peptides, opium alkaloids such as morphine and codeine, semi-synthetic opioids such as heroin and oxycodone, and fully synthetic opioids such as pethidine and methadone. The term 'opiate' is often used as a synonym for 'opioid', but is more properly restricted to the natural opium alkaloids and their semi-synthetic derivatives.
- Routes of administration: Oral, intramuscular, intravenous, subcutaneous ('skin popping'), intranasal ('snorting'). Heroin can also be inhaled ('chasing the dragon').
- Mechanism of action: Act at specific opioid receptors. Morphine and heroin are relatively selective for the μ–opioid receptor subtype.
- Effects: Euphoria, analgesia, respiratory depression, constipation, anorexia, loss of libido, pruritus, miosis (pinpoint pupils). Tolerance develops rapidly but diminishes as soon as the drug is discontinued, leading to a potentially fatal accidental overdose if the drug is restarted at the previous dose, for instance, after being discharged from hospital or prison.
- Overdose: Respiratory depression and death.
- Withdrawal syndrome: Intense craving, restlessness, insomnia, muscle pains, tachycardia, mydriasis, running nose and eyes, perspiration, piloerection (whence the expression, 'going cold turkey'), abdominal cramps, vomiting, diarrhoea. These symptoms begin about 8-12 hours after the last fix, peak at 36-72 hours, and subside over 7-10 days.
- Management/Detoxification: Stop the drug and prescribe reducing doses of a substitute such as methadone or buprenorphine (first ensure that the person really is using opioids and not just angling for a substitute drug to misuse or sell). Refer for

psychological support e.g. abstinence or rehabilitation programme, and, if need be, social support. Clonidine and lofexidine are centrally acting $\alpha 2$ agonists that can also be used for detoxification. Naltrexone, a long-acting opioid antagonist, can help to prevent relapses, but induces withdrawal if the person is still dependent.
- Management/Harm reduction and maintenance therapy: If abstinence is unrealistic, consider substitute prescribing of oral methadone or buprenorphine, with the aim of reducing injecting, stabilizing drug use and associated lifestyle, and preventing crime. Needle exchanges and drug education programmes can also be helpful, and may encourage the person into detoxification.
- Management/Overdose: Cardiorespiratory support, instil IV naloxone (not to be confused with naltrexone, see above), e.g. 0.4-2mg IV, titrated to response. As naloxone has a shorter half-life than opiates, it may need to be given often or as an intravenous infusion to prevent re-occurrence of signs and symptoms. If the person is threatening to self-discharge, it can be given IM. Naloxone may precipitate severe withdrawal in high-dose opiate users, who may be very angry at you for ruining their trip.

Benzodiazepines

- Related compounds: Other sedatives/hypnotics that are often misused include chlormethiazole, choral, and barbiturates.
- Route of administration: Oral, intravenous.
- Mechanism of action: Benzodiazepines act at the $GABA_A$-BDZ receptor complex to enhance the inhibitory action of GABA.
- Effects: Benzodiazepines have anxiolytic, hypnotic, anticonvulsant, muscle relaxant, and amnesic properties. Tolerance develops rapidly. Dependence is common: about one-third of patients taking benzodiazepines for more than six months develop dependence.
- Overdose: Over-sedation, coma, death. There are additive effects with other drugs, including opiates and alcohol.
- Withdrawal syndrome: Anxiety, irritability, tremor, disturbed sleep, altered perception, and, rarely, depression, psychosis, seizures, and *delirium tremens*.

In some cases, the withdrawal syndrome may be prolonged for several months.

- Management: Advise users not to drive or operate machinery.
- Management/Prevention: Iatrogenic dependence is the commonest form of benzodiazepine dependence, so restrict use and prescribe only short courses.
- Management/Detoxification: Switch from benzodiazepines with a short half-life to benzodiazepines with a long half-life (e.g. diazepam), and taper off over a period of several weeks or months.
- Management/Overdose: Flumazenil.

Volatile substances

- Related compounds: Household products such as spray paint, permanent markers, correction fluid, glue, lighter fluid, hairspray, and petrol containing volatile substances such as toluene, ethyl acetate, butane, and propane.
- Routes of administration: Inhalation ('huffing').
- Mechanism of action: Increases GABA-ergic neurotransmission.
- Effects: Effects are similar to those of alcohol, but more rapid in onset. They include euphoria, disorientation, nausea, vomiting, blurring of vision, slurring of speech, incoordination, staggering gait, hallucinations. There is a high risk of trauma, asphyxia, and aspiration pneumonia. Other complications include cardiac arrhythmias and respiratory depression leading to sudden death. Chronic misuse may lead to organ damage, peripheral neuropathy, and CNS neurotoxicity.
- Overdose: As above, including coma and death.
- Withdrawal syndrome: Although dependence can develop, withdrawal symptoms are unusual.
- Management: Aim to detect early and promote abstinence.

Novel psychoactive substances

Every week, several new drugs are produced with effects similar to illegal drugs such as cocaine or LSD. These are referred to as 'novel psychoactive substances' (NPS), or, more casually, 'designer drugs', 'club drugs', or 'legal highs'. Being untested, they cannot be sold for human consumption, and are often labelled as research chemicals, bath crystals, plant food, and such like, with no safeguards as to identity and purity, strength, effects, and risks.

Today, many novel psychoactive substances are controlled under the Misuse of Drugs Act 1971 (see above), including mephedrone, naphyrone, and methoxetamine. Moreover, the government can now issue a Temporary Class Drug Order (TCDO) for any new compound that raises concern. A TCDO makes it illegal to produce, supply, import, or export the compound for a period of up to 12 months, during which it is further investigated and, if need be, controlled under the Misuse of Drugs Act.

Self-assessment

Answer by true or false.

1. The recommended limit for alcohol consumption in males is 2-3 units a day.
2. A unit is about 12g of alcohol, equivalent to half a pint of ordinary beer.
3. In alcohol dependence, upregulation of GABA compensates for the CNS depressant effects of alcohol.
4. Average alcohol consumption in a given population is influenced by three principal factors: price, availability, and social attitudes to alcohol.
5. Symptoms of alcohol withdrawal are most likely to occur in the afternoon.
6. Wernicke encephalopathy is a delirious disorder characterized by fear, agitation and restlessness, vivid hallucinations and delusions, insomnia, autonomic disturbances, coarse tremor, nausea and vomiting, dehydration and electrolyte imbalances, and seizures.
7. Wernicke encephalopathy results from a deficiency in vitamin B12, most commonly secondary to alcohol dependence, and can therefore be prevented by vitamin B12 supplementation.
8. Korsakov syndrome is a long-term syndrome characterized by severe memory impairment and confabulation. Psychotic symptoms are unusual.
9. Gamma-glutamyltransferase (GGT) has the highest specificity for alcohol misuse, but is only raised in about 50% of cases.
10. An example of a detoxification regimen is chlordiazepoxide 20mg QDS reducing daily over seven days supplemented by thiamine 200mg OD.
11. After detoxification, controlled drinking has a better prognosis than total abstention.
12. Disulfiram is an 'anti-craving' drug that enhances GABA and thereby mimics the CNS depressant effects of alcohol.
13. Disulfiram can cause cardiac arrhythmias, and is contraindicated in hypertension, coronary artery disease, and cardiac failure.
14. Morphine and heroin are relatively selective for the δ−opioid receptor subtype.
15. Effects of opioids include euphoria, analgesia, constipation, anorexia, loss of libido, pruritus, and mydriasis.
16. Effects of amphetamines include increased energy and confidence, insomnia, anorexia, dry mouth and lips, mydriasis, tachycardia, hypertension, and hyperthermia.
17. Cannabis use has not been linked with an increased incidence of psychotic disorders.
18. Speed is a mixture of cocaine and heroin.
19. Prolonged use of high doses of amphetamines can lead to stereotyped repetitive behaviour and paranoid psychosis.
20. Users of ecstasy should be educated to avoid hyperthermia by replacing lost fluids and taking breaks from dancing.

Answers

1. False. 3-4 units a day in males and 2-3 units in females.
2. False. A unit is about 8g of alcohol.
3. False. There is compensatory upregulation of glutamate, not GABA.
4. True.
5. False. They are most likely to occur first thing in the morning.
6. False. This describes delirium tremens, not Wernicke encephalopathy.
7. False. Wernicke encephalopathy results from a deficiency in thiamine.
8. True.
9. False. Mean corpuscular volume (MCV) has the highest specificity for alcohol misuse.
10. True.
11. False. Total abstention has the better prognosis.
12. False. This describes acamprosate, not disulfiram.
13. True.
14. False. Morphine and heroin are relatively selective for the μ−opioid receptor subtype.
15. False. Miosis (pinpoint pupils), not mydriasis.
16. True.
17. False.
18. True.
19. True.
20. True.

Eating, sleep, and sexual disorders

Addiction, obesity, starvation (anorexia nervosa) are political problems, not psychiatric: each condenses and expresses a contest between the individual and some other person or persons in his environment over the control of the individual's body.

—Thomas Szasz

Eating disorders

Anorexia nervosa

Epidemiology

Anorexia nervosa is more common in females than in males by a ratio of about 10:1. It is also more common in middle to upper socioeconomic groups, models, gymnasts, and dancers. Mean age of onset is 15-16 years, and onset is rare after the age of 30 years. Interestingly, anorexia nervosa is far more common in occidental or occidentalized societies, in which the prevalence rate in adolescent females is around 1%. The disorder seems strongly related to occidental values such as individualism and the idealization of thinness and beauty.

Aetiology

Possible aetiological factors in anorexia nervosa are summarized in Table 12.1. From a psychodynamic perspective, the disorder has variously been understood as a struggle for control and identity, a form of escape from the challenges of adolescence, or a type of self-harm.

Table 12:1: Possible aetiological factors in anorexia nervosa

	Biological	Psychological	Social
Precipitating Factors			• Stressors such as failing an exam or changing schools
Predisposing Factors	• Family history of eating disorder, mood disorder, or substance misuse	• Poor self-esteem • Undue compliance or extreme perfectionism • Personality disorder, especially cluster C personality disorder • Premorbid anxiety or depressive disorder	• Pressure to diet in a society that emphasizes individualism and idealizes thinness as beauty • Family environment characterized by overprotection, rigidity, and deep-rooted and often unspoken conflict • Eating disorders in the peer group or in the media
Perpetuating Factors	• Starvation, leading to neuroendocrine changes that perpetuate anorexia		As above

Diagnosis and clinical features

DSM-5 diagnostic criteria for anorexia nervosa are:

- Restriction of energy intake leading to significantly low body weight for age, sex, developmental trajectory, and physical health.
- Intense fear of gaining weight or becoming fat, or persistent behaviour that interferes with weight gain (even if significantly underweight).
- Disturbed perception of body weight or shape, undue influence of body weight or shape on self-evaluation, or persistent lack of recognition of the seriousness of the low body weight.

DSM-5 specifies two types of anorexia nervosa: 'restricting type' and 'binge-eating/purging type'. With the latter, there is regular engagement in binge-eating and purging behaviour such as self-induced vomiting or the misuse of laxatives, diuretics, or enemas.

The ICD-10 criteria are very similar to the DSM-5 criteria, but also specify widespread endocrine disorder (manifest in women as amenorrhoea and in men as loss of sexual interest and potency) and delayed or arrested puberty in anorexia nervosa of pre-pubertal onset.

Complications

Possible complications of anorexia nervosa are listed in Table 12.2.

Table 12.2: Possible complications of anorexia nervosa

Metabolic	Dehydration, hypoglycaemia, impaired glucose tolerance, hypoproteinaemia, hypokalaemia, hyponatraemia, hypocalcaemia, vitamin deficiencies, hypercholesterolaemia, deranged liver function tests
Endocrine	• Decreased gonadotrophins, oestrogens, and testosterone leading to amenorrhoea in females and loss of sexual interest and potency in males • Increased growth hormone and cortisol • Decreased triiodothyronine
Cardiovascular	• ECG abnormalities and arrhythmias • Hypotension, bradycardia, peripheral oedema, congestive cardiac failure • Mitral valve prolapse
Gastrointestinal	• Parotid enlargement and erosion of tooth enamel from self-induced vomiting • Delayed gastric emptying, constipation • Peptic ulceration • Acute pancreatitis
Renal	Renal failure, partial diabetes insipidus, renal calculi
Neurological	Enlarged ventricles, seizures, peripheral neuropathy, autonomic dysfunction
Haematological	Iron-deficiency anaemia, leucopaenia, thrombocytopaenia
Musculoskeletal	Osteoporosis, muscle cramps
Other	Hypothermia, infections, dry skin, brittle hair and nails, lanugo hairs (fine, soft, unpigmented downy hairs)

Clinical skills: Eating disorders history

Before starting
- Introduce yourself to the patient.
- Explain that you are going to ask some questions about her eating habits. Most patients with eating disorders are reluctant to seek help, so it is especially important to be sensitive and non-judgmental.

Screening for an eating disorder
- Use the **SCOFF** questionnaire to screen for an eating disorder. A positive response to two or more of the four questions (or a suspicion that the patient is not being forthright) ought to trigger further questioning.
  - Have you ever felt so uncomfortably full that you have had to make yourself **S**ick?
  - Do you worry that you have lost **C**ontrol **O**ver how much you eat?
  - Do you believe yourself to be **F**at when others say that you are too thin?
  - Would you say that **F**ood dominates your life?

Weight and perception of weight
Determine:
- The patient's current weight and height.
- The amount of weight that she has lost, and over what period. Was the weight loss intentional?
- Whether she still considers herself to be overweight.
- How often she weighs herself or looks at herself in the mirror.

Diet and compensatory behaviours
Ask about:
- Amount and type of food eaten in an average day. What foods are avoided and why? Does she engage in ritualized eating behaviours such as cutting food into little pieces and prolonged mastication? Is she able to eat in front of other people? Beyond this, does she ever diet or fast?
- Binge eating: What, how much, how often. How does she feel after bingeing?
- Vomiting: How often, how it is induced. How does she feel after vomiting?
- Use of laxatives, diuretics, emetics, appetite suppressants, and stimulants.
- Physical exercise.

Impact on health and quality of life
Ask about:
- School or work.
- Housing and finances.
- Relationships.
- Psychiatric complications, especially substance misuse, depression, and self-harm, which are all common in people with eating disorders.
- Physical complications such as dizziness/syncope, peptic ulceration, constipation.
- Menstrual periods (if appropriate).

Complete with past medical, drug, and family history.

After finishing
- Ask the patient if there is anything she might add that you have forgotten to ask about.
- Determine her level of insight into her problem.
- Thank her.
- If possible, obtain a collateral history, carry out a physical examination, and order some laboratory investigations (see below).

Differential diagnosis

The differential diagnosis of anorexia nervosa is, first, from other mental disorders—particularly bulimia nervosa, depression, obsessive-compulsive disorder, social phobia, conversion disorder, body dysmorphic disorder, schizophrenia, and personality disorder—and, second, from certain medical disorders, including endocrine disorders such as diabetes mellitus, diabetic ketoacidosis, hyperthyroidism, Grave's disease, and Addison's disease, gastrointestinal disorders such as inflammatory bowel disease, gastroenteritis, malabsorption, and intestinal obstruction, and other medical disorders such as chronic renal failure, chronic anaemia, chronic infections, neoplasm, and pregnancy.

Investigations

Following the psychiatric history and mental state examination, a physical examination ought to be undertaken to ascertain the degree of emaciation, search for complications (Table 12.2), and exclude other causes for the patient's presentation. Laboratory investigations to consider include full blood count, urea and electrolytes, calcium, liver function tests, thyroid function tests, blood glucose, erythrocyte sedimentation rate, pregnancy test, urine drug screen, urinalysis, and faecal occult blood tests. Other investigations might include electrocardiogram, chest X-ray, and abdominal X-ray.

Management

- Educate the patient and family about the disorder and its treatment. In particular, carers should understand the need to be both firm and supportive.
- After having established a good rapport, negotiate a realistic treatment plan. Aim for a balanced diet of about 3000 calories a day in the form of small meals and supplementary snacks.
- Encourage the patient while gently challenging her disturbed body perception. Consider referring her for supportive psychotherapy and support groups, cognitive behavioural therapy, or family therapy.
- Monitor the patient's physical condition and treat any complications.
- Address any associated mental disorder.
- Consider hospitalization in severe and intractable cases, especially in the presence of medical complications, associated mental disorders, or poor social support. Day treatment may offer a more acceptable alternative to in-patient admission.

Force-feeding ⓘ

Compulsory admission and treatment, including force-feeding, may be necessary in severe, intractable, and life-threatening cases.

This is more controversial than in many other cases since the patient's cognitive abilities may otherwise be fully intact, and she may not lack capacity in the legal sense.

Moreover, compulsory admission and treatment can undermine the therapeutic relationship and further alienate the patient.

Prognosis

Prognosis is very variable, and a younger age of onset and shorter history are important positive prognostic factors. About half of sufferers recover completely, while a fifth experience chronic, severe illness. The remainder make a recovery of sorts, but retain abnormal eating habits and sometimes become bulimic. The long-term mortality from suicide and the complications of starvation is over 5%, higher than for any other mental disorder.

Bulimia nervosa

Epidemiology

Bulimia nervosa is more common in females by a ratio of about 10:1. It is most prevalent in models, gymnasts, dancers, and other groups that place particular value on a slim physique. The typical age of onset is in the teens and early twenties, with the disorder affecting 1-3% of females in these age groups. Like anorexia, bulimia is far more common in occidental or occidentalized societies that promote individuality and idealize thinness and beauty. Many bulimia sufferers have a history of anorexia. A 2002 study of 15- to 18-year-old high school girls in Nadroga, Fiji, by Becker et al. found that the self-reported incidence of vomiting rose from 0% in 1995, a few weeks after the introduction of television to the province, to 11.3% in 1998.

Aetiology

Generally speaking, aetiological factors are very similar to those in anorexia nervosa. Obesity is common and there may be a history of depression, anxiety disorder, personality disorder, substance misuse, physical abuse, or childhood sexual abuse.

Diagnosis and clinical features

British psychiatrist Gerald Russell (born 1928) first described bulimia nervosa in 1979. The term 'bulimia' derives from the Greek *bous* (ox) and *limos* (hunger).

Bulimia nervosa is characterized by recurrent episodes of binge-eating followed by attempts to counteract the 'fattening' effect of the food by such methods as prolonged fasting, excessive exercise, self-induced vomiting, laxative or diuretic misuse, and stimulant drug misuse. Unlike in anorexia, the patient is usually of normal weight.

DSM-5 diagnostic criteria for bulimia nervosa are:

- Recurrent episodes of binge eating together with a sense of lack of control.
- Recurrent inappropriate compensatory behaviour to prevent weight gain.
- Episodes of binge eating and compensatory behaviour both occur, on average, at least once a week for three months.
- Self-evaluation is unduly influenced by body shape and weight.
- The disturbance does not occur exclusively during periods of anorexia nervosa.

The onset of bulimia is typically preceded by a period of dietary restriction. The patient often complains of fatigue, bloating, flatulence, constipation, abdominal pain, and menstrual irregularities. Depressive symptoms are more frequent and prominent than in anorexia, and a high proportion of patients also meet the criteria for major depression.

Complications

Complications of bulimia nervosa include:

- From purging behaviour: Dehydration, malnutrition, oedema, electrolyte abnormalities, cardiac arrhythmias, renal failure, urinary tract infection, muscle paralysis, tetany, seizures.
- From induced vomiting specifically: Dental erosion, enlargement of the parotid glands ('chipmunk facies'), oesophagitis, oesophageal tears, aspiration pneumonia. The Russell sign, named for Gerald Russell, consists of the callosities, scarring, and abrasions that can form on the dorsal surface of the index and long fingers as a result of repeated self-induced vomiting.
- Drug adverse effects and overdose.

Differential diagnosis

- Anorexia nervosa.
- Binge eating disorder.
- Depressive disorder.
- Obsessive-compulsive disorder.
- Personality disorder.
- Body dysmorphic disorder.
- Medical disorders such as diabetic ketoacidosis or intestinal obstruction.
- Obesity.

Investigations

Following the psychiatric history and mental state examination, a physical examination ought to be undertaken to search for complications and exclude other causes for the patient's presentation. Laboratory investigations to consider include full blood count, urea and electrolytes, calcium, blood glucose, pregnancy test, urine drug screen, and urinalysis. Other investigations might include electrocardiogram, chest X-ray, and abdominal X-ray.

Management

- Educate the patient and family about the disorder and its treatment.
- Encourage the patient while gently challenging her disturbed body perception. Consider referring her for supportive psychotherapy and support groups, cognitive behavioural therapy, interpersonal therapy, or family therapy.

- Alternatively or in addition, selective serotonin reuptake inhibitors (SSRIs) such as fluoxetine and sertraline are sometimes prescribed.
- Monitor the patient's physical condition and treat any complications.
- Address any associated mental disorder.
- Consider hospitalization in severe and intractable cases, especially in the presence of medical complications, associated mental disorders, or poor social support.
- Prognosis is better than in anorexia, not least because bulimia sufferers are keener to seek and accept help.

Binge eating disorder

Binge eating disorder, which was approved for inclusion in DSM-5, involves recurring episodes of eating significantly more food in a short period of time than most people would eat under similar circumstances, with episodes marked by feelings of lack of control. Episodes occur, on average, at least once a week for three months. A person with binge eating disorder may eat too quickly, even when no longer hungry. She or he may eat alone owing to embarrassment, and afterward feel guilt or disgust. This psychological and social dimension is important in distinguishing binge eating disorder from a simple eating problem. In contrast to bulimia nervosa, there is no subsequent purging behaviour.

Sleep disorders

Methought I heard a voice cry 'Sleep no more!
Macbeth doth murder sleep', the innocent sleep,
Sleep that knits up the ravell'd sleeve of care,
The death of each day's life, sore labour's bath,
Balm of hurt minds, great nature's second course,
Chief nourisher in life's feast.

—Shakespeare, Macbeth

Introduction and classification

Sleep disorders are often related to another mental disorder or to a medical disorder. Such 'secondary' sleep disorders ought to be distinguished from 'primary' sleep disorders on the basis of their clinical presentation and course.

Primary sleep disorders, the subject of this section, can be divided into dysomnias (insomnia and hypersomnia), disorders of the sleep-wake schedule (sleep delay and jet lag), and parasomnias (nightmares, night terrors, and somnambulism).

ICD-10 Classification of primary sleep disorders

F51	Non-organic sleep disorders
F51.0	Non-organic hypersomnia
F51.2	Non-organic disorder of the sleep-wake schedule
F51.3	Sleepwalking (somnambulism)
F51.4	Sleep terrors (night terrors)
F51.5	Nightmares
F51.8	Other non-organic sleep disorders

Dysomnias

Insomnia

Insomnia—difficulty in initiating or maintaining sleep—affects some 30% of the population, and is more common in females and the elderly. It is only clinically significant if it occurs on most nights and leads to distress or daytime effects such as fatigue, poor concentration, poor memory, and irritability. These symptoms predispose to accidents, depression, anxiety disorders, and medical disorders such as infection, hypertension, obesity, and diabetes. Insomnia should only be diagnosed if it dominates the clinical picture.

Insomnia can result from a variety of biological, psychological, physical, and environmental factors, often acting in combination. Short-term insomnia more often results from a stressful life event, a poor sleep environment, or an irregular routine; and chronic insomnia from mental and medical disorders and drug adverse effects (Tables 12.3, 12.4).

In assessing insomnia, it is important to take a detailed history and enquire into sleep hygiene and the sleeping environment. As part of the history, aim to cover the sleep disturbance and its daytime effects, as well as the psychiatric history, medical history, drug history, and social history. An informant history from a bed-partner may be useful. If need be, a clearer picture can be obtained by asking the patient to keep a sleep diary, or, less commonly, by carrying out sleep studies (polysomnography).

Table 12.3: Some mental and medical disorders that predispose to insomnia

Mental disorders
Depressive disorder
Mania and bipolar affective disorder
Anxiety disorders
Post-traumatic stress disorder
Schizophrenia
Alcohol and drug misuse

Medical disorders
Sleep apnoea
Chronic pain, for example, from arthritis or cancer
Chronic obstructive pulmonary disease
Chronic renal failure
Neurological disorders such as Parkinson's disease and other movement disorders
Restless leg syndrome
Headaches
Fibromyalgia

Table 12.4: Some drugs that predispose to insomnia

Stimulants such as caffeine, amphetamines, and cocaine
Alcohol
Benzodiazepines
Nicotine
Selective serotonin reuptake inhibitors
Levodopa
Phenytoin
Beta blockers
Diuretics
Theophylline
Corticosteroids
Thyroid hormone

Management involves treatment of the cause (if any), advice on sleep hygiene (see clinical skills box), and behavioural strategies such as sleep restriction. Sedatives may be effective in the short-term, but are best avoided in the longer term. Even if used, they should only play a minor role in overall management. Over-the-counter sleeping remedies often contain an antihistamine, while herbal alternatives are usually based on the herb valerian, a hardy perennial flowering plant with heads of sweetly scented pink or white flowers.

Clinical skills: Counselling for people with insomnia

- Have a strict routine involving regular and adequate sleeping times (most adults need about seven hours of sleep every night). Allocate a time for sleeping, for example, 11pm to 7am, and do not use it for any other activities. Avoid daytime naps, or make them short and regular. If you have a bad night, avoid 'sleeping in' because this makes it more difficult to fall asleep the following night.
- Have a relaxing bedtime routine that enables you to relax and 'wind down' before going to sleep. This may involve breathing exercises or meditation, or simply reading a book or listening to some light music.
- Many people find it helpful to have a hot drink: if this is the case for you, prefer a herbal or malted or chocolaty drink to stimulant drinks such as tea or coffee.
- Sleep in a familiar, dark, and quiet room that is adequately ventilated and neither too hot nor too cold. Try to use this room for sleeping only, so that you come to associate it with sleep.
- If you can't sleep, don't become anxious and try to make yourself sleep. The more anxious you become, the less likely you are to fall asleep. Instead, get up and do something relaxing and enjoyable for about half an hour, and then give it another try.
- Take regular exercise during the daytime, but do not exercise in the evening or just before bedtime because the short-term alerting effects of exercise may keep you awake.
- Try to reduce your overall levels of stress by implementing some simple lifestyle changes.
- Eat an adequate evening meal containing a good balance of complex carbohydrates and protein. Eating too much can make it difficult to fall asleep; eating too little can disturb your sleep and affect its quality.
- Avoid caffeine, alcohol, and tobacco, particularly in the evening. Also avoid stimulant drugs such as cocaine and amphetamines. Whereas alcohol may make it easier to fall asleep, it makes it more difficult to *stay* asleep, and also decreases the overall quality of sleep.
- If insomnia persists despite these measures, seek advice from your doctor. In some cases, insomnia may have a clear and definite cause that needs to be addressed in itself—for instance, a physical problem or an adverse effect of medication.

Hypersomnia

In hypersomnia, the patient complains of excessive daytime sleepiness, sleep attacks, or sleep drunkenness. A diagnosis of primary hypersomnia can only be secured if these symptoms are not better accounted for by a lack of sleep or by another sleep disorder or mental or medical disorder, and if they are associated with significant distress or impairment. The condition often responds to small doses of central nervous system (CNS) stimulant drugs.

Common causes of secondary hypersomnia are listed in Table 12.5.

Table 12.5: Common causes of secondary hypersomnia

Other sleep disorders
   Insomnia
   Sleep apnoea
   Narcolepsy
Mental disorders
   Dysthymia
   Depressive disorder
   Bipolar affective disorder
Medical disorders
   Chronic pain
   Urinary tract infection
   Brain tumour, etc.
Drugs
Other, e.g. head trauma, viral infection

Kleine-Levin syndrome

Kleine-Levin syndrome ('Sleeping Beauty syndrome') is a very rare recurrent primary hypersomnia associated with behavioural and cognitive disturbances, overeating, and/or hypersexuality. Episodes last for days or weeks, and are interspersed by long periods of normality. The condition most often presents in adolescent males and resolves in early adulthood. Aetiology is unclear, but could be viral.

Narcolepsy

Narcolepsy (Ancient Greek, *seized by somnolence*) is a relatively rare disorder resulting from a disruption in the normal pattern of rapid eye movement (REM) and non-REM sleep. Onset is in adolescence or early adulthood. Clinical features include daytime somnolence and sleep attacks, cataplexy (sudden loss of muscle tone), sleep paralysis, and hypnagogic hallucinations, although not all of these symptoms need be present to secure the diagnosis. The principal differential diagnosis is from hypersomnia and epilepsy, notably petit mal absence seizures. Management involves support and counselling (such as advice on the importance of sleep hygiene and daytime naps), and drugs including CNS stimulants such as methylphenidate, modafinil, and antidepressants.

Disorders of the sleep-wake schedule

Sleep delay

In sleep delay, there is chronic difficulty initiating sleep at socially accepted times, although once asleep there is no difficulty in maintaining sleep and total sleep time is normal. The disorder is commonest in adolescents and university students, and tends not to present to medical attention. The differential diagnosis is from lifestyle choice, insomnia, and mental and medical disorders.

Jet lag

Jet lag tends to be experienced after crossing three or more time zones, and results from a mismatch between body and environmental rhythms. Symptoms include disturbed sleep, tiredness, poor concentration, and irritability. The rate of adjustment to jet lag is 1.5 hours per day following a westward flight, and 1 hour per day following an eastward flight. Management should aim at matching body and environmental rhythms (see clinical skills box). It has been reported that, in some cases, melatonin can be effective in the prophylaxis and management of jet lag.

Clinical skills: Advice for people at risk of jet leg

- If you are able to, choose a destination that involves flying westward: evidence suggests that flying westward causes less jetlag than flying eastward.
- Choose daytime flights to avoid losing sleep.
- Use sleeping aids such as blindfolds, earplugs, and neck rests to help you sleep during the flight.
- Before your departure, gradually adjust your sleep schedule so that it approximates to that at your destination. For instance, if you are due to fly eastward, try going to bed (and waking up) earlier than you normally do.
- When you arrive, immediately reset your watch and time givers to local time.
- Do as the locals do in terms of eating and sleeping. Have your meals when they do and try not to have more than one short nap during the daytime.
- Take exercise.
- Avoid caffeine and alcohol.
- Avoid sleeping tablets.

Parasomnias

Parasomnias are abnormal episodic events during sleep and include nightmares, night terrors, and sleepwalking (Table 12.6). They are part of normal development in children, but in adults usually only arise at times of stress and distress. Important differentials are epilepsy, substance misuse, and mental and medical disorders such as post-traumatic stress disorder.

Table 12.6: Parasomnias

Type	Incidence	Onset	Sleep stage	Behaviour	Recall	Treatment
Nightmares	Frequent in children	Late in sleep	REM	Easily aroused	Usual	Support
Night terrors	3% of children, commonest in ages 4-7 There is often a family history	First 1-2 hours of sleep	Non-REM stage 4	Terrified, with screaming and thrashing Cannot easily be aroused May last 10-20 minutes	None	Reassurance and practical advice for parents Behavioural waking schedule if persistent
Sleepwalking	1-15% of 8-15 years olds, but also seen in adults Associated with night terrors	First 1-2 hours of sleep	Non-REM stage 4	May last minutes to 1 hour	None	Safety precautions Avoid sleep deprivation and alcohol

12

Dream psychology

And Jacob went out from Beersheba, and went toward Haran. And he lighted upon a certain place, and tarried there all night, because the sun was set; and he took of the stones of that place, and put them for his pillows, and lay down in that place to sleep. And he dreamed, and behold a ladder set up on the earth, and the top of it reached to heaven: and behold the angels of God ascending and descending on it. And, behold, the LORD stood above it, and said, I am the LORD God of Abraham thy father, and the God of Isaac: the land whereon thou liest, to thee will I give it, and to thy seed; And thy seed shall be as the dust of the earth, and thou shalt spread abroad to the west, and to the east, and to the north, and to the south: and in thee and in thy seed shall all the families of the earth be blessed. And, behold, I am with thee, and will keep thee in all places whither thou goest, and will bring thee again into this land; for I will not leave thee, until I have done that which I have spoken to thee of. And Jacob awakened out of his sleep, and he said, Surely the LORD is in this place; and I knew it not.

—Bible, Genesis 28

In his *General Aspects of Dream Psychology*, Jung argues that dreams contribute to the self-regulation of the psyche by automatically bringing up everything that is repressed or neglected or unknown. However, he continues, their compensatory significance is often not immediately apparent because of our still very incomplete knowledge of the nature and needs of the human psyche.

Yet, some 2,000 years before the time of Jung and Freud, thinkers such as Plato, Aristotle, and the 1st century Hellenistic philosopher Philo of Alexandria already held some fairly advanced notions in the still unborn field of dream psychology. For instance, in the *Politicus*, Plato says that 'every man seems to know all things in a dreamy sort of way, and then again to wake up and know nothing'. Aristotle wrote a book called *On Divination in Sleep*, in which he argues that skilful dream interpretation calls upon the faculty of observing resemblances. He then compares dream presentations to the forms reflected in water: if the motion in the water is great, then the reflection bears little resemblance to its original, and particular skill is required on the part of the dream interpreter.

In his treatise *On Sleep*, Philo of Alexandria offers four different interpretations for the ladder to heaven that appears in Jacob's dream. I am not particularly keen on any of Philo's interpretations and much prefer the fourth century interpretation of St Gregory the Theologian and St John Chrysostom, who thought of the ladder in terms of an ascetic path of virtue along which it is possible for man to ascend from earth to heaven, 'not using material steps, but improvement and correction of manners'.

The notion of dream interpretation far antedates the birth of psychoanalysis, and probably served an important function in most, if not all, historical societies. In having lost this function, modern man has also lost the most magical part of his nature, which he obliviously passes on to the next generation of dreamers.

Sexual disorders

Sexual dysfunction

Sexual dysfunction can occur at any stage of sexual intercourse: initiation, arousal, penetration, and orgasm (Table 12.7). It can result from organic causes (such as diabetes, angina, prostate surgery, antihypertensives, antidepressants, antipsychotics) or from psychological causes (such as depression, anxiety, sexual inexperience, traumatic sexual experience, relationship difficulties, stress), or from a combination of both. In secondary dysfunction, there is a history of normal function: in primary dysfunction such a history is lacking. The epidemiology of sexual dysfunction is hard to establish, but erectile dysfunction and premature ejaculation are common in men, and anorgasmia and hypoactive sexual desire are common in women.

Table 12.7: Types of sexual dysfunction (commoner types in bold)

	Male	Female
Sexual desire disorders	Hypoactive sexual desire	**Hypoactive sexual desire (F>M)**
	Sexual aversion (rare)	Sexual aversion (rare)
Sexual arousal disorders	**Erectile dysfunction***	Failure of genital response
Sexual pain disorders	Dyspareunia	Dyspareunia (F > M)
Orgasm disorders	Ejaculatory impotence	Vaginismus[§]
	Premature ejaculation**	**Anorgasmia (F>M)**

*   Erectile dysfunction or impotence is more common in elderly males.

** Premature ejaculation is more common in young males embarking on their first sexual relationships.

[§]   Vaginismus describes involuntary vaginal contractions in response to attempts at penetration.

The sexual history is often omitted by embarrassed students, but is nonetheless an important part of the psychiatric history. This is not only because sexual problems are important in themselves, but also because they predispose to mental disorder, or result from mental disorder or its treatment. The sexual history is best taken by direct but tactful questioning at or near the end of the psychiatric history. Remain professional and formal throughout, but do not persist in your questioning if the patient becomes uncomfortable.

Presenting complaint
Ask about:
- The presenting problem (in detail). Ask specifically about erectile dysfunction and ejaculatory dysfunction in males, and hypoactive sexual desire, anorgasmia, vaginismus, and dyspareunia in females.
- The onset, course, and duration of the problem. Is the problem primary or secondary?
- The frequency and timing of the problem. Is the problem partial or situational? With situational erectile dysfunction, the patient still has morning erections.
- The effect that the problem is having on the patient's life.

Sexual history
If not already covered, ask about:
- Number of partners and nature and quality of relationships.
- Frequency of sex.
- Types of sex.
- Sexual preferences and paraphilias (see later).
- Contraceptive methods.
- Symptoms of sexually transmitted disease such as sores, discharge, bleeding, itching, rashes, dysuria, and abdominal pain.
- Sexual development: age at puberty and at first intercourse.
- Sexual experience.
- Attitudes to sex.
- History of physical or sexual abuse (avoid suggestive questioning).

To finish
Make sure you cover:
- The psychiatric history.
- The medical history.
- The drug history, including alcohol and illicit drugs.

In assessing sexual dysfunction, it is important to take a full sexual history (see clinical skills box), including details of the psychiatric and medical histories. A physical examination emphasizing the genitourinary, vascular, and neurological systems and laboratory investigations such as urinalysis and hormone levels may be required to exclude organic causes.

With sexual dysfunction arising from an organic cause, treat the cause if at all possible. With sexual dysfunction arising from psychological causes, treatment may involve simple reassurance and advice, sex therapy, and/or drug or physical treatment.

In sex therapy, the couple is usually seen together over a certain number of sessions and encouraged to discuss their sexual relationship openly. They are educated about sex and given a series of assignments to perform at home. These progress from non-genital 'sensate focus technique' (that is, non-genital caressing) to full intercourse, and are designed to rebuild the couple's sexual relationship through the behavioural technique of graded exposure. In addition, specific exercises may be taught for specific forms of dysfunction, such as Seman's technique for premature ejaculation (involves the partner squeezing the base of the penis to prevent ejaculation) and relaxation training and vaginal dilators for vaginismus. The outcome of sex therapy is generally good, except with hypoactive sexual desire.

Drugs and physical treatments for certain sorts of sexual dysfunction include phosphodiesterase type 5 inhibitors such as sildenafil (caution in heart disease), intracavernosal injections of alprostadil (prostaglandin E1), testosterone replacement, vacuum erection devices, penile prosthetic implants, and penile microrevascularization.

Paraphilias

Paraphilias are disorders of sexual preference that begin in late adolescence or early adulthood and most commonly affect males (Table 12.8). They are 'disorders' in that the principal object of sexual arousal or the principal method of achieving sexual arousal is abnormal—although note that this circular definition is heavily values loaded.

In DSM-5, paraphilias are no longer ipso facto mental disorders. Instead, a paraphilia becomes a mental disorder (a 'paraphilic disorder', e.g. 'pedophilic disorder') if it is causing distress to the individual (not merely distress resulting from society's disapproval), or if it involves another's person's psychological distress, injury, or death, or a desire for sexual behaviours involving unwilling persons or persons unable to give legal consent. Crucially, at least by DSM-5, it is now possible for an individual to engage in consensual atypical sexual behaviour without this being labelled as mental disorder.

If there is a rapid change in sexual behaviour, particularly in middle or old age, it is important to exclude mental disorders such as dementia, psychotic disorders, and affective disorders.

Table 12.8: Paraphilias

Paraphilia	Description
Transvestism	Disturbance of gender role behaviour. Transvestites intermittently or permanently assume the appearance, mannerisms, and interests of the opposite sex. Transvestism is not to be confused with transsexualism, in which the person feels trapped inside a body of the opposite sex. In DSM-5, transsexualism is no longer classed as a disorder but as 'gender dysphoria'.
Paedophilia	Sexually arousing fantasies, urges, or behaviours involving sexual activity with prepubescent children. It is estimated that about 50% of victims of abuse are relatives or friends of the abuser.
Exhibitionism	Sexually arousing fantasies, urges, or behaviours involving exposing one's genitalia to unsuspecting strangers. Offenders are typically young males, and their victims pubescent females.
Voyeurism (Scopophilia)	Sexually arousing fantasies, urges, or behaviours involving observing an unsuspecting person naked or undressing, or engaged in sexual activity.
Frotteurism	Sexually arousing fantasies, urges, or behaviours involving rubbing against or touching a non-consenting person, typically in crowded places such as a busy train carriage.
Sexual sadism	Sexually arousing fantasies, urges, or behaviours involving humiliating, or causing suffering to, others (cf. sexual masochism). Sadism is named after the 18th century writer, the Marquis de Sade.
Sexual masochism	Sexually arousing fantasies, urges, or behaviours involving being humiliated or being made to suffer. Masochism is named after the 19th century writer, Leopold von Sacher-Masoch.
Fetishism	Sexually arousing fantasies, urges, or behaviours involving non-living objects not limited to articles of clothing used in cross-dressing or to devices designated for genital stimulation.
Other paraphilias	Incest (close relatives), zoophilia/bestiality (animals), necrophilia (dead bodies), coprophilia (faeces), urophilia (urine), klismaphilia (enemas), narratophilia (obscene language), and telephone and internet scatologia (obscene language, pictures, etc. over the phone or internet).

The psychology of sadomasochism

Sadomasochism is hard to understand. Here, I propose several understandings. While some may hold in some cases or circumstances and not others, none are mutually exclusive.

Most obviously, the sadist may derive pleasure from feelings of power, authority, and control, and from the 'suffering' of his or her partner. The sadist may also harbour an unconscious desire to punish the object of sexual attraction for having aroused his desire and thereby subjugated him, or, in some cases, for having frustrated his desire or aroused his jealousy.

By objectifying his partner, who is thereby rendered subhuman, the sadist no longer needs to handle his partner's emotional baggage, and can deceive himself that the sex is not all that meaningful: a mere act of lust rather than an intimate and pregnant act of love. The partner becomes a trophy, a mere plaything, and while one can own a toy and perhaps knock it about, one cannot fall in love with it or be hurt or betrayed by it.

Sadism may also represent a kind of displacement activity or scapegoating in which uncomfortable feelings such as anger and guilt are displaced and projected onto another person.

For the masochist, taking on a role of subjugation and helplessness can offer a release from stress or the burden of responsibility or guilt. It can also evoke infantile feelings of dependency, safety, and protection, which can serve as a proxy for intimacy. In addition, the masochist may derive pleasure from earning the approval of the sadist, commanding his full attention, and, in a sense, controlling him.

For the dyad, sadomasochism can be seen as a means of intensifying normal sexual relations (pain releases endorphins and other hormones), regressing to a more primal or animal state, testing boundaries, building trust, creating intimacy, or playing. In her recent book, *Aesthetic Sexuality*, Romana Byrne goes so far as to argue that S&M practices can be driven by certain aesthetic goals tied to style, pleasure, and identity, and, as such, can be compared to the creation of art.

12

Self-assessment

Answer by true or false.

1. Eating disorders are more common in homosexual males than in heterosexual males.
2. Average age of onset for anorexia nervosa is in the mid to late twenties.
3. An important aetiological factor in anorexia is pressure to diet in a society that idealizes thinness and beauty.
4. DSM-5 specifies two types of anorexia: purging type and non-purging type.
5. Depressive symptoms are more common in bulimia than in anorexia.
6. The Russell sign refers to the enlargement of the parotid glands that results from repeated induced vomiting.
7. SSRI antidepressants can be used in the treatment of bulimia.
8. In refeeding, the patient should aim at a balanced diet of about 3000 calories a day.
9. Prognosis in bulimia is better than in anorexia.
10. Even after recovery, many people with a diagnosis of anorexia retain abnormal eating habits.
11. Insomnia is more common in males and in the elderly.
12. Sedatives should only play a minor role, if any, in the management of insomnia.
13. Narcolepsy is characterized by a tetrad of daytime somnolence and sleep attacks, cataplexy, sleep paralysis, and hypnopompic hallucinations, although not all of these features are always present.
14. In sleep delay, total sleep time is normal.
15. Nightmares, night terrors, and sleepwalking are all more common in children.
16. Night terrors occur in non-REM stage 4 sleep.
17. Erectile dysfunction and ejaculatory impotence are common in males.
18. Vaginismus describes voluntary vaginal contractions in response to attempts at penetration.
19. Transsexuals intermittently or permanently assume the appearance, mannerisms, and interests of the opposite sex.
20. Voyeurism describes sexually arousing fantasies, urges, or behaviours that involve exposing one's genitalia to unsuspecting strangers.

Answers

1. True.
2. False. Average age of onset is 15-16.
3. True. Anorexia is uncommon in societies that do not idealize thinness and beauty.
4. True. 'Restricting type' and 'binge-eating/purging type'.
5. True.
6. False. This describes 'chipmunk facies'.
7. True.
8. True.
9. True.
10. True.
11. False. Insomnia is more common in females and in the elderly.
12. True.
13. False. Hypnagogic hallucinations.
14. True.
15. True.
16. True.
17. False. Erectile dysfunction and premature ejaculation. Ejaculatory impotence is comparatively uncommon.
18. False. Involuntary vaginal contractions.
19. False. This describes transvestism.
20. False. This describes exhibitionism.

Child and adolescent psychiatry

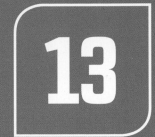

13

Introduction

Like forensic psychiatry, child psychiatry is a sub-specialism of psychiatry to which most students receive only limited exposure.

There are essentially three types or classes of childhood mental disorders:

- Developmental disorders such as autism and Asperger syndrome.
- Disorders that are more or less specific to childhood and adolescence such as ADHD, conduct disorder, and tic disorders.
- 'Adult' disorders occurring in childhood such as mood and anxiety disorders.

The practice of child psychiatry differs from that of adult psychiatry, not only in that the range of disorders is different, but also in that:

- Children's problems must be looked at in context of their developmental stage. Some issues are normal at one stage but no longer so at a later one.
- Children may not be able to express themselves as eloquently as (most) adults. This means that greater emphasis must be placed on their appearance and behaviour, and on collateral histories from guardians, siblings, teachers, social workers, and other health workers.
- Distress in children is expressed more in terms of behavioural disturbance than in terms of sharply defined symptoms. Collateral histories might differ significantly from one informant to another.
- Guardians must be closely involved in the management plan, not least because they may be contributing to the child's problems.
- Drugs should be used less frequently and more cautiously than in adult psychiatry.

Child development

Children's problems must be looked at in the context of their developmental stage, as some issues are normal at one stage but no longer so at a later one. Thus, it is necessary to have some knowledge of child development, and of the average ages at which key milestones are achieved (Table 13.1).

Table 13.1: Average age for the acquisition of milestones

Key stages	Age	Gross motor skills	Vision & fine movement	Hearing and language	Social behaviour
Newborn	Birth -1/2	Symmetrical movements, limbs flexed, head lag on pulling up	Looks at light/faces in direct line of vision	Startles to noises and voices, cries	Responds to parents, endogenous smile
Supine infant	2/12	Raises head in prone position	Eyes 'fix and follow' to midline	Coos and grunts	Exogenous smile, i.e. at faces or objects
	3-4/12	Rolls over from supine to prone, sits with support	Eyes follow past midline	Laughs	
Sitting infant	6/12	Rolls over from prone to supine, sits unsupported	Transfers objects from hand to hand	Babbles, single syllable words (yes, no)	Separation anxiety
	9/12	Crawls and, from 10/12, 'cruises' (walks holding on to furniture)	Pincer grasp	Double syllable words (mama, bye-bye)	Stranger anxiety, plays pat-a-cake and peek-a-boo
Toddler	1 year	Takes first steps	Starts to feed himself	Uses 10 words	Onlooker and parallel play
	18/12	Runs, walks carrying a toy	Stacks 3 cubes	Uses 10-20 words	Temper tantrums
	2 years	Ascends stairs in child-like manner, arm throws a ball	Copies a line, stacks 6 cubes	Uses 200 words, pronouns, 2-word sentences	Alone play
Communicating child	3 years	Climbs stairs like an adult, descends stairs in child-like manner, jumps in one place, rides tricycle, catches ball with arms	Copies a circle, stacks 9 cubes, builds bridge with cubes	Uses 900 words and understands many more, compound sentences	Knows own name and gender, understands 'taking turns', i.e. co-operates
	4 years	Climbs down stairs like an adult, hops on one foot, throws overhand	Copies a cross and, from 4.5 years, a square	Tells stories	Imitates parents, has imaginary friends
	5 years	Stands on one leg, catches ball with hands	Copies a triangle	Asks the meaning of words	Conforms with peers

Children are not mere mini-adults, but gradually develop into adults by progressing through various phases or stages of development. Stage theories of development include psychoanalytic development theories, cognitive development theories, and psychosocial development theories. Three of the most influential stage theories of development, namely, those of Freud, Piaget, and Erikson, are summarized in Table 13.2.

Table 13.2: Three influential theories of development

Age (years)	Sigmund Freud Psychosexual development	Jean Piaget Cognitive development	Erik Erikson Psychosocial development
1	**Oral stage (0-1.5)** Dependent for his/her needs Focus is on sucking (mouth) Fixation leads to dependent and passive adults	**Sensorimotor stage (0-2)** Cognition limited to physical experiences and interactions Develops object permanence Lacks symbolic representation	**Trusts *vs* mistrust (0-1.5)** Develops trust, security, and basic optimism
2	**Anal stage (1.5-3.5)** Issues of self-control and obedience Focus is on anus Fixation leads to anal retentive (rigid) or anal expulsive (disorganized) adults	**Preoperational stage (2-7)** Increasing use of symbolic representation, principally language Thinking is intuitive, egocentric, and irreversible	**Autonomy *vs* doubt (1.5-3)** Learns to be self-sufficient and in control
3			
4	**Phallic stage (3.5-6)** Issues of morality and sexual identification Focus is on penis and genital pleasure (Oedipus complex) Fixation leads to amoral or puritanical adults		**Intuitive *vs* guilt (3-6)** Inquisitive exploration of environment, e.g. through play situations, reinforces sense of purpose and independence
5			
6			
7	**Latency period (6-puberty)** Dormant sexuality Same-sex friendships		**Industry *vs* inferiority (6-12)** Competence at certain tasks builds up self-esteem and leads to acceptance by the peer group
8		**Concrete operational stage (7-11)** Logical use of symbols related to concrete objects Develops conservation of numbers	
9			
10			
11			
12		**Formal operational stage (11+)** Logical use of symbols related to abstract concepts Achieved by only 35% or so of high school graduates	
13			**Identity *vs* role confusion (12-18)** Develops a sense of identity through thoughts and ideals, and peer group
14			
15			
16	**Genital stage (from puberty)** Resurgence in sexuality Successful resolution of conflicts from this and previous psychosexual stages leads to maturity		PLUS three other adult stages: • Intimacy *vs* isolation • Generativity *vs* stagnation • Integrity *vs* despair
17			
18			

13

Attachment theory and the inheritance of loss

Inspired by the seminal work of John Bowlby (1907-1990) on attachment theory, Mary Ainsworth (1913-1999) devised a procedure called the 'Strange Situation' to observe patterns of attachment in human infants. In the Strange Situation, an infant is observed exploring toys for twenty minutes while his mother and a stranger enter and leave the room. Depending on the infant's behaviour upon being reunited with his mother, he can be classified into one of three categories: secure attachment, anxious-ambivalent insecure attachment, and anxious-avoidant insecure attachment.

In secure attachment, the infant explores freely and engages with the stranger while his mother is present. When his mother leaves, he is subdued but not distressed; and when she returns, he greets her warmly. A pattern of secure attachment is thought to arise if the mother is generally available to the infant and able to meet his needs responsively and appropriately.

In anxious-ambivalent insecure attachment, the infant is anxious of exploration and ambivalent towards the stranger, even in the presence of his mother. When his mother leaves, he is distressed; but when she returns he is ambivalent towards her. A pattern of anxious-ambivalent insecure attachment is thought to arise if the mother generally gives the infant attention, but inconsistently and according to her own needs.

In anxious-avoidant insecure attachment, the infant explores the toys but seems unconcerned by the presence or absence of either the stranger or his mother. However, he does not avoid the stranger as strongly as he does his mother. A pattern of anxious-avoidant insecure attachment is thought to arise if the mother generally disengages from the infant, such that he comes to believe that he has no influence over her.

An infant's pattern of attachment is important because it can lead to an internal model of the self as unlovable and inadequate, and of others as unresponsive and punitive. It can also help to predict a person's reaction to loss or adversity and his pattern of relating to peers, engaging in romantic relationships, and parenting children.

Through parenting children, an insecure attachment can be passed on from parent to child, and in this manner one generation's loss can be inherited by the next.

That which a child did not receive he cannot later give, or, as it says in the Talmud,

The parent who teaches his son, it is as if he had taught his son, his son's son, and so on to the end of generations.

Developmental disorders

Intellectual disability

Chapter 10.

Autism

First described by the Austrian-American psychiatrist Leo Kanner (1894-1981) in 1943, autism is a pervasive developmental disorder characterized by a triad of:

- Impairments in social interactions despite a desire for them.
- Abnormalities in patterns of communication.
- A restricted, stereotyped, and repetitive repertoire of behaviours, interests, and activities.

In addition to these specific diagnostic features, there may be a range of non-specific problems such as phobias, abnormal movements, and behavioural problems (Table 13.3). Mental retardation is present in about three-quarters of cases, and epilepsy in about one-quarter. A minority may have 'savant' skills such as calendar, mathematical, or musical abilities, but these are generally restricted to a small and specific domain.

Table 13.3: Behavioural problems in autism

- Difficulty interacting with others
- May avoid eye contact
- May not want cuddling
- May prefer to remain alone
- Difficulty expressing needs; may use gestures
- Inappropriate response or no response to sound
- Inappropriate laughing or giggling
- Echoing of words or phrases
- Unusual or repetitive play
- Inappropriate attachment to objects
- Spinning of objects or of himself
- Insistence on sameness
- Apparent insensitivity to pain
- Lacks fear in the face of danger

By definition, the onset of autism is before three years of age. Incidence is about 2 per 1000, but this figure masks a male to female ratio of about 4:1. All socioeconomic classes are equally affected. Hypotheses about the aetiology of autism—a behavioural syndrome which may well have several aetiologies—include genetics (prevalence of autism in siblings is 2-6%), obstetric complications, and infections. Theories about cold, rejecting parents ('refrigerator mothers') and the MMR vaccine have long been discredited.

The differential diagnosis of autism is principally from other developmental disorders (intellectual disability, developmental language disorder, Asperger's syndrome, Rett's syndrome, disintegrative psychosis), early-onset schizophrenia, and deafness. About 5% of children with autism also have fragile X syndrome, and another 3% have tuberous sclerosis.

There is no specific treatment for autism. Management involves neuropsychological and psychiatric testing, patient and family education and support, speech and language therapy, behavioural modification, and treatment of associated mental and medical disorders.

Asperger syndrome

First described in 1944 by the Austrian paediatrician Hans Asperger, Asperger syndrome is a pervasive developmental disorder characterized by:

- Qualitative impairments in social interaction.
- A restricted, stereotyped, and repetitive repertoire of behaviours, interests, and activities.

Unlike in autism, there is no significant delay in language or cognitive development. As intelligence is normal, presentation may be later than with autism. Individuals may appear aloof, eccentric, and clumsy. The prevalence of Asperger syndrome is difficult to establish, but it is more common than autism, and, like autism, is considerably more common in males (4:1). The differential diagnosis is principally from schizoid and anankastic personality disorders. Prognosis is better than with autism and individuals are able to lead independent, successful lives. Some are even able to make important contributions to society, particularly in the fields of engineering, mathematics, and physics. Indeed, Hans Asperger used to refer to his patients as 'my little professors'.

Autism spectrum disorder

Asperger syndrome appears to be closely related to autism. DSM-5 has brought these and other similar constructs together under a single umbrella diagnosis of autism spectrum disorder (ASD). ASD is characterized by deficits in social communication and social interaction, and restricted repetitive behaviours, interests, or activities. To secure the diagnosis, symptoms must have been present in the early developmental period, and must be causing significant impairment in functioning. They must not be better explained by intellectual disability or global developmental delay. DSM-5 specifiers for ASD include 'with or without accompanying language impairment' and 'with or without accompanying intellectual impairment'.

Behavioural disorders

Conduct disorder

Conduct disorder is characterized by a repetitive and persistent pattern of dissocial or aggressive behaviour to people and animals, destruction of property, deceitfulness or theft, and serious violation of rules. Conduct disorder is more severe than ordinary childish mischief or adolescent rebelliousness, with major violations of age-appropriate social expectations over a period of six months or more. Conduct disorder affects 5-10% of 8- to 16-year olds, and is much more common in males. Environmental factors such as large families, poor parenting, deprivation, and abuse play an important aetiological role. In securing a diagnosis, it is important to consider and rule out attention-deficit hyperactivity disorder, autism spectrum disorder, and mood and adjustment disorders.

Oppositional defiant disorder is a type of conduct disorder seen in younger children, and is thought to represent a milder form of conduct disorder. It is defined by angry and irritable mood, argumentative and defiant behaviour, or vindictiveness in the absence of the more severe dissocial or aggressive acts described above.

Management of conduct disorder involves family therapy, parenting classes for the guardians, and social skills training for the child. Prognosis is variable, and depends in part on the severity of the conduct disorder. A fair number may segue to antisocial personality disorder. Substance misuse, violence, and crime are common.

Attention-deficit hyperactivity disorder (ADHD)

In the 5th century BC, Hippocrates described people with 'quickened responses to sensory experience, but also less tenaciousness because the soul moves on quickly to the next impression'. Today, the cardinal features of ADHD (referred to as 'hyperkinetic disorder' in ICD-10) are difficulty maintaining attention and hyperactivity/impulsivity. These features arise in early childhood, are pervasive over situations, and persistent in time. Children are easily distracted, frequently shifting their attention from one task to another and unable to complete any. They appear fidgety and are unable to sit still or be quiet. Associated features include impulsive and antisocial behaviour, learning difficulties, and soft neurological signs.

Data from the US National Health Interview Survey indicate that, in 2012, 13.5% of boys aged 3-17 had received a diagnosis of ADHD, up from 8.3% in 1997. These figures are far higher than in the UK, partly because the ICD-10 criteria for hyperkinetic disorder are much more stringent, and partly because of a greater reluctance or lesser readiness to make the diagnosis. Adult ADHD, once looked upon as a rarity, is also becoming much more common, and in Canada now accounts for more than one third of all prescriptions of ADHD psycho-stimulant drugs.

ADHD is sometimes criticized for being little more than a loose and un-validated label for the consequences of poor parental attachment and childhood emotional trauma or neglect. David Neeleman, the founder and CEO of JetBlue Airways, has publicly stated that he considers his ADHD as one of his greatest assets, and many people who carry the diagnosis are similarly creative, driven, and tenacious, and, in some cases, very successful.

Pathophysiology in ADHD is thought to involve a deficiency of dopamine and noradrenaline in frontal and pre-frontal brain areas. Management is accordingly by psychostimulant drugs such as methylphenidate, amphetamine, and dextroamphetamine, or by noradrenaline reuptake inhibitors such as atomoxetine.

In the UK, drugs are generally reserved for severe or recalcitrant cases.

Other management strategies include parent training and education, behavioural modification, family therapy or interpersonal psychotherapy, school-based interventions, remedial education, social skills training, physical exercise, and, more controversially, various dietary modifications such as the addition of omega-3 or the elimination of artificial colours and flavours. Prognosis is mitigated and in a majority of cases symptoms (especially attention-deficit) persist into adolescence and adult life.

Emotional disorders

Affective disorders

Adult-type depressive disorders are thought to occur in adolescents, pre-pubertal children, and even pre-school children. According to estimates, the point prevalence of depressive disorders in adolescents is about 4%, dropping to less than 1% in preschool children. Clinical features are similar to those in adults, but relapse is more common and prognosis poorer. Hypomanic or manic episodes are very unusual in pre-pubertal children, but 'masked' symptoms may include irritability, agitation, impulsivity, and severe temper tantrums.

Anxiety disorders

Anxiety disorders of childhood (sometimes referred to as 'emotional disorders' to distinguish them from anxiety disorders of adulthood) should be distinguished from anxieties that might be considered a normal part of child development. Prevalence is probably around 5%, and, unlike with adults, males and females are more or less equally affected. In separation anxiety disorder of childhood, the child fears that harm is going to befall him or his attachment figures, preventing them from being reunited. This manifests as distress and physical symptoms on separation, fear of being left alone, reluctance to go to school or separate at night, and nightmares. Other childhood anxiety disorders specifically recognized by ICD-10 include phobic anxiety disorder of childhood, social anxiety disorder of childhood, and sibling rivalry disorder. Management is similar to that of adult anxiety disorders, except that drugs are seldom used. Prognosis is good.

Enuresis

Enuresis is the repeated involuntary voiding of urine in the absence of an organic cause, after the chronologic and mental age of five years. Organic causes include constipation, structural abnormalities of the urinary tract, urinary tract infection, diabetes, epilepsy, neurological abnormalities, and drugs such as diuretics.
Enuresis can be:

- Nocturnal, diurnal, or both.
- Primary (if continence has never been achieved) or secondary (if incontinence has been preceded by a period of continence).

Enuresis, particularly nocturnal enuresis, is common, and by age seven years still affects about 7% of boys and 3% of girls. In most cases, it is a manifestation of delayed maturation of the nervous system, although psychological factors may also be responsible. Perhaps surprisingly, a family history can be found in around 70% of cases.

Management involves exclusion of organic causes, reassurance and explanation, bladder training, 'bed and pad' or enuresis alarms, positive reinforcement systems such as star charts, and, if still necessary, drugs such as desmopressin (a synthetic drug that mimics the action of antidiuretic hormone/vasopressin) and imipramine (a tricyclic antidepressant). In particular, parents must be explained that the condition is common, that the voiding of urine is not intentional, and that no one is to blame. Prognosis is good.

Encopresis

According to DSM-5, encopresis is the repeated voluntary or involuntary passage of faeces into inappropriate places, such as clothing or the carpet. For a diagnosis to be made, at least one such event must occur every month for at least three months, the behaviour must not owe to the effects of a substance or medical condition (with the exception of a mechanism involving constipation), and the child must be at least four years old.

Encopresis affects 1-2% of children under the age of 10, and is much more common in boys. Retentive encopresis with overflow is more common than non-retentive encopresis, and can result from both physical and psychological causes (Figure 13.1). Primary non-retentive encopresis typically results from poor social training. Secondary non-retentive encopresis (that is, non-retentive encopresis preceded by at least one year of faecal continence) typically results from emotional stress or defiance, and is more likely to be situational and/or accompanied by other regressive behaviours.

Children with encopresis are likely to suffer from hostile attitudes and behaviours on the part of parents and teachers, and may come to feel unloved and unwanted. Management involves excluding physical causes such as anal fissure and Hirschsprung's disease; explanation and reassurance; stress reduction; stool softening agents and cleaning out; dietary modifications; and retraining.

Elective mutism

In elective mutism or selective mutism, the child is unable to speak in certain, defined situations (most commonly at school) but is able to do so normally in others. The child may also limit his or her participation in non-verbal activities such as playing. Elective mutism affects about 1 in 150 children, and is slightly more common in girls. Onset is usually at the time of entering school. Affected children tend to have an overprotective mother and to be confident and talkative inside the home, but shy, anxious, and isolated outside. Other anxiety disorders and behavioural disorders are common, particularly social phobia. Parents and teachers need to be educated about the problem and reassured: although the condition may persist for months or years, it has a good long-term prognosis. Management involves behavioural therapy and stress and anxiety reduction.

Tic disorders

Tics are repetitive, stereotyped, and purposeless movements and vocalizations. They can be voluntarily suppressed, but this leads to a build up in tension and anxiety (in that much they are rather like compulsions).

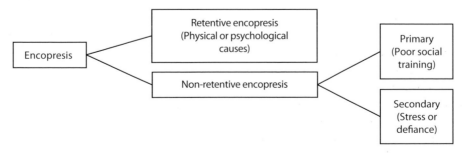

Figure 13.1: Types of encopresis and their common causes. Mixed types are common.

Tics affect up to 20% of all children in the first decade of life, and are three times more common in boys. The most frequent tics are simple motor tics involving a group of functionally related muscles, for instance, blinking, grimacing, and shoulder shrugging. Other types of tic include complex motor tics such as jumping, hitting oneself, and gesturing obscenities (copropraxia); simple vocal tics such as throat-clearing, sniffing, and barking; and complex vocal tics such as repeating one's own utterances (palilalia), repeating other people's utterances (echolalia), or shouting out obscenities (coprolalia). Tics are exacerbated by stress and attenuated by sustained concentration. Their differential diagnosis is essentially from other disorders of movement. In most cases, they are mild and transient and do not require any treatment.

Gilles de la Tourette syndrome (Tourette syndrome)

Tourette syndrome is a tic disorder involving multiple motor tics and at least one vocal tic. The syndrome can be mimicked by certain conditions, including stroke, encephalitis, and carbon monoxide poisoning; and by certain drugs, including stimulants, levodopa, and carbamazepine ('tourettism'). First described by Jean Itard (1774-1838) and then by George Gilles de la Tourette (1857-1904), Tourette syndrome is thought to have affected such luminaries as Samuel Johnson and André Malraux. Incidence is about 1 in 2000, but boys are more frequently afflicted than girls by a ratio of 3-4:1. Onset is before age 18, with a mean of age 7 for motor tics and age 11 for vocal tics. The number, location, and severity of the tics vary over time, and they often resolve by early adulthood. Coprolalia occurs in about 30% of cases, and is largely responsible for the public notoriety of the syndrome.

Both genetic and environmental factors play an aetiological role, and symptoms are thought to result from dysfunction in the frontal cortex, thalamus, and basal ganglia. Co-morbid mental disorders, particularly ADHD and obsessive-compulsive disorder (OCD), are common, and may eclipse and/or survive the tic disorder.

Management involves education of patient and family, and one or more of behavioural therapy, drugs (commonly clonidine, baclofen, or an antipsychotic), and treatment of co-morbid mental disorders such as OCD and ADHD. Note that the use of stimulants, for instance, in the treatment of comorbid ADHD, is likely to aggravate any tic disorder.

Self-assessment

Answer by true or false.

1. Stranger anxiety develops at around 6-9 months of age.
2. Pincer grasp develops at around 18 months of age.
3. According to Freud, fixation at the anal stage leads to an amoral or puritanical adult.
4. Thinking in Piaget's pre-operational stage is logical as opposed to intuitive.
5. 90% of high school graduates are at Piaget's formal operational stage.
6. Erikson described eight stages of cognitive development.
7. In autism, male to female ratio is about 10:1.
8. Autistic spectrum disorder is characterized by deficits in social communication and social interaction, and restricted repetitive behaviours, interests, or activities.
9. Aggressive behaviour, destruction of property, and theft are not ordinary features of oppositional defiant disorder.
10. Pathophysiology in ADHD is thought to involve a deficiency of dopamine and noradrenaline neurotransmitters in the frontal and pre-frontal brain areas.
11. Primary enuresis is diagnosed if incontinence has been preceded by a period of continence.
12. A family history can be found in about 90% of cases of enuresis.
13. Secondary non-retentive encopresis is typically the outcome of poor social training.
14. Elective mutism is often associated with other anxiety disorders.
15. Tourette syndrome is characterized by multiple motor or vocal tics.

Answers

1. True.
2. False. Around 12 months of age.
3. False. Fixation at the phallic stage.
4. False. Logical thinking develops at the concrete operational stage.
5. False. Only 35%!
6. True. Three of the eight are adulthood stages.
7. False. The male to female ratio is about 4:1.
8. True.
9. True.
10. True.
11. False. Secondary enuresis.
12. False. About 70% of cases.
13. False. Primary non-retentive encopresis.
14. True.
15. False. Multiple motor and at least one vocal tic.

13

So why a career in psychiatry?

Know then thyself, presume not God to scan
The proper study of mankind is man
Placed on this isthmus of a middle state
A being darkly wise, and rudely great
With too much knowledge for the sceptic side
With too much weakness for the stoic's pride
He hangs between, in doubt to act, or rest
In doubt to deem himself a God, or Beast
In doubt his mind or body to prefer
Born but to die, and reasoning but to err
Alike in ignorance, his reason such
Whether he thinks too little, or too much
Chaos of thought and passion, all confused
Still by himself abuse, or disabuse
Created half to rise, and half to fall
Great lord of all things, yet a prey to all
Sole judge of truth, in endless error hurled
The glory, jest, and riddle of the world.

—Alexander Pope (1688-1744), *An Essay on Man*

HEAVEN
THE PSYCHOLOGY OF THE EMOTIONS
AND HELL

DR NEEL BURTON

This book proposes to do just that, examining over 25 emotions ranging from lust to love and humility to humiliation, and drawing some useful and surprising conclusions along the way.

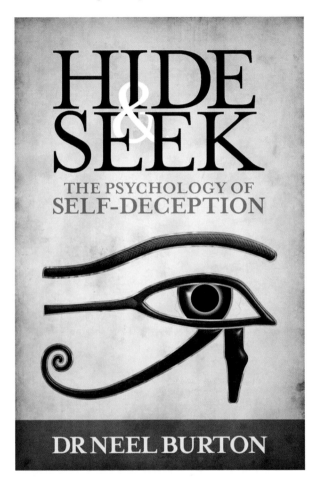

Heaven and Hell, The Psychology of the Emotions
ISBN 978-0-9929127-2-7

Today more than ever, the education doled out in classrooms is cold and cognitive. But, once outside, it is our uneducated emotions that move us, hold us back, and lead us astray. It is, at first and at last, our emotions that determine our choice of profession, partner, and politics, and our relation to money, sex, and religion. Nothing can make us feel more alive, or more human, than our emotions, or hurt us more.

Yet many people lumber through life without giving full consideration to their emotions, partly because our empirical, materialistic culture does not encourage it or even make it seem possible, and partly because it requires unusual strength to gaze into the abyss of our deepest drives, needs, and fears.

Hide and Seek, The Psychology of Self-Deception
ISBN 978-0-9560353-6-3

Self-deception is common and universal, and the cause of most human tragedies. Of course, the science of self-deception can help us to live better and get more out of life. But it can also cast a murky light on human nature and the human condition, for example, on such exclusively human phenomena as anger, depression, fear, pity, pride, dream making, love making, and god making, not to forget age-old philosophical problems such as selfhood, virtue, happiness, and the good life. Nothing could possibly be more important.

EMQ 1. Descriptive psychopathology: Disorders of perception

A. Hypnagogic hallucination
B. Hypnopompic hallucination
C. Thought echo
D. Extracampine hallucination
E. Pseudo-hallucination
F. Delusional perception
G. Synaesthesia
H. Derealization
I. Déjà vu
J. Illusion

For each of the following situations, select the most appropriate term.

1. A teenager who has lost his way in the woods becomes anxious, and, as night falls, begins to see 'shapes' in the trees and bushes.
2. On further questioning, a 27-year-old lady with mild to moderate depressive disorder reveals that she sometimes hears her name being called out just before falling asleep.
3. A 33-year-old lady with a personality disorder complains of hearing the voice of the devil telling her that she is going to join him in hell. On further questioning, she reveals that she experiences this voice inside her head, and is able to blot it out at any time.
4. A 26-year-old gentleman with schizophrenia hears the voice of his dead grandmother coming from 'beyond the grave'.
5. A 19-year-old student with a first episode of psychosis is distressed because he saw the stripes on a medical student's tie. According to him, the stripes mean that the student is 'one of them' and 'out to get me'.

EMQ 2. Descriptive psychopathology: Delusional themes/types of delusion

A. Thought broadcasting
B. Thought echo
C. Delusional perception
D. Delusion of reference
E. Idea of reference
F. Capgras syndrome
G. Fregoli syndrome
H. Cotard syndrome
I. De Clérambault syndrome
J. Othello syndrome
K. Folie à deux

6. A 45-year-old lady, who works as the secretary to the director of a large and successful company in the City of London, fixedly believes that her boss secretly loves her.
7. A 28-year-old gentleman with a diagnosis of schizophrenia refuses to see his psychiatrist, because he believes that the psychiatrist has been replaced by an identical looking imposter who is none other than a Russian secret agent.
8. After the sudden death of his parents in a car crash, a 21-year-old psychology student begins experiencing the feeling that people are talking about him behind his back, and that what he reads in textbooks and journals may well have been written with him in mind.
9. The sister and long-term carer of a 38-year-old gentleman with a long history of schizophrenia shares his delusion that the ghosts of their ancestors are trying to have them killed.
10. A patient who was admitted to a psychiatric hospital four weeks ago with features of a severe and treatment-resistant depressive disorder no longer wants to eat in the presence of other patients. When asked about this, she says that her insides are rotting, and her breath smells so bad as to put people off their food.

EMQ 3. Descriptive psychopathology: Disorders of movement

A. Catalepsy
B. Catatonia
C. Cataplexy
D. Retardation
E. Stupor
F. Dystonia
G. Akathisia
H. Parkinsonism
I. Tardive dyskinesia
J. Negativism

11. A 19-year-old lady with new onset psychosis is started on a small dose of risperidone. After just a few hours, the duty psychiatrist is called to see her because 'she can no longer move her eyeballs'. The duty psychiatrist prescribes a small dose of procyclidine, to which the patient makes an excellent response.
12. A 19-year-old gentleman with new onset psychosis is started on a small dose of risperidone. After just a few days, he is noted to be even more restless and agitated, and apparently unable to sit still. The duty psychiatrist increases the dose of the risperidone, but this only makes matters worse.

13. A patient with severe depression is admitted to a psychiatric hospital because she is immobile and mute. As she is not eating and drinking and is visibly dehydrated, she is started on a course of electroconvulsive therapy.
14. A 25-year-old gentleman with schizophrenia is admitted to a psychiatric hospital after he is found in the street, standing on one leg and immobile.
15. Once in hospital, the psychiatrist examining this gentleman finds that his limbs can be placed in any posture, after which they are maintained in that posture for several minutes at a time.

EMQ 4. Mental health services
A. Crisis team
B. Liaison psychiatry
C. Community Mental Health Team
D. Early Intervention Service
E. GP practice and Accident & Emergency
F. Day hospital
G. Rehabilitation
H. Assertive Outreach Team

16. Engages 'revolving door' patients in treatment and supports them in their day-to-day.
17. Improves the short- and long-term outcomes of schizophrenia and other psychotic disorders through a three-pronged approach involving preventative measures, earlier detection of untreated cases, and intensive treatment and support in the early stages of illness.
18. Is at the centre of mental healthcare provision.
19. Provides psychiatric services in a general hospital setting, both for in- and out-patients.
20. Acts as a gatekeeper to a variety of psychiatric services, including admission to a psychiatric hospital.

EMQ 5. Psychiatric ethics
A. Competence
B. Capacity
C. Bolam v Friern Hospital Management Committee (1957)
D. Tarasoff v Regents of the University of California (1976)
E. Gillick v West Norfolk and Wisbech Area Health Authority (1985)
F. Re. F (1990)
G. Re. C (1994)

21. The legal presumption that adult persons have the ability to make decisions.

22. The clinical determination of a patient's ability to make decisions about his or her treatment.
23. Established that a patient with a severe mental disorder can retain the capacity to make certain decisions about his or her treatment.
24. Ruled that physicians have a duty to breach confidentiality if maintaining confidentiality may result in harm to the patient or community.
25. Ruled that a child can be competent to consent to treatment if he or she fully understands the treatment proposed.

EMQ 6. The Mental Health Act
A. Section 2
B. Section 3
C. Section 4
D. Section 5(2)
E. Section 5(4)
F. Section 17
G. Section 35
H. Section 36
I. Section 37
J. Section 41
K. Section 58
L. Section 117
M. Section 135
N. Section 136

26. Emergency admission for assessment.
27. Doctor's emergency holding power.
28. Removal by the police of a person with a suspected mental disorder from a public place to a place of safety.
29. Detention and treatment of a person convicted of an imprisonable offence.
30. Restriction order.

EMQ 7. First rank symptoms of schizophrenia
A. Third person auditory hallucination
B. Running-commentary
C. *Gedankenlautwerden*
D. *Echo de la pensée*
E. Thought insertion
F. Thought withdrawal
G. Thought broadcasting
H. Passivity of affect
I. Passivity of volition
J. Passivity of impulse
K. Somatic passivity
L. Delusional perception
M. None of the above

31. A patient complains that his thoughts are being vaporized, and that people are catching them in butterfly nets and pinning them into photo albums.
32. A patient complains of hearing several voices telling her to slit her wrists.
33. A patient complains of hearing her own thoughts at the same time as she is having them.
34. A patient who tried to strangle himself with his shoelaces maintains that it had nothing to do with him.
35. A patient who sees you looking at your watch in yet another endless team meeting says that her time has come to leave this madhouse.

EMQ 8. Organic differential of schizophrenia
A. Cannabis misuse
B. Hallucinogen misuse
C. Stimulant misuse
D. Head injury
E. Central nervous system infection
F. Brain tumour
G. Temporal lobe epilepsy
H. Delirium
I. Dementia
J. Cushing's syndrome
K. Porphyria
L. Systemic lupus erythematosus

36. An agitated 23-year-old student is brought to A&E with visual and auditory hallucinations, paranoid ideation, itching, and formication. On physical examination, his pupils are noted to be dilated, his pulse rate is 110 bpm, his blood pressure is 170/140 mmHg, and his temperature is 37.9°C.
37. A 73-year-old lady is admitted to hospital following an overdose of eight tablets of temazepam 10mg following the death of her dog three months ago. During the evening shift she becomes particularly agitated and claims that she is seeing spiders on the curtains. Urinary dipstick uncovers a urinary tract infection.
38. A 28-year-old lady seen in psychiatry out-patients describes discrete episodes involving a sense of jamais-vu, distortion of the shapes and sizes of objects, and olfactory and gustatory hallucinations.
39. A 22-year-old lady presents to A&E with recent-onset severe abdominal pain accompanied by hallucinations and paranoid delusions. A urine sample is noted to become dark on standing.
40. A 42-year-old lady develops paranoid delusions shortly after being started on prednisolone for the treatment of her rheumatoid arthritis.

EMQ 9. Psychiatric differential of schizophrenia
A. Schizophrenia
B. Manic psychosis
C. Depressive psychosis
D. Schizoaffective disorder
E. Drug-induced psychosis
F. Schizotypal disorder
G. Persistent delusional disorder
H. Brief psychotic disorder
I. Induced delusional disorder
J. Puerperal psychosis

41. Following the death of her father in a car crash, a 26-year-old office worker soon begins to experience florid psychotic symptoms. The symptoms resolve within ten days.
42. Three years after losing the custody of her 3-year-old son, a 42-year-old in-patient continues to believe that the government conspired to have the child removed from her. She also believes that the doctors and nurses are government agents tasked with preventing her from seeing her son by locking her up and drugging her under the pretext of mental disorder.
43. A 19-year-old student in his first year at university is admitted to a psychiatric hospital one Saturday night. By the ward round on Sunday morning, he is back to his normal self and ready for discharge.
44. After her husband leaves her for a man, a 36-year-old GP is admitted with tearfulness and prominent psychomotor retardation. After a few days, she develops a number of psychotic symptoms, some of which are first rank symptoms of schizophrenia.
45. A 17-year-old is referred to psychiatric services because his parents are concerned that he is a 'loner'. He remains guarded and suspicious throughout the interview, but does inadvertently reveal a number of odd beliefs, such as the belief that his parents will die unless he keeps his hair long.

EMQ 10. Differential diagnosis of depression
A. Bipolar I disorder
B. Bipolar II disorder
C. Cyclothymia
D. Mild depressive disorder
E. Moderate depressive disorder
F. Severe depressive disorder
G. Adjustment disorder
H. Bereavement
I. Abnormal bereavement reaction
J. Dysthymia

46. A 32-year old lady complains of low mood, poor concentration, fatigue with early-morning waking, and loss of appetite. In the last few days, her partner has had to do all the school runs.

47. A 26-year-old lady with prominent psychomotor retardation complains of low mood. Both her speech and her movements are retarded.

48. Three months following her husband's death, a 45-year-old lady with prominent psychomotor retardation says that she would rather be dead.

49. A 36-year-old gentleman moved to the UK from the United States four months ago. While succeeding at his new job, he complains of being unable to cope. His wife tells you that, since moving to the UK, he has been uncharacteristically irritable with occasional angry outbursts.

50. A 40-year-old gentleman has a long history of recurrent depressive episodes and hypomania, but has never suffered a full-blown manic episode.

51. Three months following the death of her husband in a knife attack, a 32-year-old lady confides that she has made plans to be with him.

EMQ 11. Antidepressant drugs
A. Citalopram
B. Fluoxetine
C. Paroxetine
D. Amitriptyline
E. Lofepramine
F. Venlafaxine
G. Reboxetine
H. Mirtazapine
I. Trazodone
J. Lamotrigine

52. Discontinuation of this SSRI is most likely to result in the SSRI discontinuation syndrome.

53. This drug is so widely used that trace quantities have been found in tap water.

54. This drug is a relatively good choice in a patient with moderate depression and prominent weight loss.

55. These two drugs are a relatively good choice for the treatment of bipolar depression (two marks).

56. These three drugs are a relatively good choice for a patient with moderate depression and prominent sleep disturbance (three marks).

57. These two drugs should be avoided in patients who are at high risk of suicide (two marks).

58. This drug is a secondary amine.

59. This drug is a noradrenergic and specific serotonergic antidepressant (NaSSa).

60. This drug is a noradrenaline reuptake inhibitor (NARI).

61. This drug requires blood pressure monitoring.

EMQ 12. Differential diagnosis of anxiety
A. Panic disorder
B. Agoraphobia
C. Social phobia
D. Post-traumatic stress disorder
E. Hyperthyroidism
F. Substance misuse
G. Obsessive-compulsive disorder
H. Anankastic personality disorder
I. Conversion disorder
J. Somatoform disorder (Briquet syndrome)
K. Cerebrovascular accident
L. Hypochondriacal disorder
M. Factitious disorder
N. Malingering

62. After losing her mother in a car crash, a 25-year-old lady suddenly loses the function of her right arm.

63. A consultant cardiologist is increasingly frustrated by a 35-year-old lady with a long history of multiple and severe physical symptoms which cannot be accounted for by a physical disorder.

64. A 45-year-old businessman who travels frequently presents to his GP with anxiety, sweating, tremor, and nausea. He has no past psychiatric history.

65. A 35-year-old depressed company director complains of being overworked. During a follow-up appointment, he appears upset that his psychiatrist, who is very experienced, is not adhering to the latest guidelines for the management of moderate depressive disorder.

66. A 29-year-old lady experiences palpitations about three or four times a month. As they come on unexpectedly, she feels unable to leave her home alone or go to places such as cinemas and crowded shopping centres where help may be difficult to obtain.

67. A 29-year-old woman brings her toddler into A&E for the third time this month. Blood tests reveal that the toddler has a high sodium level, but no cause can be found.

EMQ 13. Ego defence mechanisms
A. Compensation
B. Denial
C. Displacement
D. Distortion
E. Idealization

F. Intellectualization
G. Manic defence
H. Projection
 I. Rationalization
J. Reaction formation
K. Repression
L. Sublimation

68. A woman whose husband has left her still sends him text messages as though he were only on a business trip.
69. After a horrific year, a person throws a lavish party for New Year's Eve and dances all night like he has never danced before.
70. When asked about the banking crisis by the Leader of the Opposition, the Prime Minister replies, "We saved the world... er, the banks."
71. A person who is heavily in debt builds a complex spreadsheet of how long it would take to repay his debts using different payment options and interest rates.
72. A young man makes advances on an older woman. He claims she never called him back because 'she has issues with an ex'.
73. An abducted hostage develops sympathy for her hostage-taker. Even after being rescued, she remains concerned for his wellbeing and loyal to his cause.

EMQ 14. Intellectual disability
A. Mild intellectual disability
B. Moderate intellectual disability
C. Severe intellectual disability
D. Psychotic disorder
E. Hypomania
F. Depression
G. Attention-deficit hyperactivity disorder
H. Conduct disorder
 I. Autism
J. Down's syndrome—trisomy 21
K. Down's syndrome—Robertsonian translocation
L. Fragile X syndrome
M. Phenylketonuria
N. Neurofibromatosis type I (Von Recklinghausen syndrome)
O. Tuberous sclerosis

74. A 24-year-old man with an IQ of 67 is able to hold down a job in a supermarket. However, he needs help from his brother to organize his finances.
75. A 16-year old boy with severe intellectual disability suffers a progressive deterioration in his level of functioning. At times, he is noted to become very agitated and bang his ears.

76. A 16-year-old boy with severe intellectual disability suffers from prominent loss of appetite and sleep disturbance, and no longer enjoys interacting with his carers or listening to music as he once did.
77. A two-month-old boy with a karyotype 46, XY, t(12;21) is noted to have Brushfield spots on his irises.
78. A four-year-old boy with intellectual disability has an elongated face, large and protruding ears, prognathism, macroorchidism, and hypotonia. DNA testing reveals more than 200 CGG trinucleotide repeats in the FMR1 gene.

EMQ 15. Psychotropic drugs
A. Chlordiazepoxide
B. Chlormethiazole
C. Lorazepam
D. Diazepam
E. Temazepam
F. Haloperidol
G. Phenelzine
H. Moclobemide
 I. Venlafaxine
J. Mirtazapine
K. Trazodone
L. Donepezil
M. Zopiclone

79. A 73-year-old lady is seen in the dementia clinic. One week ago she got lost in her neighbourhood and almost got hit by a motorbike. Her Folstein Mini-Mental State Examination (MMSE) score is 19/30.
80. A 73-year-old gentleman with a long history of binge drinking is diagnosed with alcohol dependence. His GP prescribes thiamine and recommends a detoxification programme.
81. A 24-year-old gentleman with paranoid schizophrenia who has been admitted to hospital becomes extremely agitated, smashing windows and threatening members of staff and fellow patients. As he does not respond to de-escalation techniques, rapid tranquillization is required.
82. A 49-year-old lady with moderate-to-severe depression and a history of hypertension has not responded to an adequate trial of an SSRI. Her sleep and appetite are severely disturbed.
83. A 55-year-old gentleman with a long history of moderate-to-severe depression has failed to respond to a variety of antidepressants. His psychiatrist therefore decides to start him on a reversible monoamine oxidase inhibitor (RIMA).

84. The above gentleman is asking for one of these two drugs to help him sleep (two marks).

EMQ 16. Adverse effects of psychotropic drugs
A. Chlorpromazine
B. Risperidone
C. Olanzapine
D. Clozapine
E. Fluoxetine
F. Paroxetine
G. Venlafaxine
H. Amitriptyline
 I. Lithium
J. Semisodium valproate
K. Lorazepam
L. Disulfiram
M. Acamprosate

85. Dry mouth, blurred vision, glaucoma, constipation, urinary retention, sedation, weight gain, sexual dysfunction, cardiac arrhythmias, neurotoxicity.
86. Weight gain, sedation, anticholinergic side-effects, orthostatic hypotension, increased risk of convulsions at higher doses, agranulocytosis.
87. Prominent hyperprolactinaemia.
88. Nausea, tremor, sedation, weight gain, alopecia, blood dyscrasias, hepatotoxicity, pancreatitis.
89. Long-term adverse effects include weight gain, oedema, goitre and hypothyroidism, hyperparathyroidism, cardiotoxicity, irreversible renal damage, nephrogenic diabetes insipidus, and a raised leukocyte and platelet count.
90. Discontinuation syndrome consists of headache, dizziness, shock-like sensations and parathesiae, gastrointestinal symptoms, lethargy, insomnia, and changes in mood (depression, anxiety/agitation).

EMQ 17. Child psychiatry
A. Intellectual disability
B. Autism
C. Asperger's syndrome
D. Conduct disorder
E. Oppositional defiant disorder
F. Hyperkinetic disorder
G. Complex vocal tics
H. Tourette's syndrome
 I. Childhood depressive disorder
J. Elective mutism
K. Enuresis
L. Encopresis
M. Part of normal development

91. A three-year-old girl regularly wets her bed, much to the frustration of her parents who take her to see their GP.
92. An 11-year-old boy is brought to his GP after developing socially embarrassing vocal tics, often involving the shouting out of obscenities. On further questioning, the GP uncovers an earlier history of multiple motor tics. He refers the child to a neurology clinic.
93. A three-year old girl is noted to be confident and talkative inside the home, but shy, anxious, and isolated outside. When she starts school, she does not speak in class.
94. A five-year-old boy's behaviour is consistently defiant, disobedient, and provocative. However, he has never caused any serious destruction of property or harm to others.
95. A six-year-old boy is noted to be aloof, eccentric, and clumsy. His IQ is 112 and there are no significant delays in language or cognitive development.

Answers
1. J
2. A
3. E
4. D
5. F
6. I
7. F
8. E
9. K
10. H
11. F
12. G
13. E
14. B
15. A
16. H
17. D
18. C
19. B
20. A
21. B
22. A
23. G
24. D
25. E
26. C
27. D

28. M	62. I
29. I	63. J
30. J	64. F
31. G	65. H
32. M	66. A
33. C	67. M
34. J	68. B
35. L	69. G
36. C	70. D
37. H	71. F
38. G	72. I
39. K	73. J
40. J	74. A
41. H	75. D
42. G	76. F
43. E	77. K
44. C	78. L
45. F	79. K
46. E	80. A
47. F	81. C
48. I	82. J
49. G	83. H
50. B	84. E, M
51. I	85. H
52. C	86. D
53. B	87. B
54. H	88. J
55. G, J	89. I
56. D, E, I	90. F
57. D, E	91. M
58. E	92. H
59. H	93. J
60. G	94. E
61. F	95. C

Index

abnormal bereavement reaction, 110

abstention from alcohol, 153

abuse of psychiatry, 69

acamprosate, 153

acute stress reaction, 111

adjustment disorder, 110

affect, 19

aftercare, 45

agoraphobia, 107-108

AIDS dementia complex, see *HIV-related dementia*

Ainsworth, Mary, 176

alcohol, 147-154

alcoholic hangover, see *veisalgia*

Alcoholics Anonymous, 153

Alice in Wonderland Syndrome (AIWS), 1

Alzheimer's disease, 134-135

amnestic syndrome, 137

amphetamine(s), 154, 157

anankastic personality disorder, 107, 124, 177

Ancient Greece, 3

Ancient Rome, 3-4

anhedonia, 19, 20

anorexia nervosa, 161-164

anticholinergics, 65

antidepressants, 82-84, 90, 91, 112, 152

antipsychiatry movement, the, 6, 37

antipsychotics, 2, 22, 37, 56, 57, 60, 62, 63, 64-67, 90-91, 112, 138

antisocial personality disorder, 122

Anton syndrome, 133

anxiety, definition (see also, *existential anxiety*), 105

anxiety disorders, 105-110

Aquinas, St Thomas, 4

Aristotle, 3, 4, 71, 116, 169

Asclepiades, 3

Asperger's syndrome, 89, 177

assertive outreach, 40

assisted suicide, 95

attachment theory, 176

attempted suicide, 95

attention deficit hyperactivity disorder (ADHD), 89, 177-178

atypical antipsychotics (see also, *antipsychotics*), 65

autism, 176-177

autism spectrum disorder, 177

avoidant personality disorder, 123

bad faith, 117

Baillarger, Jules, 87

Balint syndrome, 133

Beck, Aaron, 47, 80

behavioural disorders, 177

belle indifférence, la, 114

benzodiazepines, 64, 67-68, 91, 110, 111, 152, 153, 158, 158-159, 166

bereavement, 110

Bethlehem, the, 4

Bible, the, 3, 77, 81

binge eating disorder, 165

biological psychiatry, 5

bipolar disorder, 73, 74-75, 86-93

bipolar II disorder, 74, 89

Bleuler, Eugen, 9, 53

blood tests in alcohol misuse, 153

body dysmorphic disorder, 115

Bolam's test, 44

borderline personality disorder, 122

Bowlby, John, 176

breeder hypothesis, 60

Breuer, Josef, 6

brief psychotic disorder, 70

bulimia nervosa, 112, 164-165

Cade, John, 91

CAGE questionnaire, 152

cannabis, 62, 156

capacity, 42-43, 164

Capgras syndrome, 21

carbamazapine, 92

care co-ordinator, 41

care programme approach, 40-41

catalepsy, 18

cataplexy, 18, 167

catatonia, 5, 18, 53, 58, 112

catharsis, 6

Celsus, 4

Charcot, Jean-Marie, 6

charities, 40

charming psychopath, 122

child development, 173-176

chlordiazepoxide, 153

chlorpromazine, 5, 64

cholinesterase inhibitors, 138

Christianity, 4, 95-96

Christie, Agatha, 115

Cicero, 3-4, 4, 71

circumstantiality, 18, 19

Class A, B, C drugs, 155

classifications of mental disorder, 28-30

clomipramine, 113

clonidine, 158

clozapine, 64, 65, 66, 67, 68

cocaine, 154, 157

Coehlo, Paulo, 123

cognitive assessment, 24-26

cognitive behavioural therapy, 47-48, 68, 80, 109, 113

cognitive distortions, 80

collective unconscious, 9

common law, 44

community care, 37

community mental health team, 39

competence (see also, *capacity*), 42

complex needs service, 124-125

compulsion, 112

conduct disorder, 177

confabulation, 150

confidentiality, 41-42

controlled drinking, 153

controlled substances, 155

conversion disorders, see *dissociative disorders*

copycat suicide, 99

Cotard syndrome, 22

counter-transference, 7

counselling, 47

Crane, Hart, 95

creativity, 61, 79, 89, 91, 93

Creutzfeldt-Jakob disease, 136-137

criminal sections, 46

crisis team, 39-40, 101

culture-bound syndromes, 102, 111-112, 161, 164

cyclothymia, 74

Dali, Salvador, 155

David (Biblical character), 3

day hospital, 40

death, 97, 116-117

debriefing, 111

de Clérambault syndrome, 22, 70

deep breathing, 113

démence précoce, 5, 53, 87

deliberate self-harm, 95, 102-103

delirium, 129-132

delirium screen, 131

delirium tremens, 149-150

delusions, 5, 20-22, 56-57, 144

delusional themes, 21-22

dementia, 132-138

dementia with Lewy bodies, see *Lewy body dementia*

dependent personality disorder, 123-124

depot preparations, 64

depression, 3, 53, 56, 57, 60, 73-85, 111, 113, 137

Deprivation of Liberty Safeguards, 43

de Quincey, Thomas, 156

descriptive psychopathology, 5, 11-12, 13, 16-26

designer drugs, see *novel psychoactive substances*

detoxification from alcohol, 153

developmental disorders, 176-177

dhat, 111

diagnostic hierarchy, 27, 29

diagnosis in psychiatry, 59

dialectical behavioural therapy, 48, 124

diamorphine, see *heroin*

Diana, Princess, 112

Diderot, Denis, 4

Diogenes syndrome, 132

disability, 144

disorganized symptoms, 56

dissociative disorders, 113-115

dissociative fugue, 114, 115

disulfiram, 153

dopamine hypothesis, 62, 64

Down's syndrome, 142

dream interpretation, 6, 7, 8, 169

dream psychology, see *dream interpretation*

drift hypothesis, 60

drinking guidelines, 147

driving guidelines, 46

drugs, see *recreational drugs*

DSM-IV, 59, 74, 89, 111, 141

DSM-5, 5, 29, 111

dual diagnosis, 148

dysthymia, 74

early intervention services, 40

ecstasy, 154, 157

ego, 7

ego defences, 7, 121, 124, 126-127

Ekbom syndrome, 22

elective mutism, 179

electroconvulsive therapy, 63, 84-85

Elephant Man, 143

emotionally unstable personality disorder, see *borderline personality disorder*

encopresis, 179

Enlightenment, the, 4, 6

entheogens, 70

enuresis, 178-179

Erikson, Erik, 173, 175

Esquirol, JED, 5, 141

ethics, 41-46, 95-97

euthanasia, 95, 96

evolutionary psychiatry, 22, 61, 89, 105, 108

exhibitionism, 171

existential anxiety, 116-117

existentialism, 81, 96

expressed emotion, 62

extrapyramidal side-effects, 64-65

factitious disorders, 116

Falret, Jean-Pierre, 87

false epidemics in psychiatry, 89

family therapy, 48, 68

Faulkner, William, 76

fetishism, 171

fever therapy, 63

first rank symptoms, 54-55

flumazenil, 159

fluoxetine, 83

folie à deux, 70-71

forensic psychiatry, 125

formulation, the psychiatric, 12, 13, 26-28

Foucault, Michel, 6, 79

fragile X syndrome, 142

Frankl, Victor, 81

free association, 6, 7

Fregoli syndrome, 21

Freud, Anna, 7

Freud, Sigmund, 5, 6-8, 9, 39, 81, 169, 173, 175

frontotemporal dementias, 135

frotteurism, 171

fugue, see *dissociative fugue*

functional mental disorders, 129

Galen, 3

Galileo, 4

Ganser syndrome, 114

gender dysphoria, see *transsexualism*

generalized anxiety disorder, 109, 110

Gerstmann syndrome, 133

Greece, see *Ancient Greece*

hallucinations, 23-24, 57, 67, 71, 144

hallucinogens (see also, *entheogens*), 157-158

haloperidol, 65, 131

handicap, 144

hangover, see *veisalgia*

hebephrenia, 5, 53, 58

Hemingway, Ernest, 15

heretics, 4

heroin, 154

hierarchy of needs, Maslow's, 116

Hippocrates, 3, 4, 108, 177

histrionic personality disorder, 123

HIV-related dementia, 136

Hofman, Albert, 154-155

Homer, 3

homosexuality, 30, 126

Hume, David, 96

humoural theory, 3, 4

Huntington's disease, 135-136

Husserl, Edmund, 11

hypersomnia, 167

hypnosis, 6

hypochrondriacal disorder, 115

hypomania, 74

hysteria, 6, 8, 112, 114

ICD-10, 5, 19, 111

id, 7

imipramine, 82

impairment, 144

individuation, 9

induced delusional disorder, 70-71

insomnia, 166-167

institutionalization, 37-38

intellectual disability, 141-144

interpersonal therapy, 48

iproniazid, 82

IQ scoring, 141

Islam, 4

Jacob's dream, 169

James, William, 124

Jamison, Kay Redfield, 86, 89

Jaspers, Karl, 5, 11

jet lag, 168

jokes, 7

Jung, Carl Gustav, 8-10, 107, 169

ketamine, 63
Kierkegaard, Soren, 119
Kitanaka, Junko, 111
Kleine-Levin syndrome, 167
Kleist, Karl, 87
Klüver-Buçy syndrome, 133
Korsakov syndrome, see *Wernicke-Korsakov syndrome*
Kraepelin, Emil, 5, 53, 59, 87, 119
Krafft-Ebing, Richard von, 9

language, 61
late paraphrenia, see *paraphrenia*
legal highs, see *novel psychoactive substances*
Leonhard, Karl, 87
leucotomy, see *lobotomy*
Lewis Carroll, 1
Lewy body dementia, 135
liaison psychiatry, 40
libido, 7
lilliputian hallucinations, 1
lithium, 90, 91-92
lobotomy, 63, 67
lofexidine, 158
lorazepam, 64, 67-68, 91
Locke, John, 4
logico-deductive approach, 14
logotherapy, 81
LSD, 63, 154

Macdonald's triad, 122
malingering, 116
mania (see also, *bipolar disorder*), 86-93
manic-depressive illness (see also, *bipolar disorder*), 87
Marchiafava-Bignami disease, 151
Maslow, Abraham, 116
masochism (sexual masochism), 171
maternity blues, 85
meaning, 81, 116
melancholy, see *depression*
memantine, 138
Mental Capacity Act, the, 42-43
Mental Health Act, the, 43, 44-46, 156, 164
mental health services, 38-41
mental state examination, 4, 12, 13, 16-26
methadone, 158
Middle Ages, the, 4
migraine, 1
mild cognitive impairment, 137
milieu therapy, 124
Mill, JS, 20
mindfulness, 48

mixed dementia, 136
Molière, 4
monasteries, 4
Moncrieff, Joanna, 92
monoamine hypothesis, 80-81, 90
monoamine oxidase inhibitors, 82
mood stabilizers, 90, 91-93
moral treatment, 4, 5
motivational interviewing, 154
multiple personality disorder, 114
Munchausen syndrome, see *factitious disorders*

Nagel, Thomas, 97
naloxone, 158
naltrexone, 153, 158
narcissistic personality disorder, 123
narcolepsy, 167
Nash, John, 61
negative symptoms, 56, 62
neurofibromatosis, 143
neuroleptic malignant syndrome, 67, 83
neurology, 129
neuronal loop model of OCD, 113
neurosis, 6, 7, 107, 117
neurosurgery, 113
Nietzsche, Friedrich, 89
nightmares, 168
night terrors, 168
normal pressure hydrocephalus, 136
novel psychoactive substances, 159

obsession, 112
obsessive-compulsive disorder, 112-113, 113
Oedipus complex, 8
One Flew Over the Cuckoo's Nest, 38
Open Dialogue, 67
opiates, 158
opioids, 158
opium, 154, 158
oppositional defiant disorder, 177
organic mental disorders, 129
Othello syndrome, 22, 70, 151

paedophilia, 171
panic disorder, 108-109, 110, 113
paranoia, 5, 53, 58
paranoid personality disorder, 121
paraphilias, 170-171
paraphrenia, 70
parapraxes, 7
parasomnias, 168

parasuicide, 95
pathological intoxication, 151
persistent delusional disorder, 70
persistent somatoform pain disorder, 115
personality disorder clusters, 120
personality disorders, 119-125
personality disorder, definition, 120
phencyclidine, 63
phenomenology, 5
phenylketonuria, 142
Philo of Alexandria, 169
Phineas Gage, 133
phobic anxiety disorders, 107-108, 110, 113
physical examination in psychiatry, 26
Piaget, Jean, 173, 175
Pick's disease, 135
Pinel, Philippe, 4, 5, 119
Pirsig, Robert, 71
Plato, 3, 4, 46, 71, 117, 169
pleasure principle, 7
Pliny the Elder, 97
Poe, Edgar Allen, 89
police sections, 46
positive symptoms, 56, 62, 64
postnatal depression, 85
post-traumatic stress disorder, 111
pregnancy, 152
pre-morbid personality, 16
Prichard, JC, 119
prion diseases, 136-137
prodromal phase of schizophrenia, 57
projection, 6, 121, 126
psychiatric history, the, 4, 12-13, 14-16
psychiatric hospitals, 4, 5
psychiatric imperialism, 111-112
psychoanalysis (see also, *psychodynamic psychotherapy*), 5, 6-10
psychodynamic psychotherapy (see also, *psychoanalysis*), 47
psychological medicine, see *liaison psychiatry*
psychological treatments, 46-48
psychopathy, 119, 122, 124
psychosexual development, 7-8
psychosis, 3, 4, 9, 10, 23, 53-71, 144
puerperal disorders, 85
puerperal psychosis, 85

Rajneesh, 22
rapid cycling, 90, 92
Re C, 43
recreational drugs, 154-159
rehabilitation, 40, 68
Renaissance, the, 4

Renton, 148
repression, 6, 7, 126
resistance, 7
Rilke, RM, 91
risk assessment, 27
Rome, see *Ancient Rome*
Rosenhan experiment, 22, 69
rule of thirds, the, 68
Ruskin, John, 86
Russell, Gerald, 164
Russell sign, the, 165

sadism (sexual sadism), 171
sadomasochism, see *sadism* and *masochism*
safety, 14
safety plan, 101
Saul (Biblical character), 3
Sartre, Jean-Paul, 96, 117
schizoaffective disorder, 70
schizoid personality disorder, 121
schizophrenia (see also, *psychosis*), 5, 6, 9, 22, 53-69, 121
schizophreniform disorder, 70
schizotypal (personality) disorder, 61, 70, 121
Schneider, Kurt, 54, 119
Schopenhauer, Arthur, 7
SCOFF questionnaire, 163
seasonal affective disorder, 80
seasonality of births, 60
sedatives, see *benzodiazepines*
selective serotonin reuptake inhibitors (SSRIs), 83-84, 113, 165
self-actualization, 116
self-deception, see *ego defences*
serotonin syndrome, 83
sexual disorders, 169-171
sexual dysfunction, 169-170
Shakespeare, 71, 75, 80, 129, 165
Shorter, Edward, 112
shyness, 108
sleep delay, 168
sleep disorders, 165-169
sleep hygiene, 167
sleep walking, 168
smoking in schizophrenia, 68
social phobia, 108
social skills training, 68, 153
societies, see *charities*
Socrates, 117
somatization disorder, 115
somatoform disorders, 115-116
specific phobia, 108
splitting, 124, 126

SSRI discontinuation syndrome, 83
stage theories of development, 174-175
Steinbeck, John, 143
stigma, 11, 37, 87
Strange Situation, the, 176
street names for drugs, 155
stress-vulnerability model, 61
structural model of the mind, 7
Styron, William, 76
suicide, 69, 85, 93, 95-101
suicide contagion, 99
Sunday neurosis, 81
sundowning, 130
superego, 7
Supervised Community Treatment, 45
supported accommodation, 68
supportive therapy, 47
syllogomania, 132
symptom pool, 112
synaesthesia, 24, 157
Szasz, Thomas, 6, 161

Talmud, the, 176
tangentiality, 18, 19
Tarasoff case, 42
tardive dyskinesia, 66
Tennyson, Lord, 18
Theophrastus' 30 personality types, 119
therapeutic community, 124-125
thought avoidance paradox, 112
thought disorder, 56

tic disorders, 179-180
Tillich, Paul, 117
topographical model of the mind, 7
Tourette's syndrome, 113, 180
transference, 6
transsexualism, 171
transvestism, 171
tuberous sclerosis, 143
Tukes, the, 4
traditional societies, 69, 79, 127
tricyclic antidepressants, 82-83
typical antipsychotics (see also, *antipsychotics*), 65

unconscious, the, 7, 9

valproate, 90, 92
values, 30, 41
vascular dementia, 136
veisalgia, 149
Vesalius, 4
volatile substances, 159
voyeurism, 171

Watters, Ethan, 112
Wernicke-Korsakov syndrome, 150
Werther effect, the, 99
Weyer, Johann, 4
Woolf, Virginia, 93

Yerkes-Dodson curve, the, 106
York Retreat, the, 4